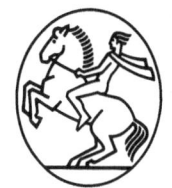

Processes
of the Cranial Midline

International Symposium
Vienna, Austria, May 21–25, 1990

Edited by
W. Koos and B. Richling

Acta Neurochirurgica
Supplementum 53

Springer-Verlag Wien New York

Univ.-Prof. Dr. Wolfgang Koos and
Univ.-Prof. Dr. Bernd Richling
Department of Neurosurgery, University of Vienna Medical School, Vienna, Austria

With 153 partly coloured Figures

Typesetting: Thomson Press, New Delhi, India

Printed on acid-free paper

ISSN 0065-1419

ISBN-13:978-3-7091-9185-9   e-ISBN-13:978-3-7091-9183-5
DOI: 10.1007/978-3-7091-9183-5

Preface

On the occasion of the 25th anniversary of the founding of the Vienna School of Neurosurgery at the University of Vienna an international symposium on the anatomy, the approaches to, and the treatment of pathologic processes of the cranial midline, and on the results obtained, was held in Vienna in May 1990.

This book contains selected papers on the diagnostics and therapy of processes of the cranial midline. The topics range from processes of the anterior cranial fossa via pterional approaches and processes of the cavernous sinus to lesions in the area of the pituitary, the third ventricle, the midbrain, and the posterior cranial fossa. Issues like approaches to the clivus, to the supratentorial and infratentorial petrous bone and to the brain stem are addressed and techniques like stereotactic endoscopic interventions or the endovascular treatment of cerebral vascular malformations are discussed.

The present book is intended to provide a survey of the complexity of cranio-cerebral processes of the cranial midline and their diagnostics and treatment and informs on the state of the art.

Wien, November 1991   The Editors

Contents

Listed in Current Contents

Acta Neurochirurgica, Suppl. 53, 1–6 (1991)
© by Springer-Verlag 1991

Lipoma of the Corpus Callosum Associated with Frontal and Facial Anomalies

J. C. de Villiers[1], P. F. de V Cluver, and **J. C. Peter[2]**

[1]Department of Neurosurgery, University of Cape Town Medical School, and [2]Department of Paediatric Neurosurgery, Red Cross War Memorial Children's Hospital, Cape Town, South Africa

Summary

Seven patients with a corpus callosum lipoma associated with a frontal cranial defect with or without a superficial lipoma or a fronto-nasal dysplasia, were encountered over a period of 12 years. This group of patients is reported as these associated lesions may provide a lead to the cause of lipomas of the corpus callosum as well as of the different lesions in the fronto-facial region.

From our experience and that of others, the frontal lesion may be an extracranial lipoma, a frontal bone defect, with or without an external lipoma, a lipomeningocele connecting the extracranial lipoma through a frontal defect with the corpus callosum lipoma, a frontal encephalocele. Fronto-nasal dysplasia associated with a corpus callosum lipoma, seems to form an independent group although some of these patients may have other extracranial lesions as well.

It is suggested by the authors that as the primitive mesenchyme gives rise to the meninx primitiva as well as to the fronto-facial skeleton a disturbance of the neural crest may give rise to these combined lesions. Further analysis of similar cases may indicate the timing of these events, and perhaps reveal a common causative factor.

Keywords: Corpus callosum lipoma; frontal encephalocele; frontal lipoma; fronto-nasal dysplasia.

Introduction

In a review of congenital anomalies involving midline structures of the scalp and skull encountered in our teaching hospitals, occipital and sincipital encephaloceles were found to comprise the majority of these lesions with bregmatic dermoids forming the third significant group. Seven patients with frontal lesions of the scalp and skull, associated with a lipoma of the corpus callosum managed by us, stimulated this report and review of the literature.

Lipomas of the corpus callosum are still uncommon lesions even though the diagnosis of even small lesions by means of CT and MRI has become easier. An association between such a lipoma and an extracranial frontal lesion is even more of a rarity. A frontal lipoma, extending through a defect in the frontal bone in continuity with a lipoma of the corpus callosum, was first described by Arnold in 1868[2]. Since then a relatively small number of reports of lipoma of the corpus callosum with frontal lipomas and other frontal lesions, have followed. These case descriptions comprise a heterogeneous group of conditions which can be broadly classified as follows:

a) A lipoma of the corpus callosum in continuity with an extracranial lipoma through a frontal defect or wide metopic suture – a lipomeningocele[2,12,7].

b) The corpus callosum lipoma may be connected to an extracranial lipoma by a thin fibrous stalk[3,16,1].

c) The corpus callosum lipoma may be associated with a non-lipomatous frontal encephalocele. (case 11)[8]; (case 1)[24]; (case 16 and 41)[22].

d) The intra- and extracranial lipomas may be independent and not connected in any way[15,9,6,4,24*,11,19]. (*case 2).

e) A corpus callosum lipoma may be associated with fronto-nasal dysplasia of varying degree but with a frontal bone defect and, at times a frontal extracranial lipoma[19,18].

A lipoma of the corpus callosum may be associated with, but not connected to, an occipital bone defect[25] or a parietal bone defect[17].

Materials and Methods

Information was extracted from the departmental records and hospital folders of patients admitted to the Department of Neurosurgery at Groote Schuur Hospital and the Red Cross War Memorial Children's Hospital in Cape Town.

During the period 1979 to 1990 only four patients were admitted to either of these hospitals. Since our study commenced, an adult was referred to us by colleagues in Port Elizabeth and two more children were referred to us by the cranio-facial unit at Tygerberg Hospital. As these patients are drawn from a very large geographic area with a population of complex ethnic structure, our observations are made on a sample of unknown bias so that valid epidemiological conclusions can not be drawn from these findings.

Findings

Table 1 indicates the relevant features of these seven patients.

Age at Presentation

All our patients presented within the first year of life with a local obvious anomaly: a frontal mass or a facial cleft. Of the reported cases most presented before the age of 1 year and even those who presented with a problem as teenagers such as our cases 1 and 5, an operation had often been done on a frontal or facial lesion at an earlier age.

Sex Incidence

The Female:Male ratio in this series was 3:5 while reported F:M ratio is 13:7, but in some reports the sex is not indicated.

The Frontal Mass

Our patients had a frontal mass or a mass overlying the anterior fontanelle or fronto-nasal dysplasia, with or without a frontal bone defect. Our case 4 had a mid-frontal dermal sinus, which seems to be unique (Fig. 1). In some instances such a mass had abnormal

Table 1

	Patient sex/age	Frontal lesion	Facial features	Other clinical features	Plain X-rays	C.T. scan	M.R.I.
1	D.N. M 28 yrs	Midline bone defect	Fronto-nasal dysplasia Hypertelorism	Mental defect Seizures Poor vision	Midline cleft Calcification of C. C. Lip.	C. C. Lip. calcification Bony defect Bony spur	Not done
2	J.M. F 2 mths	Meningocele at ant. fontanelle	Normal	Nil	Encephalocele at ant. fontanelle on A.E.G. No I.C. clacification	C. C. Lip. extending to dura at ant. fontanelle	Not done
3	Van W. F 5 wks	Lipoma over ant. fontanelle	Normal	R. fronto-temporal naevus	C. C. Lip. with low density calcification	C. C. Lip. Lat. Vent. Lip. + Lip. over ant. fontanelle No connection	C. C. Lip. + Lip. in lateral ventricles and over ant. fontanelle
4	Z.T. M 6 mths	Mid-frontal dermal sinus	Normal	Nil	Small mid-frontal bone defect	C. C. Lip. + ant. inter-hemispheric dermoid	Not done
5	B.C.	No bony or soft tissue abnormality	Fronto-nasal dysplasia Mild hypertelorism	Coloboma and dermoid of L. eye Nasal dermoid	?	C. C. Lip. + calcification	C. C. Lip. Ant. situated Agenesis of C. C.
6	S.S. M	Large fronto-nasal encephalocele	Fronto-nasal dysplasia Hypertelorism	Nil	?	R. frontal men. encephalocele Small C. C. Lip.	Large R. frontal mening. encephalocele C. C. Lip. (small)
5	F.N. M. 11 yrs	Frontal bone defect Local bulge of meninges No encephalocele	Fronto-nasal Hypertelorism	Nil	?	Frontal defect C. C. Lip. extending to defect Bony spur	C. C. Lip. extending to defect

A.E.G. = Airencephalogram.
C. C. Lip. = Corpus callosum lipoma.

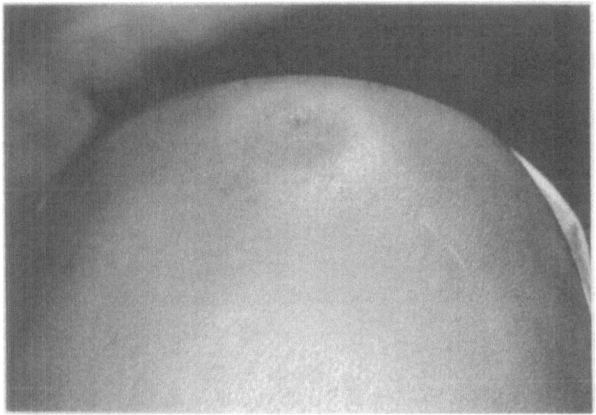

Fig. 1. Case 4. Frontal soft tissue depression with midline dermal sinus

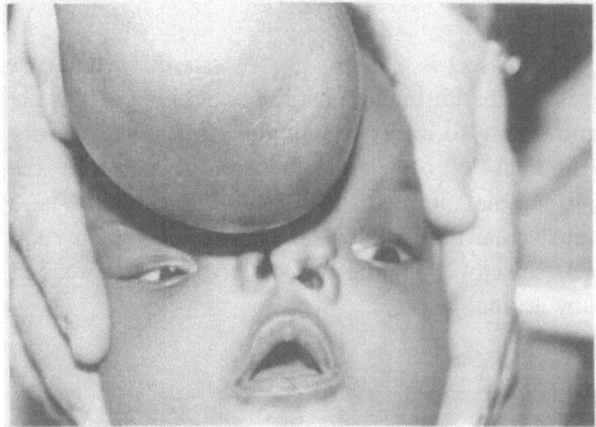

Fig. 2. Case 6. Larger frontal encephalocele. Fronto-nasal dysplasia. Hpertelorism

hairy skin covering it[24,7], while others were described as a birthmark[12]. Our case 3 had a naevus lateral to the mass.

Pascual-Castroviejo et al.[19] regard the presence of a frontal extracranial lipoma and a midline intra-cranial bony spur in contact with the frontal bone as indicative of a co-existent lipoma of the corpus callosum. These findings were present in our cases 1 and 7.

Skull Defect

A widely patent metopic suture is obvious (case 1) as is the defect associated with a frontal encephalocele but it may be minute or even absent in the presence of a frontal extracranial lipoma. A widely patent metopic suture was described by Hyashi et al.[7]. A small defect transmitting only a minute stalk joining a subcutaneous- with an intracranial lipoma, was found by Nordin et al.[16] and Bailey[3].

Hypertelorism

This was present in four of our seven patients with fronto-nasal dysplasia (Fig. 2). Although Arnold's[2] description antedated this concept, hypertelorism is clearly demonstrated in the illustration of his patient. It is not only associated with fronto-nasal dysplasia but also with other low mid-frontal lesions[9,13,12,24,7]. In some reports this feature is not mentioned.

Median Facial Cleft (Fronto-nasal Dysplasia)

Four of our patients (nos. 1, 5, 6 and 7) had fronto-nasal dysplasia (Fig. 3). A saddle-nose deformity was

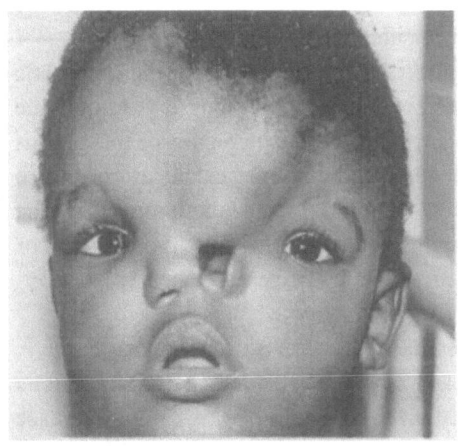

Fig. 3. Case 7. Fronto-nasal dysplasia with frontal bone defect and local bulge. Hypertelorism

noted in the patient of Kushnet and Goldman[12] and Zee et al.[24]. The association between lipoma of the corpus callosum, fronto-nasal dysplasia with or without frontal extracranial lipoma noted by Pascual-Castroviejo et al.[19] is confirmed by our findings. In the earlier descriptions it may not have been possible to demonstrate the association between a median facial cleft, a frontal extracranial lipoma and a lipoma of the corpus callosum because of radiographic limitations[5].

Neurological State

Overt neurological deficit was not a feature of any of our patients, neither is it noted in the reported cases. Seizures occurred in our case 1 and is a common feature in other case reports, as one would expect in patients with lipomas of the corpus callosum.

Mental State

Our case 1 is mentally grossly retarded while case 5 is of superior intellectual ability but the others were too young to assess meaningfully for subtle defects. The lack of correlation between the size of the intracranial lipoma, the facial abnormality and intellectual development, was indicated by Pascual-Castroviejo[19], but the IQs of their patients were at low normal levels.

Radiology

In our earlier cases, as in those reported before the advent of CT scanning, plain x-rays of the skull suggested the presence of a corpus callosum lipoma in most of the patients old enough to show the characteristic calcification[4].

With computerized tomography, the characteristic features of this syndrome comprising a frontal bone defect, a low-density mass in the region of the corpus callosum with surrounding dense calcification and in some instances, a lipomatous stalk connecting the corpus callosum lipoma with the subcutaneous one or an independent encephalocele, are clearly demonstrable[9,12,24] (Fig. 4).

MRI studies have only been done on our cases 3, 5, 6 and 7. Case 3 (Fig. 5) showed the characteristic hyper-intensity on short T_1 weighting and a decrease in signal intensity with increased T_2 weighting so

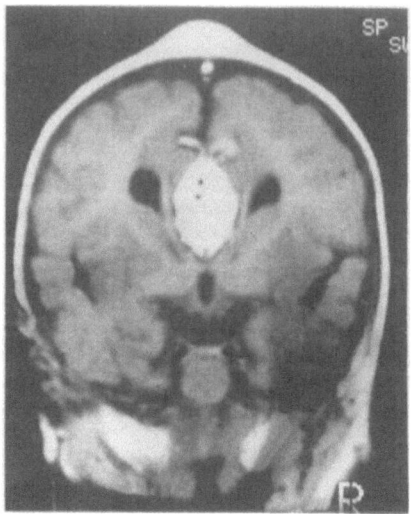

Fig. 5. Case 3. Coronal MR scan (T_1 weighted) showing a lipoma of the corpus callosum and over the anterior fontanelle

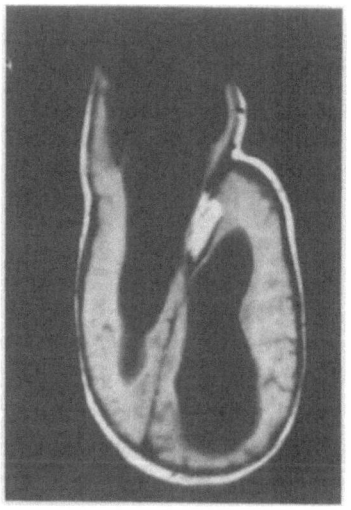

Fig. 6. Case 6. (Same patient as Fig. 2.) MR scan (T_1 weighted) showing a large frontal encephalocele associated with a lipoma of the corpus callosum

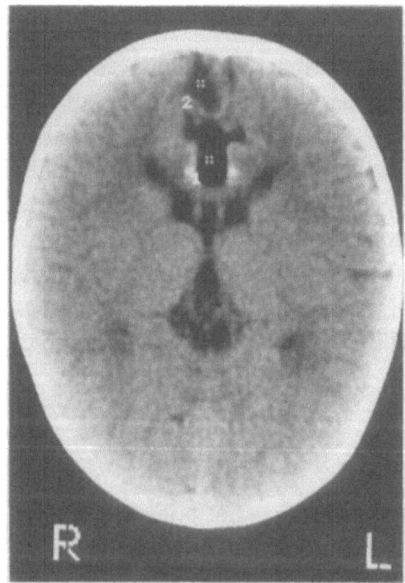

Fig. 4. Case 4. (Same patient as Fig. 1.) CT scan. Lipoma of corpus callosum (*1*). Interhemispheric dermoid cyst (*2*)

characteristic of fat in the corpus callosum, lateral ventricles and over the anterior fontanelle. Case 6 showed a massive right frontal encephalocele and a small lipoma of the corpus callosum (Fig. 6).

The MR features of intracranial lipomas have been adequately reviewed by Truwit and Barkovich[22]. That lipomas of the corpus callosum can now be detected even when very small, has been indicated by Pascual-Castroviejo[19]. They also demonstrated in some of their cases the ability of CT scanning to show up such a lesion in patients where previous air encephalography and arteriography had failed to do so.

Management

In the first instance, the subcutaneous mass should be removed for cosmetic reasons. A dural defect, if present, is always closed and the skull defect may be closed, depending on its size and the age of the patient. Excision of the subcutaneous mass was carried out in our patient 2 and the dermal sinus and cyst of the patient 4 removed, but the corpus callosum lipoma left undisturbed.

There is no indication for surgical removal of a lipoma of the corpus callosum. Attempts at removal are hazardous due to the relationship of the lipoma to the anterior cerebral arteries and even if removed, the epilepsy which is so often a feature, will not be affected.

If hydrocephalus should develop, this should be treated appropriately.

Corrective surgery for the facial deformity should be done as soon as it is feasible but particular difficulties may be encountered due to the bony spurs encountered in the fronto-basal region when a corpus callosum lipoma is associated with a frontal lipoma[7]. Expansion of the skull to accommodate a large cerebral hernia was done in our case 6 and described also by Zee et al.[24].

Pathology

Of the patients reported in the literature, only three have died (all following surgery of the corpus callosum lipoma) and a post-mortem examination was only carried out on the first[2] and third[9] cases. Arnold's patient showed a subcutaneous lipoma extending through a defect in the frontal bone and dura to become continuous with a lipoma of the corpus callosum while the patient of Kinal et al.[9] had two unconnected lipomas.

Discussion

Before the advent of CT scanning and MRI, small lipomas of the corpus callosum were probably overlooked[19].

The lesions of the skull and scalp associated with a corpus callosum lipoma are almost without exception, frontally situated. As indicated, they range from a lipoma extending from the corpus callosum through a defect in dura and skull to a frontal extracranial lipoma associated with but unconnected to a lipoma of the corpus callosum, despite the fact that there may

be a frontal bone defect. A frontal bone defect in association with a corpus callosum lipoma may transmit a frontal encephalocele without any lipomatous element in it.

All these lesions may occur in association with different variants of fronto-nasal dysplasia. It is possible that an analysis of these associated lesions could cast some light on the pathogenesis of corpus callosum lipoma and the other conditions described with it.

There can be little doubt that Krainer's[10] suggestion that persistence of some part of the meninx primitiva, which for some reason or other is caused to differentiate into adipose tissue, is the most acceptable explanation for intracranial lipoma. It adequately accounts for the subarachnoid cisternal situation of intracranial lipomas, which no other theory does and also for the frequent occurrence of such lipomas in relationship to the corpus callosum.[22]

The development of fat in the meninx primitiva is best accounted for by the suggestion of Wasserman[23] that the primitive perivascular reticulo endothelium, which usually serves a haemopoietic function, becomes specialised in the storage of fat. Such perivascular reticulo endthelium is also present in the primitive meninx so that it can explain the presence of fatty tissue here.

Occurrence of meninx primitiva within the banks of the lamina reuniens which should serve as the bridge for the ingrowth of the fibres of the corpus callosum, could interfere with the proper development of the corpus callosum i.e. agenesis. The degree of callosal agenesis, and the size and position of the corpus callosum lipoma, would be related to the timing of the non-differentiation of the meninx primitiva[22]. Pascual-Castroviejo et al.[19] indicated that the lipomas of the corpus callosum associated with fronto-nasal dysplasia were always anteriorly situated and this was certainly true in our cases as well.

A corpus callosum lipoma as well as one in the subcutaneous tissues may occur when a midline cranial defect allows extension of the meninx primitiva through it into an extracranial position. Should the skull defect remain, the intracranial lipoma will be continuous with a subcutaneous lipoma, while closure of the skull around such an initial defect would lead to the intracranial and extracranial lipomas being isolated completely or being connected by a rudimentary stalk.

There must, however, be another factor which causes the differentiation of the meninx primitiva and this has been blamed on developmental disturbance of the neural crest[14] but the nature of this disturbance is, as yet, unknown.

Mesenchyme of neural crest origin gives origin to much of the skeletal and connective tissue surrounding the inferior aspect of the fore-brain as well as the skeletal and connective tissues of the midface forming the bony and cartilagenous skeleton[20]. Sedano *et al.*[21] indicated that failure of the nasal capsule to develop, will give rise to the various features of fronto-nasal dysplasia of which ocular hypertelorism is the most constant feature. As the neural crest may also, in part, give rise to the meninx primitiva, the cause for the cranio-meningeal dysplasia may be seen as a form of rostral neural crest disturbance.

Whatever the aetiological agent, the time at which it acts upon the developing cranium and face can probably explain the variability of the clinical manifestations[21] and requires further study.

Acknowledgements

Drs. R. Keeley and F. van Aarde of Port Elizabeth for referring case 5 to us. Dr. J. Lotz for radiological studies, paticularly the MRI interpretations of our patients. Professor B. Zeeman of the Cranio-facial Unit of the Tygerberg Hospital for information about cases 6 and 7.

References

1. Addlestone R, Workman JB (1974) Lipoma of the corpus callosum. J Nucl Med 15: 714–716
2. Arnold J (1868) Ein Fall von angeborenem Teratom der Stirngegend. Virchows Arch (A)43: 181–196
3. Bailey I (1987) Lipoma of the corpus callosum presenting as a forehead swelling. Saudi Med J 8: 633–638
4. Cant WHP, Astley R (1952) Lipoma of the corpus callosum. Arch Dis Child 27: 478–479
5. De Meyer W (1967) The median cleft face syndrome. Neurology 17: 961–971
6. Groff RA, Liu CT, Leopold RL (1951) Lipoma of the corpus callosum: survey of the literature and report of two cases. Arch Neurol Psychiat 65: 253–254
7. Hyashi T, Kadowaki T, Shyojima K, Honda E (1986) Fronto-ethmoidal lipomeningocele. Childs Nerv System 2: 37–39
8. Kazner E, Stochdorph O, Wende S, Grumme T (1980) Intracranial lipoma – diagnostic and therapeutic considerations. J Neurosurg 52: 234–245
9. Kinal ME, Rasmussen G, Hamby WB (1951) Lipoma of the corpus callosum. J Neuropath Clin Neurol 1: 168—178
10. Krainer L (1935) Die Hirn- und Rückenmarkslipome. Virchows Arch 295: 107–142
11. Kudo H, Sakamoto K, Kobayashi N (1984) Lipomas of the corpus callosum and the forehead, associated with a frontal bone defect. Surg Neurol 22: 503–508
12. Kushnet MW, Goldman RL (1978) Lipoma of the corpus callosum associated with frontal bone defect. Am J Roentgenol 131: 517–5180
13. Kuwabara T, Yoshioka M, Akashi K (1963) A case of intracranial lipoma. Clin Neurol 3: 485–486
14. List CF, Holt JF, Everett M (1946) Lipoma of the corpus callosum. Am J Roentgen 55: 125–134
15. Luten J (1951) Lipomen van het corpus callosum. Ned Tijdschr Geneeskd 97: 1416–1421
16. Nordin WA, Tesluk H, Jones RK (1955) Lipoma of the corpus callosum. Arch Neurol Psychiat 74: 300–307
17. Oftedal S-I (1959) Anomalies of the midline structures of the brain. Acta Psychiat Neurol Scand 34: 451–463
18. Pai GS, Leukoff AH, Leithisen RE (1987) Median cleft of the upper lip associated with lipomas of the central nervous system and cutaneous polyps. Am J Med Genet 26: 921–924
19. Pascual-Castroviejo I, Pascual-Pascual SI, Perez-Higueras A (1985) Frontonasal dysplasia and lipoma of the corpus callosum. Eur J Pediatr 144: 66–71
20. Ross RB, Johnston MC (1972) Cleft lip and palate. Williams & Wilkins, Baltimore.
21. Sedano HO, Cohen M, Jirasek J, Gorlin RJ (1970) Frontal dysplasia. J Pediatr 76: 906–913
22. Truwit CL, Barkovich AJ (1990) Pathogenesis of intracranial lipoma: An MR study in 42 patients. AJNR 11: 665–674
23. Wassermann F (Quoted by List *et al*)
24. Zee C-S, McComb JG, Segall HD, Tsai FY, Stanely P (1981) Lipomas of the corpus callosum associated with frontal dysraphism. J Comput Assist Tomogr 5(2): 201–205
25. Zettner A, Netsky MG (1960) Lipoma of the corpus callosum. J Neuropath Exp Neurol 19: 305–319

Correspondence: Prof. J. C. de Villiers, Department of Neurosurgery, Medical School, University of Cape Town, Cape Town, Observatory 7925, South Africa.

Acta Neurochirurgica, Suppl. 53, 7–13 (1991)
© by Springer-Verlag 1991

Anterior Skull Base Tumour. The Choice Between Cranial and Facial Approaches, Single and Combined Procedure. From a Series of 78 Cases

B. George[1], S. Clemenceau[1], J. Cophignon[1], P. Tran ba Huy[2], B. Luboinski[3], K. L. Mourier[1], and G. Lot[1]

[1]Department of Neurosurgery, Hôpital Lariboisiere, Paris, France, [2]Department of Otorhinolaryngology, Hôpital Lariboisiere, Paris, France, [3]Department of Otorhinolaryngology, Institut G. Roussy, Villejuif, France

Summary

In order to define the most adequate surgical procedure to apply on anterior skull base lesions, we reviewed 78 cases of either benign (43 cases) or malignant (35 cases) tumours; they were treated either by a single surgical approach including transfacial approach (TF) in 9 cases, transbasal approach (TB) in 15 cases and fronto-orbital ridge deposition (FORD) in 16 cases or by a combined procedure: TB + TF (28 cases), TB + FORD (10 cases). In 7 cases, a pterional approach was associated to one of these combined procedures.

A classification is proposed, based on the tumour extension along the anteroposterior axis: I) anterior to the crista galli; II) anterior to the anterior clinoïd process; III) posterior to the anterior clinoïd process; and along the vertical axis A: below the bone level; B: below the dura level; C: at and above the dura level. This classification appears very useful to choose among the surgical procedures which one is the more appropriate. In type A tumour (N = 8), TF is sufficient while in type B (N = 38) and C (N = 32) a cranial route is always necessary; among the latter, a combined procedure is frequently asked for posterior tumours type II (N = 29) and III (N = 24). However, others parameters such as tumour consistency, vascularization and need for en-bloc removal are also relevant in this choice

Keywords: Anterior skull base tumour; skull base; cribriform plate; clivus; transbasal approach; transfacial approach.

Skull base anterior fossa tumours are border lesions between neurosurgery and otorhinolaryngology. Different transcranial and transfacial techniques in single or combined procedure have been proposed to treat them[1-4,8,9,14-18]. However, it has not yet been established how to choose the most adequate technique in each case. This report is an attempt of classification based on the possibilities of each main surgical techniques we used in 78 cases of anterior skull base lesions, so to establish which type of tumour, each surgical protocole is the most appropriate to deal with.

Material

Over the last 9 years, 78 cases of anterior skull base lesions were treated by different techniques. Age ranged from 2 to 80 years (average 38.5 years). There were 62 males and 16 females. Pathology is listed in Table 1. Benign lesions were observed in 43 cases with juvenile nasopharyngioma as the most frequent type and malignant tumour in 35 cases with mainly adenocarcinomas. Complete resection was achieved in 66 cases; removal was intentionally limited in 3 benign bone tumours (one osteoma and 2 fibrous dysplasia) and subtotal in 7 cases of extensive malignant tumour; in the last 2 cases of juvenile nasopharyngioma, a small remnant of the tumour was discovered on post-operative MRI or CT scan control, which asked for a re-operation (Table 1).

Surgical Techniques

Three main surgical techniques were applied alone or in combination: Fig. 1

i) *transfacial approach* (TF) with a paralateronasal skin incision and facial bone flap including on one or both sides the nasal bone, inferior wall of the orbit beyond the infraorbicularis nerve groove and anterior wall of the maxillary sinus. This bone flap is generally replaced after tumour removal except in case of invasion by the tumour,

Table 1. *Pathology*

Benign		Malignant	
Juvenile nasopharyngioma	17	Adenocarcinoma	15
Mucocele	10	Epidermoïd carcinoma	6
Meningioma	7	Sarcoma	4
Osteoma	3	Esthesioneurocytoma	5
Fibrous dysplasia	3	Chordoma	3
Others	3	Cylindroma	2
Total	43		35

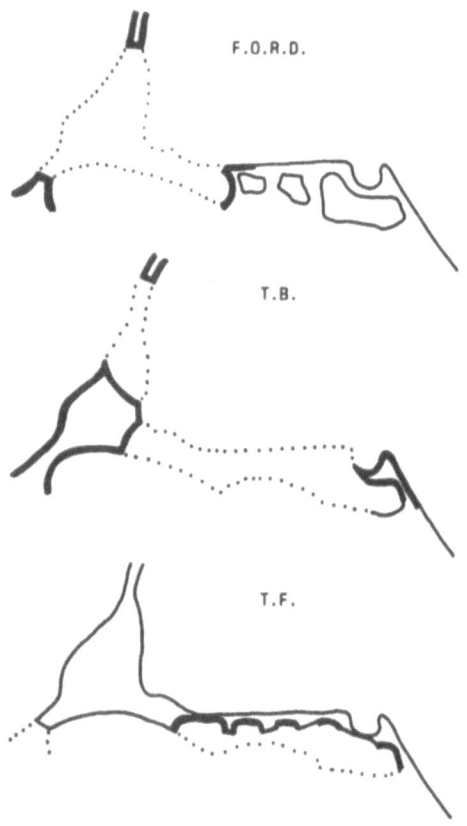

Fig. 1. Opening and access to the skull base given by the three main surgical techniques. *FORD* fronto-orbital ridge deposition, *TB* transbasal approach, *TF* transfacial approach

ii) *transbasal approach* (TB) as described by Derome[8] with bicoronal incision and free bifrontal bone flap passing through the frontal sinuses. The cribriform plate is bilaterally exposed after section of the olfactory nerves. Exposure of the anterior fossa is more or less extended posteriorly as far as the anterior clinoïd processes according to the site of the tumour. Reconstruction is generally performed with irradiated bone graft and autologous split bone flap pieces then covered by a pediculated pericranium graft. This pericranium graft is split from the deep aspect of the skin flap with which it has been elevated during opening, so to keep an anterior vascular supply; it is placed over the dura of the anterior fossa and sutured to it. In case of large dural defect, a piece of dura from the frontal convexity is cut keeping a vascular pedicle and turned down and sutured over the dura of the frontal base; the convexity defect is then closed using temporalis fascia or pericranium,

iii) *fronto-orbital ridge deposition* (FORD) we reported (Cophignon *et al.*) in 1983[6], with removal of the medial part of the fronto-orbital rim. It is more of less extended laterally; it generally includes the orbital ridges until the supraorbicularis nerve, the frontal ridge with the anterior wall of the frontal sinus down to the root of the nose and the anterior part of the ethmoïd with the crista galli. It is removed in one piece and repositioned and wired at the end of the procedure, (Fig. 5).

Tumoural Classifications (Fig. 2)

Each tumour were classified according to its anatomical extension along the vertical and anteroposterior axis as following:

– vertical grading:
  A. if space is left between tumour and bone,
  B. if space is left between tumour and dura,
  C. if the tumour reaches the dura whether it is firmly adherent or it invaded it and eventually the brain,
– anteroposterior grading:

  I.   if the lesion does not extend posteriorly beyond the crista galli,
  II. if the lesion does not extend posteriorly beyond the jugum sphenoïdale,
  III. if the lesion extends posteriorly beyond the jugum sphenoidale towards the clivus.

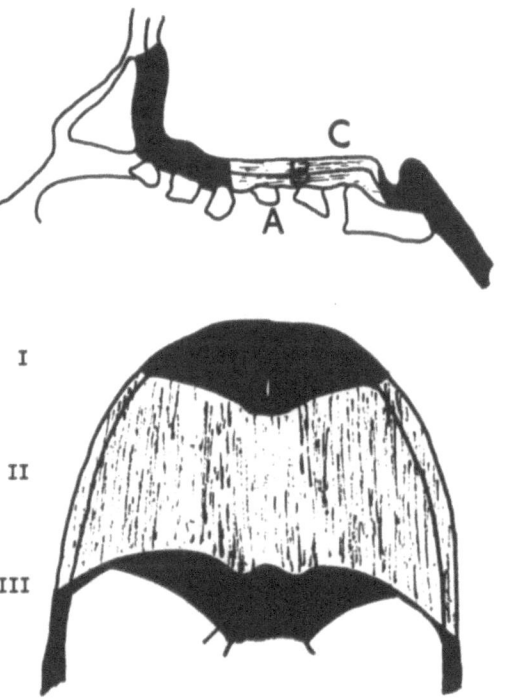

Fig. 2. Tumoural classification along the vertical axis (*A*) and horizontal axis (*A* and *B*)

CT scan and MRI were used to grade the tumours and this was then checked during surgery.

Results

A single surgical technique was used in 40 cases while in 38 cases, a combined procedure was applied including 28 TB + TF and 10 TB + FORD (Table 2).

In 7 cases, a pterional approach was associated to these procedures (5 TB + TF, 1 TB + FORD, and 1 TB). Intradural exposure had to be performed in 20 cases to remove a type C extension; it was realized in the same surgical procedure in 14 cases and separately in 6. In the 12 other type C tumours, either the dural invasion was pretty limited and could be resected by the extradural approach, or the tumour was only adherent to the dura and could be separated from it.

Tumour classification indicates 8 type A, 38 type B 32 type C for vertical extension and 17 type I, 32 type II and 29 type III for anterio-posterior extension (Figs. 3 and 4). Table 3 shows the distribution of tumours according to this classification.

Surgical techniques performed in each type of tumour are listed in Tables 4 and 5.

Single TF approach was mainly used for type A (8 type A and 1 type B); FORD was only proposed in type B and TB approach in 12 type C and 3 type B. Combined procedure was applied only in type B and C with equal frequency: 20 type C and 18 type B. Pterional approach was only indicated in type CIII tumour with adherence to the inferior or lateral aspect of the cavernous sinus including 4 juvenile nasopharyngioma, 1 chordoma, 1 adenoma and 1 meningioma.

- Type A tumours whatever its antero-posterior extension (grade II or III) required TF.
- Type B tumours anteriorly located (grade I) were treated by FORD, while more posterior ones needed TB or combined techniques.
- Type C of any grade were mostly treated by TB or combined procedures.

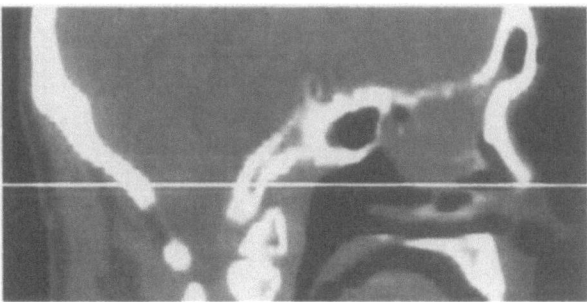

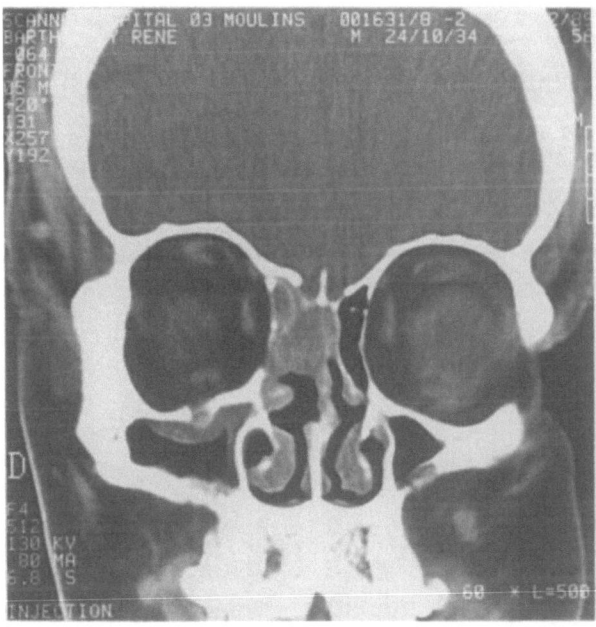

(b)

Fig. 3 a, b. Type B2 tumour: adenocarcinoma

Death undergoing during the one month post-operative period was observed in 2 cases of carcinoma; one remains unexplained since this patient was in a deep coma immediately after surgery with a normal post-operative CT scan and intracranial pressure; the other died from pneumonia on the sixteenth post-operative day. There were two local suppurations (1 cylindroma, 1 meningioma) treated by antibiotics irrigation and one persistent CSF leakage requiring a lumboperitoneal shunting.

Discussion

The best way to deal with skull base anterior fossa tumour is still a matter of debate. As early as 1941, Dandy[7] indicated the possibility of surgical attack on the base of the skull. Then multiple reports have emphasized the interest of both cranial and facial routes.

Table 2. *Surgical Technique*

	Alone	Combined + TF	+ FORD	+ Pterional
TB	15	28	10	7
TF	9			
FORD	16			
Total	40	38		

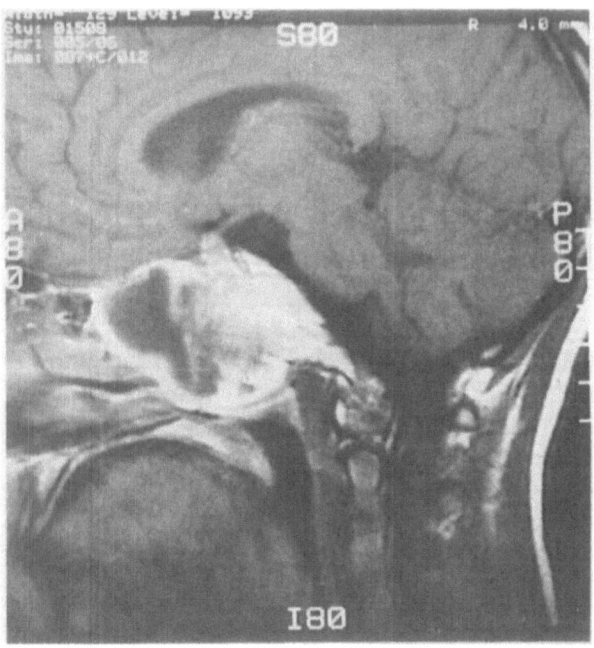

Fig. 4 a. Type C3 tumour: fibroma

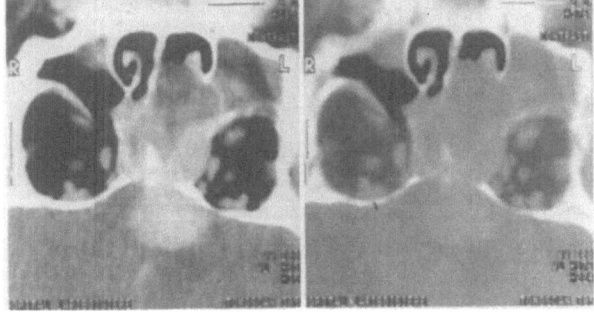

Fig. 4 b. Type C3 tumour: adenocarcinoma

Table 3. *Antero-posterior Extension*

Vertical extension	I	II	III
A N = 8	–	3	5
B N = 38	17	13	8
C N = 32	–	16	16
Total	17	32	29

Table 4. *Surgical Technique and Tumour Type*

	A	B	C
TF	8	1	–
FORD	–	16	–
TB	–	3	12
TB + TF	–	13	15
TB + FORD	–	5	5

Table 5. *Surgical Technique and Tumour Type*

	I	II	III
TF	–	4	5
FORD	16	–	–
TB	1	9	5
TB + TF	–	15	13
TB + FORD	–	4	6

Combined techniques were proposed as soon as 1954[18]. The facial approach is generally a lateral rhinotomy more or less extended[2,15,16]. The cranial opening varied with the authors from a single burr hole[4,9,20] to a bifrontal bone flap. Some advocated very low craniotomy limited to the opening of the frontal sinuses[13]; others preferred a supra-orbital bone flap[4,10–12]. With an appropriate technique, there is no reason to limit the cranial opening either to the frontal bone above the frontal sinuses or to the sinuses alone. As described by Derome[8] and improved by others[5,13,15,17], a bifrontal bone flap passing through the sinuses gives a wide exposure on the anterior skull base with good results regarding cerebrospinal fluid leakage and cosmetic aspects as well. Reconstruction includes bone grafting covering the defect from the sphenoïdal to the frontal sinuses and direct dural repair associated with a free or pediculated periosteal flap.

FORD is a technique derived from maxillo-facial techniques as those described by Tessier[19]. It directly opens the fronto-ethmoïdal part of the anterior fossa. So it is sufficient alone to treat tumour located anterior to the posterior ethmoïd. Combined or not with the transbasal approach, it provides a very low access, below the level of the anterior fossa; as consequences, it enlarges the angle of view and reduced markedly the need for brain retraction. Even in case of tumoural extension down to the lower clivus, the retraction is almost none. The FORD nicely gives the plane of nasal mucosae and more interestingly exposes the olfactory nerves in their extradural portion permitting to ligate and to cut them without any CSF leakage.

The choice between all these techniques lies upon several factors among them the tumoral extension is the most important. This is now well-defined by the new imaging tools CT scan and MRI. MRI gives a very nice definition of every tumoral extension towards the brain, orbits, nasal fossae and pharynx; in most cases, using gadolinium injection, it can be demonstrated if the dura is invaded or only displaced by the

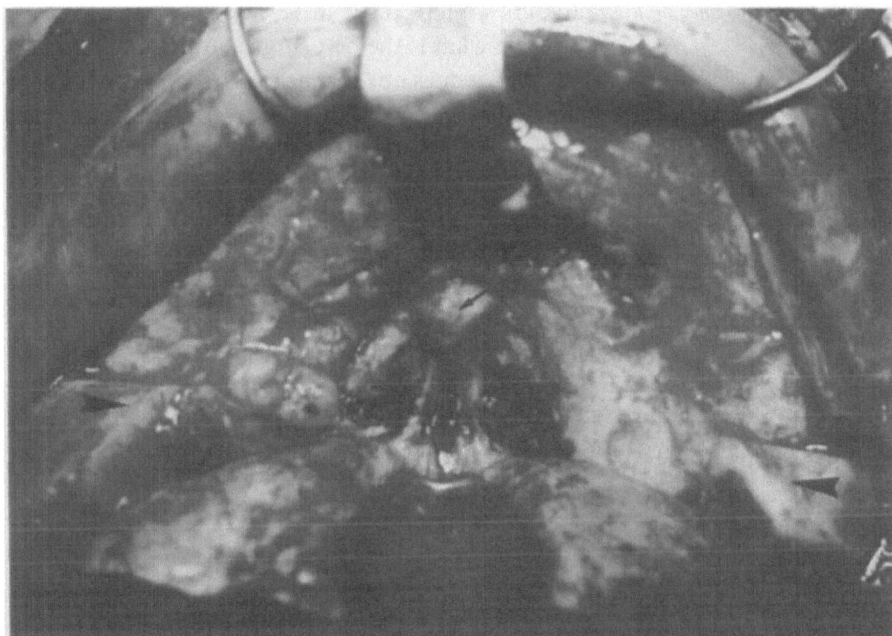

Fig. 5 a. Operative view after FORD. Large arrows: orbital ridge. Small arrow: root of the nose. Notice the olfactory nerve

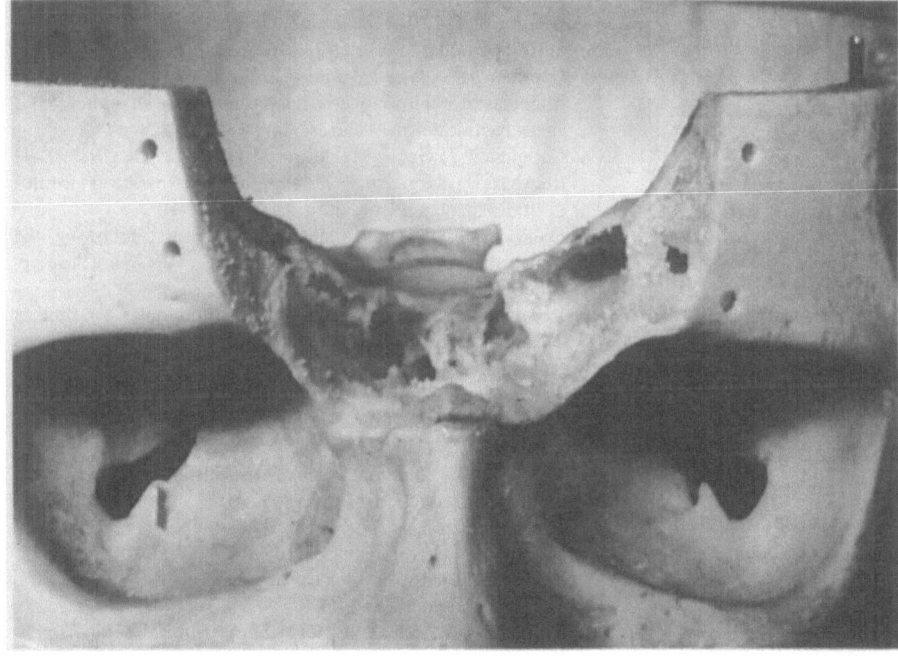

Fig. 5 b. Anatomic specimen showing the inferior enlargement given by the FORD. Notice that the access is lower than the level of the anterior fossa

tumour. CT scan remains useful in every cases for bone invasion is often better appreciated on CT coronal views than on MRI. In type CIII tumour, angiography is always necassary to appreciate the relation between the tumour and the cavernous sinus.

Transfacial approach is sufficient in type A tumour, while in tumour reaching or overtaking the skull base (type B), this technique cannot deal safely with the upper extent, which cannot be seen. Therefore, type B

and C tumours require a single or combined procedure but always including a cranial approach. In case of anterior tumour (grade I), the FORD technique is sufficient; conversely, grade II and III tumours need at least a transbasal approach; in these cases, a combined technique is to be discussed; the more posterior the tumour extension, the more the combined techniques are to be recommended (Table 6).

The alternative in combined techniques is either

Table 6. *Best Choices Among the Different Single or Combined (C) Techniques According to the Tumour Extension*

	I	II	III
A	TF	TF	TF
B	FORD	TB or C	C
C	FORD (or TB)	TB or C	C + Pterional

transbasal approach plus FORD or transbasal plus transfacial approaches. The answer is not given by the anatomical definition of the tumour but mainly by two other factors which are the tumour consistency and the need for an en-bloc resection. TB plus FORD do not permit to remove a tumour as a whole; so progressive debulking has to be done. In case of soft consistency, the tumour can be easily followed even if it extends very far laterally and posteriorly. In other cases, though ultrasonic aspirator greatly helps in tumour resection, the TB + TF procedure is generally more suitable. This combined technique is also mandatory if one contemplates to perform an en-bloc resection. In this procedure, the transbasal approach permit to split out the superior tumoral limits from the dura, ethmoïdal mucosae and lateral walls of the orbit and to push the whole tumour down towards the nasal fossae from which it is extracted by the TF opening. There are two main reasons to decide an en-bloc resection; one is the highly vascular feature of the tumour what is particularly the case in juvenile nasopharyngioma. The other is carcinologic to avoid tumoral cells seeding. In carcinoma, the best is to remove in one piece the tumour and the first surrounding normal tissue which may include the mucosae and/or the bony environment. This actually means that limited carcinomas are preferentially treated by combined TF + TB approaches while paradoxically, extensive forms (type C) are more likkely resected by TB approach alone or TB + FORD since dural invasion generally prevent from large and en-bloc resection.

Type C tumour with subdural or intracerebral extension raises the question of a one or two stages procedure. In general, at the level of the anterior skull base like on any other part, we prefer not to perform in the same time the extra and intradural resection so to reduce the infectious risks. Finally, the association with a pterional approach is discussed in type CIII tumour to permit exposure of the lateral aspect of the cavernous sinus.

Therefore, the classification of anterior skull base

tumours we have used in 78 cases, seems very useful to decide what is the best surgical technique to apply. However, it does not answer to all the questions; other parameters like consistency, vascularization and histological type are also to be taken into account. This classification also permits to discuss the results of treatment for each type of tumour with more accuracy.

Acknowledgements

We are very grateful to Miss Judith Andrens for help in the translation and preparation of this report.

References

1. Bebear JP, Bagot D' Arc M (1982) L' ethmoïdectomie totale par voie mixte: frontale extra-durale et paralatéro-nasale. Rev Laryngol 193: 179–188
2. Bridger GP (1980) Radical surgery for ethmoïd cancer. Arch Otolaryngol 106: 630–634
3. Cantrell RW, Ghorayeb BY, Filtz-Hugh GS (1977) Esthesioneuroblastoma: diagnosis and treatment. Ann Otol Rhinol Laryngol 86: 760–765
4. Clifford P (1977) Transcranial approach for cancer of the antro-ehtmoïdal area. Clin Otolaryngol 2: 115–130
5. Colohan ART, Jane JA, Park TS, Persing JA (1985) Bifrontal osteoplastic craniotomy utilizing the anterior wall of the frontal sinus: technical note. Neurosurgery 16: 822–824
6. Cophignon J, George B, Marchac D, Roux FX (1983) Voie transbasale élargie par mobilisation du bandeau fronto-orbitaire médian. Neurochirurgie 29: 407–410
7. Dandy WE (1941) Orbital tumours, results following the transcranial operative attack. Oskar Piest, New-York, 168 pp. Cited by Van Buren JM
8. Derome P (1972) Les tumeurs sphéno-ethmoidales. Possibilités d'exérèse et de réparation chirurgicale. Neurochirurgie 18, [suppl] 1: 1–164
9. Ketcham AS, Chretien PB, Van Buren JP (1973) The ethmoïd sinuses: a re-evaluation of surgical resection. Am J Surg 126: 469–476
10. Mc Carthy JG, Zide BM (1984) The spectrum of calvarial bone grafting: introduction of the vascularized calvarial bone flap. Plast Reconstr Surg 77: 10–18
11. Morley TP (1973) Tumours of the cranial meninges. In: Youmans JR (ed) Neurological surgery, Vol III. WB Saunders, Philadelphia, pp 1388–1411
12. Odom GL, Woodhall B (1966) Supratentorial skull flaps. J Neurosurg 25: 492–501
13. Persing JA, Jane JA, Levine PA, Cantrell RW (1990) The versatile frontal sinus approach to the floor of the anterior cranial fossa. J Neurosurg 72: 523–516
14. Peynegre R, Keravely, Raulo Y (1984) Traitement chirurgical des tumeurs naso-sinusiennes envahissant l' étage antérieur de la base du crane. Ann Otolaryngol 101: 169–175
15. Roux FX, Brasnu D, Laccoureye H, Fabbre A, Chodkiewicz JP (1987) Les adénocarcinomes ethmoïdaux opérés en un temps par voie trans-faciale et sous-frontale après chimiothérapie d' induction. Neurochirurgie 33: 365–370
16. Schramm VL, Myers EN (1978) How I do it: head and neck. A targeted problem and its solution. Lateral rhinotomy. Laryngoscope 89: 1077–1091

17. Schwaab G, Marandas P (1983) Les problèmes du traitement chirurgical des tumeurs malignes de l' ethmoïde par abord mixte endocrânien et facial. Ann Otolaryngol 100: 159–161

18. Smith RR, Klopp CT, Williams JM (1954) Surgical treatment of cancer of the frontal sinus and adjacent areas. Cancer NY 7: 991–994

19. Tessier P (1971) Relationship of craniostenosis to facial dysostosis and to faciostenosis. Plant Reconstr Surg 48: 224–237

20. Van Buren JM, Ommaya AK, Ketcham AS (1968) Ten years experience with radical combined craniofacial resection of malignant tumours of the paranasal sinuses. J Neurosurg 28: 341–350

Correspondence: Dr. B. George, Neurochirurgie, Hôpital Lariboisière, 2 rue Ambroise Paré, F-75010 Paris, France.

Acta Neurochirurgica, Suppl. 53, 14–18 (1991)

Surgical Treatment of Olfactory Groove Meningiomas Using the Pterional Approach

W. Hassler and J. Zentner

Department of Neurosurgery, Medical School, University of Tübingen, Tübingen, Federal Republic of Germany

Summary

We present our experience with the surgical treatment of olfactory groove meningiomas using a pterional approach. This approach provides the advantages of previous techniques, such as preserving the frontal brain and superior sagittal sinus, early devascularization of the tumour, and late dessection of tumour borders. Moreover, it also compensates for the shortcomings of other techniques, e.g., compression of frontal bridging veins, late dissection of dorsal tumour aspects involving vessels and optic nerves as well as facultative infection and cerebrospinal fluid fistula-related complications caused by opening of frontal sinuses. To date, 11 patients were treated in this way. As we encountered no surgical complications in our series we are encouraged to present our procedure.

Keywords: Olfactory meningioma; pterional approach.

Patients and Methods

Eleven patients with olfactory groove meningiomas were treated. There were 7 men and 4 women with ages between 38 and 67 years. The diameters of the tumours varied between 4 and 6 cm. All patients had suffered hyposmia or anosmia on at least one side for 3 months to 2 years. Additionally, in 9 patients personality changes and in 3 visual field defects were observed.

The procedure is as follows. Trephination is performed pterionally, preserving the frontal sinus[6,13] (Fig. 2 A). After the dura is opened, the sylvian fissure is dissected. Following the middle cerebral artery (MCA), the internal carotid artery (ICA) is reached and next to it the posteriolateral aspect of the tumour. Thus, in the first step of surgery, essential structures such as homolateral ICA, MCA, anterior cerebral artery (ACA), and optic nerve are exposed. By removal of posterior tumour parts, the chiasm, optic nerves, and ACA are decompressed (Fig. 2 B). In a second step the hyperostotic tumour nidus in the region of the planum sphenoidale is coagulated and drilled off, so that the tumour is largely devascularized. Care must be taken in order to avoid opening of ethmoidal cells with subsequent cerebrospinal fluid leakage (Fig. 2 C). The third step of surgery consists of partial resection of the cerebral falx and crista galli, thus facilitating hollowing of contralateral tumour parts (Fig. 2 D). In the meantime, haemorrhage subsides and the upper tumour parts drop successively into the resection cavity. Consequently, local pressure diminishes, and

the tumour's borders and connections to the distal contralateral ACA can now be easily dissected with no damage to the surrounding brain (Fig. 2 E).

Results

In all patients the tumour was completely removed (Fig. 3). We encountered no intraoperative complications. The postoperative course was uneventful in all but 1 patient. This patient died 10 days after surgery as a result of a fulminant pulmonary embolism, but was in good neurological condition. Psychoorganic syndromes observed preoperatively in 9 patients disappeared. In 2 patients the contralateral olfactory nerve was preserved with good postoperative function. The period of postoperative hospitalization ranged from 8 to 14 days.

Discussion

Olfactory groove meningiomas belong to those tumours in which the changes in surgical strategy over the years can be studied. It is obvious that strategy results not only from the specific features of these tumours such as their usually large size, high vascularization, perifocal edema, and the close anatomical relationship to basal arteries an optic nerves, but also from the technical possibilities available in a specific time period. This is especially evident in the case of Cushing[1]. In his first patient, a university professor, he tried to remove the tumour by applying a modern strategy: using an extradural, frontobasal approach and preserving the frontal brain, he tried to devascularize the tumour, followed by extensive tumour hollowing. Dissection from the

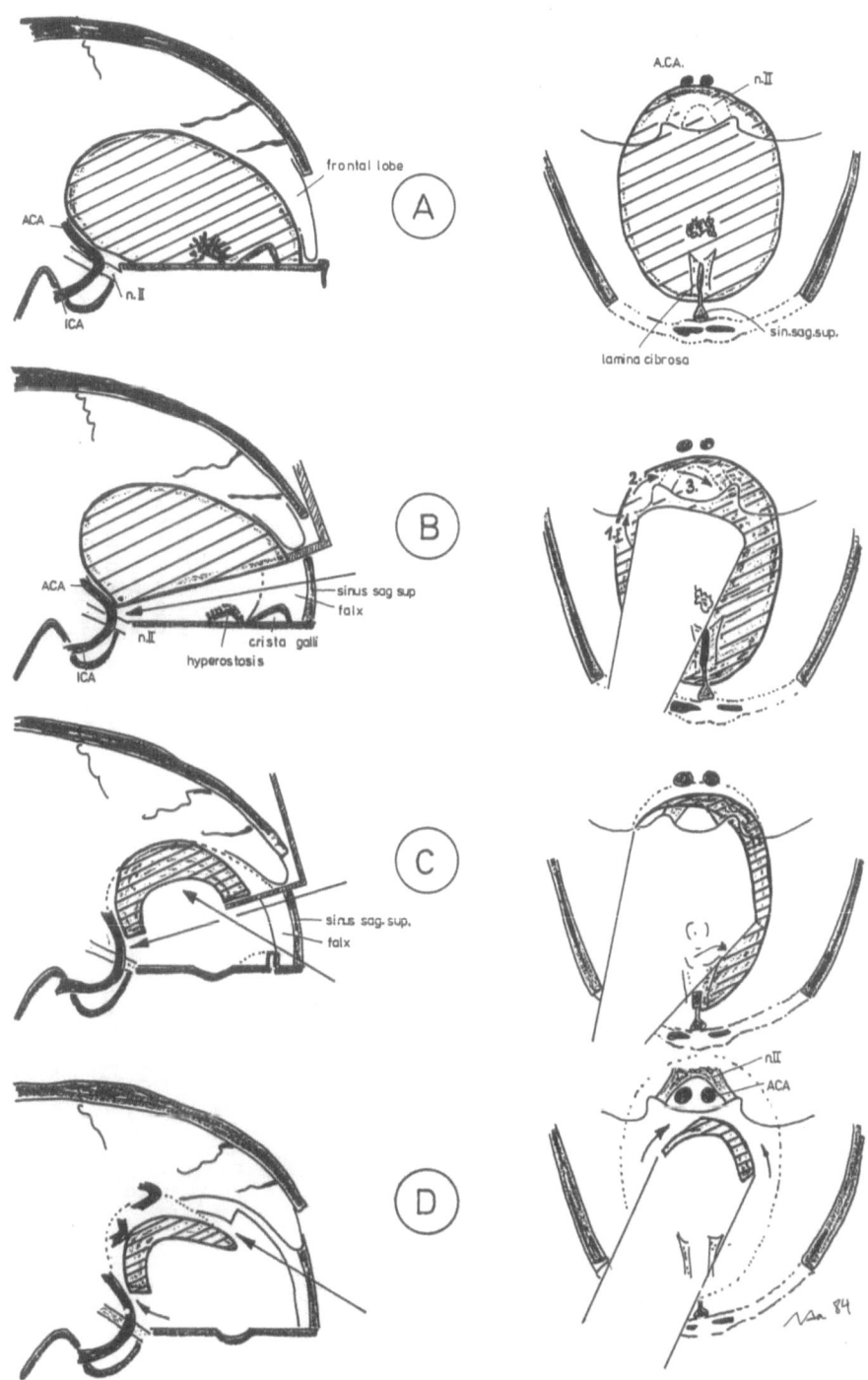

Fig. 1. Microsurgical strategy for frontobasal meningiomas as described by Seeger[10]. Bifrontal trephination (A). Unilateral basal approach, elevation of frontal pole and hollowing of the tumour (B). Decompression of optic nerves and proximal anterior cerebral artery (ACA) (C). Dissection of tumour borders (D)

surrounding brain was only performed after local pressure was reduced. Cushing failed because of the limited technical possibilities (macrosurgical operation techniques) of his time: a vessel in the depths (probably the ACA), which he could not see, was injured, and the patient died. As a consequence, Cushing later[2] exposed these tumours more extensively by polar frontal lobectomy and obtained good results with regard to survival of his patients.

With the introduction of microsurgical operation techniques, Seeger's method[10] of bifrontal trephination, unilateral frontal approach, and partial resection of the falx provided the essential advantages of early tumour devascularization, preservation of the frontal brain, and late dissection of tumour boundaries from the surrounding brain when local pressure is already reduced following extensive hollowing of the tumour. Problems resulting from this procedure

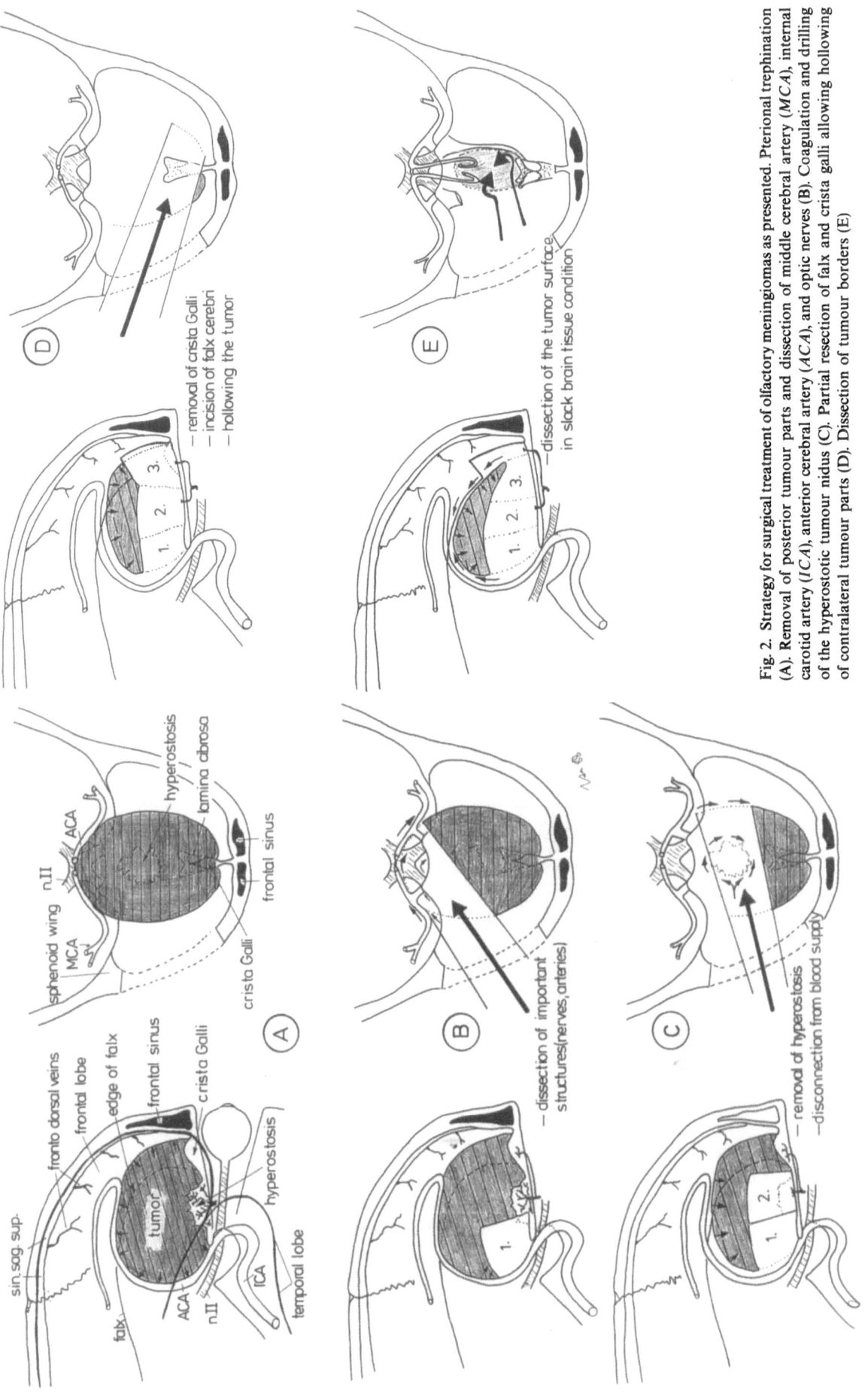

Fig. 2. Strategy for surgical treatment of olfactory meningiomas as presented. Pterional trephination (A). Removal of posterior tumour parts and dissection of middle cerebral artery (*MCA*), internal carotid artery (*ICA*), anterior cerebral artery (*ACA*), and optic nerves (B). Coagulation and drilling of the hyperostotic tumour nidus (C). Partial resection of falx and crista galli allowing hollowing of contralateral tumour parts (D). Dissection of tumour borders (E)

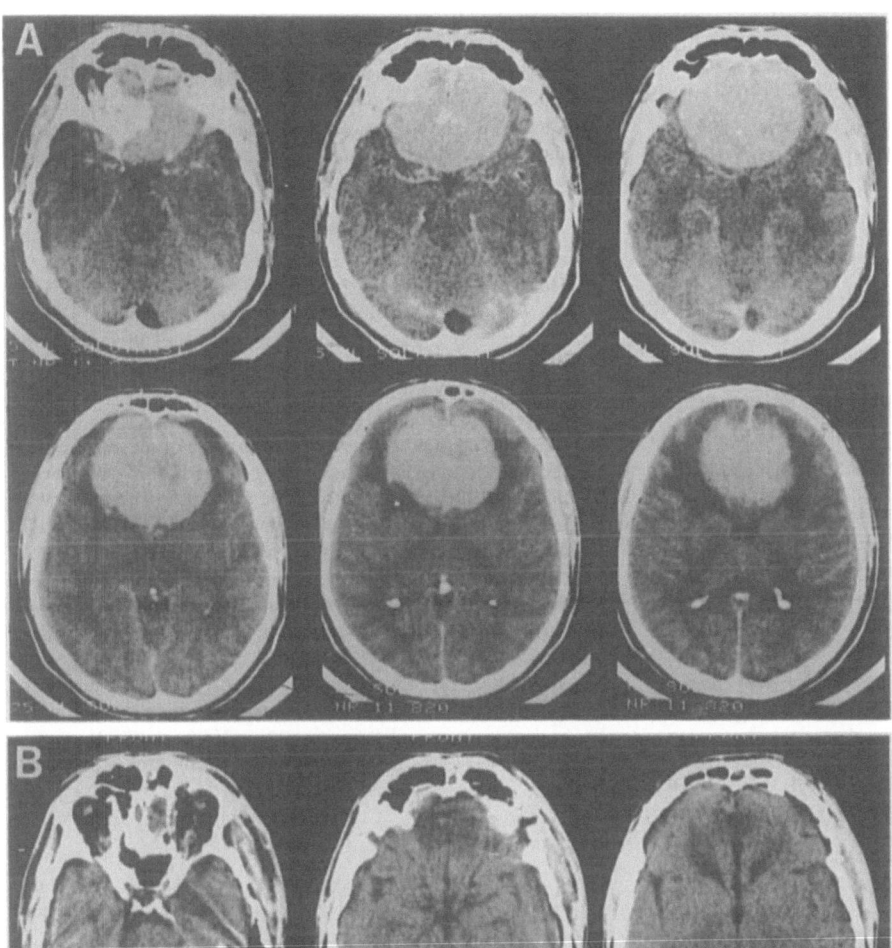

Fig. 3. A 38-year-old man with an olfactory groove meningioma. Pre-operative contrast-enhanced computed tomographic scans show large tumour with typical bifrontal edema (A). The tumour was removed completely via a right-sided pterional approach. Computed tomographic scans without contrast enhancement performed 1 week after surgery show hypodense frontobasal defects with enlarged anterior horns of the ventricles (B)

involve frontal bridging veins, which are compressed for a long time when the frontal lobes are elevated. Furthermore, essential structures such as the ACA, ICA, and optic nerves are only exposed at a late phase of surgery when the surgeon is already quite tired and his concentration is reduced. Minor disadvantages of this method include the risk of local infection caused

by opening of the frontal sinuses and of cerebrospinal fluid fistula.

The pterional approach for olfactory groove meningiomas presented here provides the advantages of Seeger's method, but compensates for its short-comings. The frontal veins are not compressed as the frontal lobes are not elevated, thus venous drainage remains intact throughout the surgical procedure. Furthermore, the most dangerous aspects of the tumour – its dorsal parts involving vessels and optic nerves – are exposed and detached in an early phase when the surgeon is at his best. To show these essential anatomical relationships more clearly, Kempe[7] had already extended unilateral frontal trephination to the temporal region in tumours with mainly posterior extension. However, he continued to apply frontal lobectomy to large tumours.

The problems involved with basal hyperostosis were discussed by Derome and Guiot[4]. As the ethmoidal cells often extend to the base of the hyperostosis, its radical removal involves a risk of cerebrospinal fluid fistula. Therefore, we drill off hyperostosis only in part and cover the bone with periosteum. In contrast to placode meningiomas, partial removal of the hyperostosis in olfactory meningiomas is justified as it is usually not infiltrated by tumour in these lesions.

To conclude, the pterional approach allows early dissection of dorsal tumour aspects involving vessels and optic nerves. Frontal bridging veins are not compressed. The contralateral parts of the tumour can be easily reached after falx resection with preservation of the contralateral olfactory nerve. Since frontal sinuses are preserved, corresponding infection and cerebrospinal fluid fistula-related complications are avoided. We encountered no surgical complications in the 11 patients treated so far with this approach. Therefore, we recommend this procedure for surgical treatment of olfactory groove meningiomas.

References

1. Cushing H (1927) Meningiomas arising from olfactory groove and their removal by aid of electrosurgery. Lancet 1: 1329–1339
2. Cushing H, Eisenhardt L (1938) Meningiomas. The olfactory meningiomas with primary anosmia. Charles C Thomas, Springfield, Ill, pp 250–282
3. Dandy WE (1938) Hirnchirurgie. Barth, Leipzig
4. Derome PJ, Guiot G (1978) Bone problems in meningiomas invading the base of the skull. Clin Neurosurg 25: 435–451
5. Durante F (1885) Estirpazione di un tumore endocranio. Arch Soc Ital Chir 2: 252–255
6. Hamby WB (1964) Pterional approach to the orbits for decompression or tumor removal. J Neurosurg 21: 15–18
7. Kempe LG (1968) Operative neurosurgery, vol 1. Springer, New York, pp 104–108
8. Ojemann RG (1982) Surgical management of meningiomas of the tuberculum sellae, olfactory groove, medical sphenoid wing, and floor of the anterior fossa. In: Schmidek HH, Sweet WH (eds) Operative neurosurgical techniques. Indications, methods, and results. Grune & Stratton, New York, pp 535–559
9. Olivecrona H, Urban H (1935) Über Meningeome der Siebbeinplatte. Brun's Beitr Klin Chir 161: 224–253
10. Seeger W (1983) Microsurgery of the cranial base. Springer, New York
11. Symon L (1977) Olfactory groove and suprasellar meningiomas. In: Krayenbühl H, et al (eds) Advances and technical standards in neurosurgery, vol 4. Springer, New York, pp 67–91
12. Tönnis W (1938) Zur Operation der Meningeome der Siebbeinplatte. Zentralbl Neurochir 3: 1–6
13. Yaşargil MG, Fox JL (1975) The microsurgical approach to intracranial aneurysms. Surg Neurol 3: 7–14

Correspondence: W. Hassler, M.D., Department of Neurosurgery, Medical School, University of Tübingen, Hoppe-Seyler-Strasse 3, D-7400 Tübingen, Federal Republic of Germany.

Acta Neurochirurgica, Suppl. 53, 19–22 (1991)

Combined Stereotactic and Microsurgical Approach to Cerebral Lesions

F. Alesch[1], **C. B. Ostertag**[2], and **W. Th. Koos**[1]

Neurochirurgische Universitätsklinik [1]Wien, Austria, and [2]Freiburg, Federal Republic of Germany

Summary

A description is given of the technique of a combined CT-stereotactic and microsurgical approach for removal of small cerebral lesions. Its usefullness in 21 cases is demonstrated.

Keywords: Small cerebral lesions; microsurgery; CT-stereotactic localization; combined approach.

Introduction

Modern high-resolution imaging techniques such as CT scanning and magnetic resonance imaging (MRI) are able to demonstrate intracerebral lesions smaller than 5mm in diameter. Such lesions, though now easy to image, still pose localization problems during an open operation. This applies not only to small lesions, but also to those that are located deep in the brain parenchyma. The identification of cortical anatomic sites can be difficult and searching in the neighboring subcortical structures risks causing damage. The risk is increased when the lesion is located in or involves functionally important regions such as the motor speech area or the motor strip. Under these circumstances the most direct and cautious surgical approach must be taken.

Despite the progress microneurosurgery has made[2], it is still not able to solve all localizing problems. CT-guided stereotaxy provides precise anatomic localisation of the lesion, but not a way to remove it. We therefore have used a method combining stereotactic and microneurosurgical techniques to be able to pinpoint the lesion and then remove it under direct visual control[3,5,6], thus minimizing the damage to critical nervous tissue during operations in subcortical regions.

Technique

A combined CT-stereotactic and microsurgical approach along a precalculated stereotactic trajectory was used in 21 patients who harbored small lesions in critical cerebral areas (Table 1). Riechert's* Stereotactic System was used in 19 patients and the Brown-Roberts-Wells** System in two patients. In the following the procedure using Riechert's Stereotactic System is described.

The coordinate frame is a circular aluminium alloy ring which has 3 axes (Fig. 1). The x-axis of the ring is parallel to the coronal plane, the y-axis is parallel to the sagittal plane and the z-axis corresponds to the patients longitudinal axis. Using these 3 axes every intracranial point can be precisely defined with an accuracy of ± 1 mm. On its outer diameter the ring has base plates at 0, 90, 180 and 270 degrees, which serve as bearings for an aiming bow. The aiming bow can be moved in each direction and can be tilted in such a way that it does not interfere with the microsurgical removal of the lesion. The base plates also serve as reinforcements for the grip of the clamp

Table 1. *Identification of Tumours in the Patients Treated by Combined Stereotactic and Microsurgical Approach (n = 21)*

Metastases	12
Cavernomas	4
Astrocytomas (WHO II)	3
Oligodendroglioma (WHO II)	1
Ependymoma (WHO II)	1

---

* Distributed by Codman GmbH, Hamburg, Germany.
** Distributed by Radionics Inc, Burlington, Massachusetts, USA.

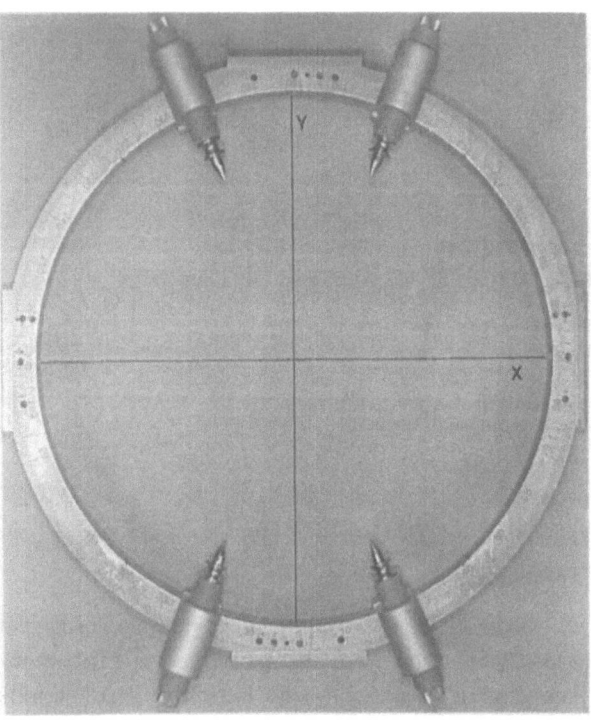

Fig. 1. Head ring of Riechert's Stereotactic System. The ring has three axes which provide a spatial definition of any point of the patient's head. X- and Y-axes are marked here. The ring has special base plates for the fixation of the aiming bow and the Mayfield head clamp holder

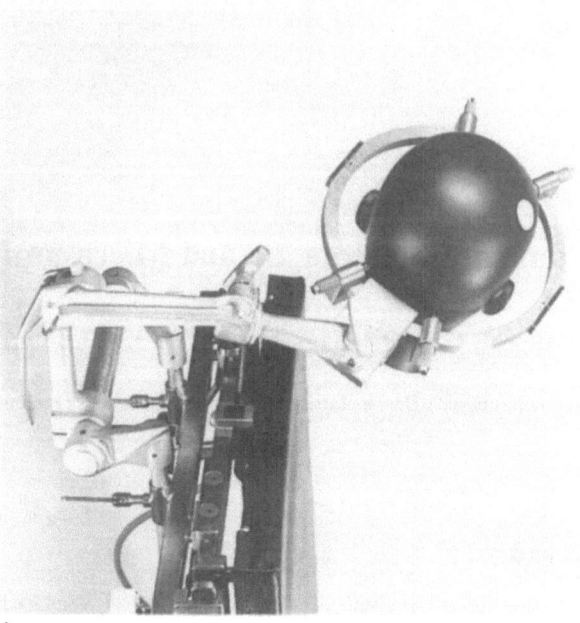

Fig. 2. The head ring is attached to the operation table using the Mayfield head clamp holder. So the patient's head can be fixed in any required position without the need of the stereotactic floorstand

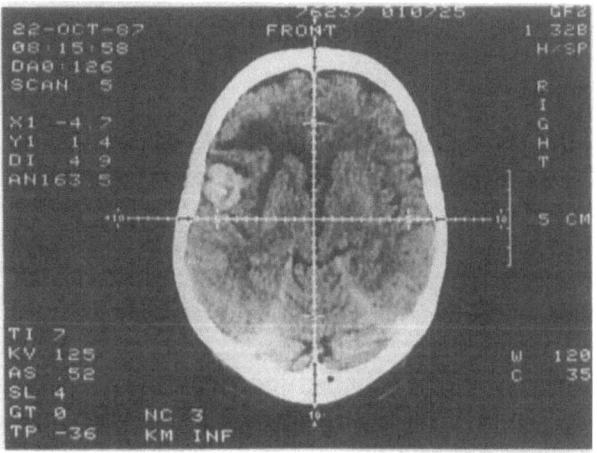

Fig. 3. Small metastatis from a pancreatic tumor which was located directly in the cortex. The CT-software allows a direct transfer of the coordinates without any modification once the CT image cross hair and the head ring are made to coincide. The Z-coordinate corresponds to the table incrementation

adapter of the Mayfield skull clamp holder. This makes it easy to fix the ring on the well-known and widely used Mayfield system (Fig. 2). The patient's head with the ring attached can be fixed in any required position without the need of the stereotactic floorstand. The head ring itself is mounted on the patient's skull using four plastic posts, each one holding a steel Mayfield pin.

Target localization is carried out in the same manner as for stereotactic biopsy. The patient is brought to a CT-scanner. The ring is clamped to the CT-table using a specially designed ring holder. Then contrast-enhanced CT is performed. Once the CT image cross hair and the head ring are made to coincide (Fig. 3), the CT-software allows a direct transfer of the coordinates without any modification.

After CT scanning, the patient is taken back to the operation theatre, where, if required, cerebral angiography under stereotactic conditions is performed. In 15 cases we also carried out stereoscopic angiography under stereotactic conditions. By using CT and angiographic data the exact lesion site can be determined. Then the entry point for the least hazardous approach must be calculated. It should be

as close as possible to the target, thus minimizing the distance of the stereotactic trajectory. The approach taken should rule out the risk of damage to adjacent cortical or subcortical vessels. Based on the angiographical data, an outline can be drawn of the vessels surrounding the lesion. This has proved to be very useful for planning the approach to make sure that no vessels are on the pre-planned trajectory. In paramedian lesions bridging veins can thus be spared.

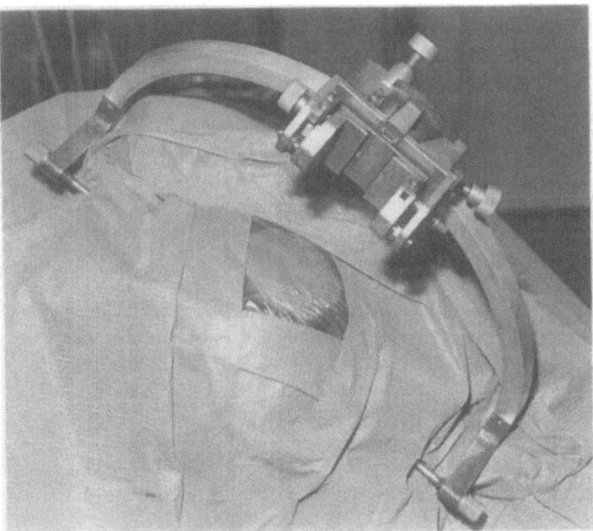

Fig. 4 a. The aiming bow is attached to the head ring under aseptic conditions. It can be tilted so that it does not obstruct microsurgery

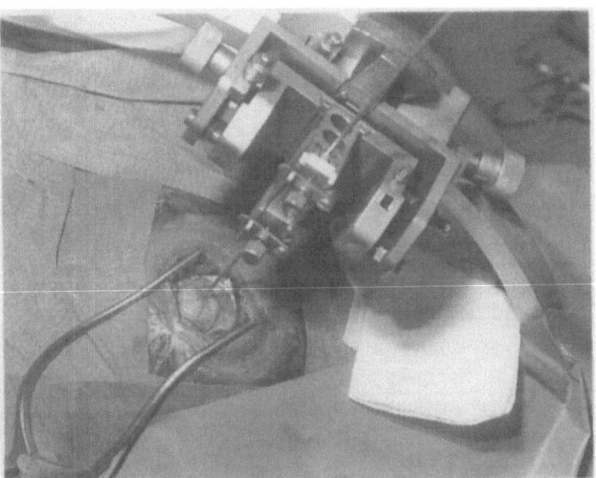

Fig. 4 b. During the operative procedure the lesion can be repeatedly pinpointed with a stereotactic cannula to confirm in which direction and at what distance the lesion is located

After the diagnostic procedures, the patient's head is secured on the operating table using the Mayfield system. The head remains stable in any desired position for craniotomy permitting unhindered access to the cranial vault or to the base of the skull. The ring is protected with a sterile foil to guarantee attachment of the aiming bow to the ring under aseptic conditions (Fig. 4a).

A linear or slightly bowed skin incision is made, usually not longer than 8cm. The location for the skin incision is marked with a stereotactic cannula, which is held by a special guide rail fixed on the aiming bow. The aiming bow can be tilted so that it does not

obstruct the microsurgery. If there is any doubt about the histological nature of the lesion and thus about the indication for open surgery, we first perform a stereotactic biopsy using a 6mm burrhole. The latter can be used for the excision of the bone flap. The diameter of the bone flap rarely exceeds 5cm.

The cortex is exposed and then, again with the help of the stereotactic device, the precise point for the cortical incision is pinpointed (Fig. 4b). The cortical incision can be kept small, as there is no doubt about the exact site of the lesion. When the lesion is located more deeply, we use the stereotactic cannula for further dissection into the brain parenchyma. In this case an inflatable rubber balloon can also be used to separate the white matter fibres[3, 7].

The rest of operation is then done by microsurgery. The lesion can be repeatedly pinpointed to confirm in which direction and at what distance the lesion is located.

Discussion

Despite advances made in neuroimaging techniques, the transfer of CT or MRI data to open surgery continues to remain a problem, especially if the lesion is small or deep seated in the brain parenchyma. Minute cortico-subcortical lesions often do not provoke macroscopic changes on the brain's surface and consequently may be difficult to find at surgery. Stereotaxy can be used to solve this problem as it allows the target to be defined and the ideal approach calculated with an accuracy of $\pm 1\,mm$[1]. In addition, the data of angiography performed under stereotactic conditions offer excellent landmarks for the removal of space-occupying lesions without causing injury to vessels. Vessels which in a planar image appeared to interfere with the lesion or the trajectory often turned out not to do so in the three-dimensional view[4]. The computer software used with Riechert's system allows an exact calculation of the stereotactic trajectory, which can then be transferred onto the CT slices.

The high accuracy of the method enables the surgeon to minimize the cortical incision as well as the bone flap and the skalp incision. This not only shortens the procedure, but also enhances patient safety and surgical efficiency. None of the 21 patients showed evidence of additional postoperative neurological deficits.

Stereotaxy is a simple and effective tool in the microsurgical treatment of small or deep-seated cerebral lesions.

References

1. Apuzzo MLJ, Chandrasoma PT, Cohen D, *et al* (1987) Computed imaging stereotaxy: Experience and perspectives related to 500 procedures applied to brain masses. Neurosurgery 20: 930–937
2. Haßler W, Harders A, Seeger W (1985) Microsurgical management of gliomas. In: Voth D, Krauseneck P (eds) Chemotherapy of gliomas. W. de Gruyter, Berlin, pp 177–187
3. Hirsch JF, Sainte Rose Ch, Pierre-Kahn A, Renier D, Hoppe-Hirsch E (1989) Stéréotaxie à crâne ouvert dans le traitement des lésions expansives du cerveau. Neurochirurgie 35: 164–168
4. Moringlane JR, Lippitz B, Ostertag CB (1988) Cerebral angiography under stereotactic conditions. Acta Neurochir (Wien) 91: 147–150
5. Ostertag CB (1988) New head fixation for the Riechert stereotaxic system. Technical note. Acta Neurochir (Wien) 94: 88–92
6. Riechert T (1982) Combined open-stereotaxic procedures. In: Schaltenbrand G, Walker AE (eds) Stereotaxy of the human brain. G. Thieme, Stuttgart New York, pp 449–456
7. Shahbabian S, Keller JT, Gould H J (1983) A new technique for making cortical incisions with minimal damage to cerebral tissue. Surg Neurol 20: 310–312

Correspondence: Dr. F. Alesch, Neurochirurgische Universitäts-klinik, Währinger Gürtel 18–20, A-1090 Wien, Austria.

Acta Neurochirurgica, Suppl. 53, 23–32 (1991)

Stereotactic-endoscopic Procedures on Processes of the Cranial Midline

D. Hellwig[1], B. L. Bauer[1], E. List-Hellwig[2], and H. D. Mennel[3]

[1] Department of Neurosurgery, [2] Department of Radiology, [3] Department of Neuropathology, Philipps-University Marburg, Federal Republic of Germany

Summary

The term "midline tumour" is defined partly from the topographic and from the pathogenetic point of view. Problems of modern imagegenerating procedures in establishing the diagnosis of cerebral midline lesions are described. The role of stereotactic diagnostic and therapeutic interventions is emphasized.

Stereotactic brain tumour biopsy, installation of shunts and reservoirs under visual control are performed. Interstitial radiotherapy is carried out for low-grade gliomas.

As an important innovation, stereotactic procedures are combined with endoscopic techniques.

Particular diagnostic and therapeutic difficulties of typical midline tumours such as craniopharyngeoma, germinoma, glioma and primary cerebral lymphoma as a local extension are discussed.

A reasonable concept in diagnosis and therapy of cerebral midline lesions is proposed.

Keywords: Endoscopy; interstitial irradiation; midline tumours; stereotaxy; craniopharyngeoma; germinoma; primary cerebral lymphoma.

Introduction

The term "midline tumour" is a topographical description. Midline tumours exhibit a wide spectrum of appearances and could be classified according to their localization or pathogenesis.

From the pathogenetic point of view this group could be defined as a relatively uniform group, because these processes include a high proportion of so called dysgenetic tumours, for example germinomas or craniopharyngeomas.

The pilocytic astrocytoma of childhood is another important tumour which probably belongs to this group. It derives from the subependymal glia and from some aspects of its growth-kinetics it could be considered as dysgenetic[12].

Beside these tumours with accepted malformation-character, lesions defined as so-called "local extensions"[28] affect the cerebral midline, as it is the case with lymphomas, gliomas, metastases.

There are many difficulties in managing midline-processes by open neurosurgery[27]. To choose the appropriate treatment, the exact diagnosis is required since some midline tumours do respond to other less invasive regimens than resection.

Image-generating methods such as CT or MRI often fail as diagnostic tools. On the other hand the so called explorative craniotomy has many risks and must be considered obsolete.

Today, stereotactic procedures play an important role in diagnosis and treatment of processes of the cranial midline. The results of the application of stereotactic operations in these lesions are encouraging.

The establishment of the histological diagnosis by stereotactic biopsy is very safe and accurate concerning smear preparation diagnosis[18].

Depending on the diagnosis, therapeutic interventions take place either directly after biopsy in the form of stereotactic interstitial irradiation or installation of shunts and reservoirs or secondarily as resection and/or external irradiation.

As an important innovation stereotactic procedures are combined with endoscopic techniques. In this way operations are performed under visual control and gain in security.

This is an overview about the present possibilities of stereotactic operation-techniques on cerebral midline lesions.

Material and Methods

1. Stereotactic Instrumentation

We used the CT-compatible instrumentation of Mundinger and Birg[32]. The biopsy specimens are obtained with special biopsy forceps, which were designed for use through the endoscope-working-channel. The diameters of the forceps ranged from 0.8 to 1.0 mm.

For endoscopy we developed a guiding-system, which is adapted to the stereotactic frame.

The endoscope guide cannula is a teflon tube, this tube is transparent to give a direct view of the route of entry to the desired target region.

For free-hand ventriculoscopy we took a special device which can be fixed on the self-retractor-system.

2. Endoscopes

We used flexible, steerable endoscopes with diameters from 1.5 to 3.3 mm.

A new prototype of flexible endoscope was constructed especially for the application in stereotactic neurosurgery (Olympus Inc. Tokyo). The main specifications are:

Outer diameter 3.3 mm, working length 300 mm, field of view 90°, direction of view 0°, depth of field 1–50mm, range of tip bending 180° up and 100° down. There is one working channel with a diameter of 1.2 mm for biopsy procedures and for application of laser-beam-therapy. This endoscope XURF P2–30 is used for stereotactic interventions on brain tumours, cystic midline processes and for ventriculoscopy.

3. Videorecording and Display

The ultralight Olympus OTV-S2 Medical-TV-Camera optimized intra-operative picture recording. The weight of this camera is only 25 g which reduces the physical strain of the endoscopist and gives a good manoeuvrability. The camera is easy compatible with a colour image-recorder.

The video recording-system also provides the possibility of documentation.

4. Operation-Technique

Stereotactic operations were performed under local anaesthesia with slight sedation. In children and for operations of the posterior-fossa general anaesthesia was employed.

The target point calculation was carried out with the computer-program TARGETRM (Fischer MET, Freiburg).

For supratentorial midline lesions we used the transfrontal approach, infratentorial lesions were operated on by the suboccipital transcerebellar approach. (Fig. 1 a, b).

5. Neuroradiological Equipment

CT-examinations were carried out with Somatom DR 3. (Siemens Inc.). For MRI Siemens Magnetom with 0.5 and 1.5 Tesla was used.

6. Histopathological Examinations

Morphological diagnosis was performed intra-operatively by smear-preparation technique or postoperatively by conventional histopathological examination.

Tissue specimens were obtained in mm-steps from the marginal areas to the center of the lesions. In this way we got an overview about the histopathological structure of the process as a whole.

7. Application of Drainages and Reservoirs

Cystic midline tumours were punctured stereotactically under endoscopic control. The total evacuation of the cysts was achieved by rinsing and suction through the endoscope-working channel. Thereafter drainages were installed and connected with a subcutaneous Omaya- or Rickham-reservoir. In this way a repeated puncture of the cysts was possible without any additional operational procedure.

For cystic craniopharyngeoma the catheter was guided through the ventricular-system, to drainage the contents of the cyst.

8. Interstitial Curietherapie

Interstitial irradiation was carried out with 125-Iodine. Dosimetry was calculated with a special three-dimensional program using the

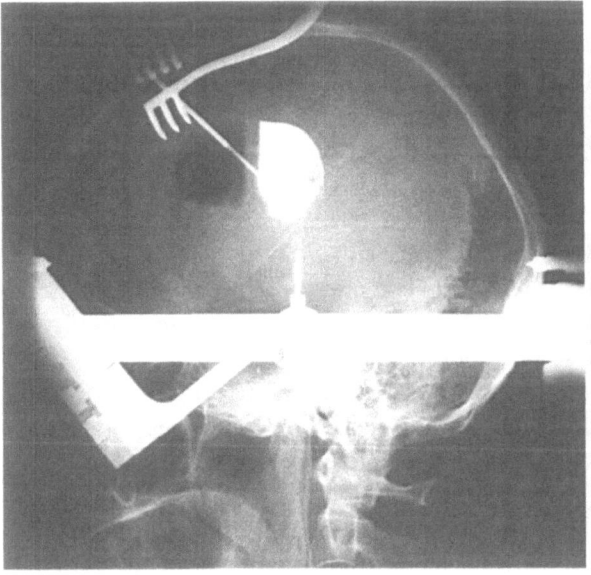

(a)

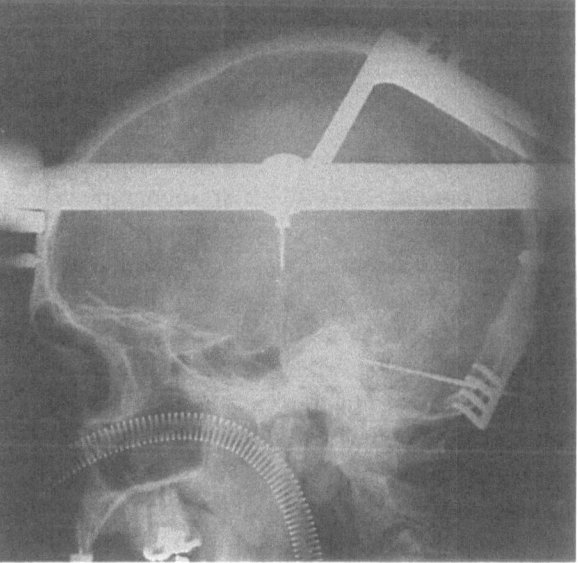

(b)

Fig. 1. Stereotactic approaches to midline tumours a) transfrontal, b) suboccipital, transcerebellar

EVADOS-system (Siemens Inc.). The peripheral tumour-dose was fixed at about 75 Gray.

The seed-application was performed with the seed-applicator-set of Fischer-MET, Freiburg.

Results

From June 1988 to August 1990 we have operated on 108 undiagnosed intracerebral lesions in "critical" localization stereotactically. 22 of these patients suffered from cerebral midline processes.

The age distribution of this group ranged from 12–77 years. 8 patients were female, 14 male (Table 1).

1. Neuroradiological Findings

MRI-examination was very sensitive and reveals pathological findings in all 8 cases, in which it was applied. This was in contrast to CT, where in 2 of 22 cases (9%) the midline lesion could not be found (Fig. 2a-d).

In 6 cases (27%) a definitive diagnosis was made on the basis of CT or MRI. These diagnosis were confirmed by smear-preparation examinations. In 16 cases (73%) it was not possible to establish the diagnosis on neuroradiological findings

Table 1. *Diagnosis and Therapy of Midline Tumours*

No.	Age	Sex	CT/MRI	Histopath. diagnosis	Therapy
1	71	f	CT: s	glioblastoma	irradiation
2	36	m	CT: s	anapl. glioma	irradiation chemotherapy
3	49	f	CT: sp	craniopharyngeoma	cysto-ventricular shunt, reservoir
4	40	m	CT: ns MRI: s	anapl. glioma	resection, irradiation chemotherapy
5	41	m	CT: s	metastasis dd: glioblastoma	irradiation chemotherapy
6	53	m	CT: s	cystic metastasis	irradiation chemotherapy
7	60	f	CT: s	primary cerebral lymphoma	cortico-steroids irradiation
8	52	m	CT: ns MRI: s	low-grade astrocytoma dd: gliosis	none
9	60	m	CT: s	anapl. glioma	irradiation chemotherapy
10	12	m	CT: sp MRI: sp	pilocytic astrocytoma	interstitial irradiation
11	51	m	CT: sp	anapl. glioma	irradiation chemotherapy
12	54	f	CT: sp MRI: sp	oligodendroglioma	interstitial irradiation
13	77	f	CT: s MRI: s	haemorrhage	none
14	41	m	CT: s	cystic astrocytoma	cyst-drainage
15	33	m	CT: sp MRI: sp	germinoma	irradiation
16	69	f	CT: s	primary cerebral lymphoma	cortico-steroids irradiation
17	73	f	CT: sp	glioblastoma	irradiation chemotherapy
18	18	m	CT: s	anapl. glioma	irradiation
19	41	m	CT: s	no diagnosis	cyst-drainage
20	68	m	CT: s	glioblastoma	irradiation
21	71	f	CT: s	cystic glioma	drainage irradiation
22	63	m	CT: s MRI: sp	oedema, necrosis infection	antibiotic therapy

ns = not sensitive, no lesion found. s = sensitive, no diagnosis possible. sp = specific, diagnosis is possible. dd = differential diagnosis.

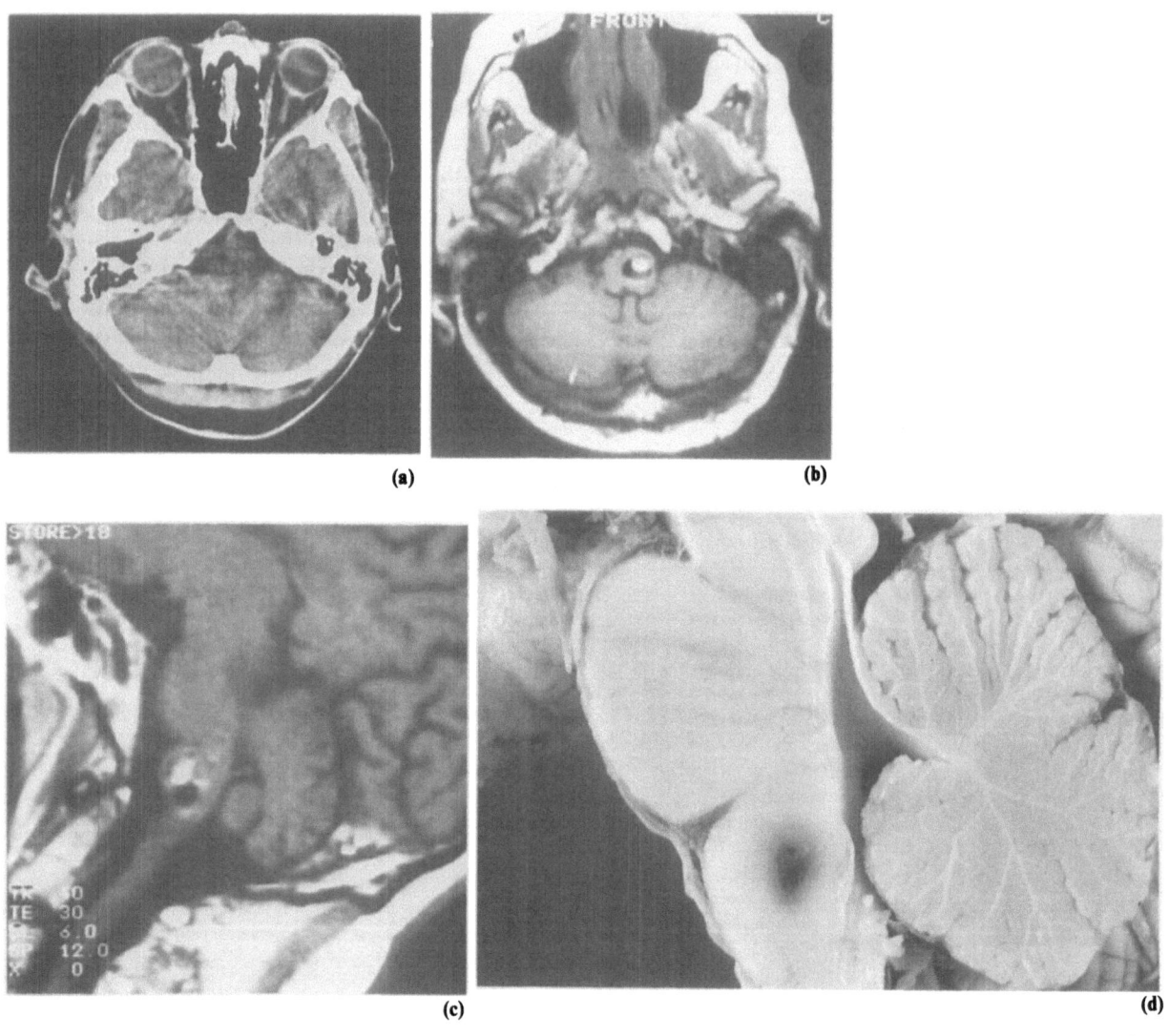

Fig. 2. Low-grade astrocytoma of the brain stem diagnosed by stereotactic biopsy. a) CT-examination does not demonstrate the tumour, while b) axial and c) sagittal MRI sections show the tumour in its topographical relationships; d) in comparison a post-mortem section

2. Endoscopic Stereotactic Biopsy and Histopathological Diagnosis

Stereotactic biopsies were performed under endoscopic control. With this technique postbiopsy bleeding was recognized immediately and could be staunched.

Vessels in the target point region caused us to choose another less dangerous region for the removal of a tissue biopsy.

In this way intra-operative complications were reduced. The postoperative morbidity was zero for stereotactic interventions on midline tumours and 2% for the total number of stereotactic interventions. The mortality for both groups was zero.

Intra-operative smear-preparations confirmed the diagnosis of midline lesions in 86%. In 3 cases no definite histopathological diagnosis was possible, even with conventional diagnostic tools. The distribution of tumour types is given in Table 1.

3. Interstitial Radiotherapy

Interstitial Curietherapy with permanent 125-Iodine application was executed for therapy of low-grade gliomas, not only in the cerebral midline but also for tumours in other critical areas. 15 radionuclid-implantations were carried out. Before these procedures morphological diagnosis was confirmed by intra-operative smear-preparation. Peri- and postoperatively no complications occured. The patients were discharged from hospital six days after intervention.

At present long-term results of our therapy-group are not available. But our follow-up with a maximum period of 3 years suggests a positive outcome.

Only one patient with a thalamic glioma died one year after isotope-implantation. Some patients suffered from an enlarged perifocal oedema induced by irradiation, which could be managed with steroids.

The major part of the patients showed decreased neurological symptoms with a good social re-entry.

4. Application of Cyst-Drainages and Reservoirs

Cystic midline lesions were emptied under endoscopic control. In tumours with rapid growth we placed a catheter at the bottom of the cyst, which was connected with a subcutaneous reservoir (Rickham, Omaya).

In this way a repeated cyst-evacuation was possible without any additional operative procedure.

For the treatment of cystic craniopharyngeoma we installed a cystoventricular shunt. This stereotactic procedure is an elegant minimal invasive method with good results (Fig. 3 a–c).

Discussion

1. Neuroradiological Findings

As our results demonstrate, neuroradiological examinations such as CT or MRI have many inherent

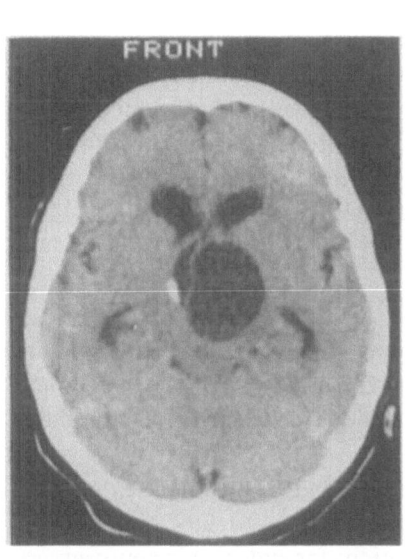

(a)

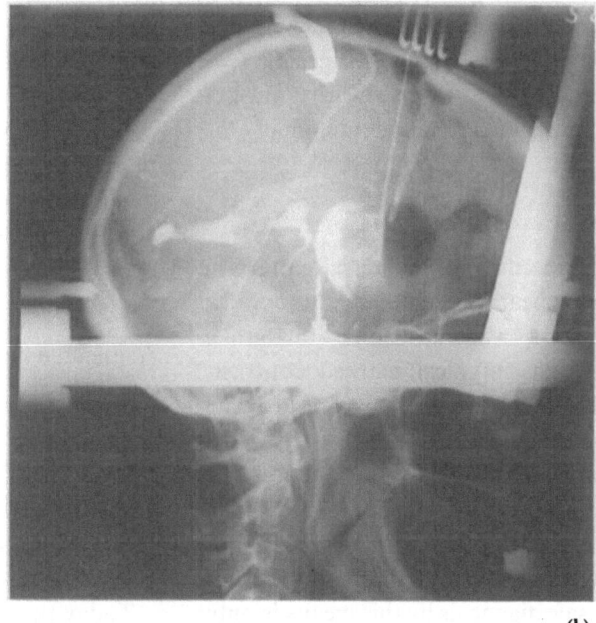

(b)

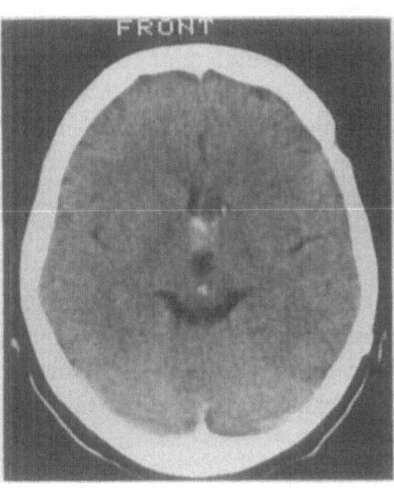

(c)

Fig. 3. Cystic craniopharyngeoma. a) Two cysts with a calcification in the wall of the smaller part. b) Insertion of a cysto-ventricular shunt and connection with an Omaya-reservoir. c) Tumour after follow-up of three years

difficulties in achieving the diagnosis of midline tumours.

One of the few exceptions is the cystic craniopharyngeoma which is easily detected by CT and MRI.

Other typical dysgenetic tumours as well as gliomatous tumours and "local extensions" of the cerebral midline could not always be diagnosed by this means.

Germinoma

Germinomas are the most common tumour of the pineal region[25]. CT reveals an isodense in some parts hyperdense and contrastenhancing tumour. A pathognomomic image-representation is not possible. The appearance is clearly heterogenic. There is no positive correlation between CT- and histopathological findings[35]. In MRI T1-weighted pictures show isointensive, T2-weighted hyperintensive characteristics. The contrast-enhancement is strong[14] (Fig. 5 a).

Altogether CT and MRI are very sensitive but not specific in the diagnosis of cerebral germinomas[7].

Glioma

Gliomas have no specific morphological pattern in CT or MRI. The appearance of these tumours in midline localization is various. Some low-grade astrocytomas show an untypical marked contrast-enhancement on CT[40], while other invasive growing malignant astrocytomas do not.

There does not appear any relationship between the degree of enhancement and histological malignancy in these tumours[46].

Errors in diagnosis of malignant gliomas by CT are not uncommon. A safe diagnosis by this means is only possible in one of five patients. In all other patients where the clinical situation demands it, especially in tumour-localization in the cerebral midline, biopsy remains the only means of obtaining a definite diagnosis[8].

MRI is more sensitive in demonstrating the extension of gliomas and of tumour response to treatment but not specific for exact histopathological diagnosis especially for tumour-grading[38].

Primary Cerebral Lymphoma

A typical local extension which is related to the cranial midline is the primary cerebral lymphoma. With increasing incidence recently[4] primary cerebral lymphomas gain in importance.

CT and MRI-imaging is not uniform for these tumours. With CT-examination three growing-types can be differentiated:

1. Slight hyperdense tumours with homogeneous contrast-enhancement (Fig. 6 a).
2. Diffuse periventricular and subependymal proliferations.
3. Encephalitic like lesions with diffuse edema[6].

For differential-diagnosis meningeomas, anaplastic astrocytomas, metastasis, meningeosis carcinomatosa, and focal infectious lesions have to be considered[24].

The T2-weighted MRI-examination shows hyperintensive demarcated tumours with increased signal intensity after Gd-DTPA application[26], which is not only specific for lymphomas[44].

The assessment of the neuroradiological findings in the referred cases leads us to the conclusion that CT and MRI are useful for tracing out cerebral midline lesions and for image-guidance of the stereotactic operation.

Improved MRI-techniques with increased contrast resolution seem to be more sensitive for demonstrating midline tumours[47], abnormal MRI findings, however, are not sufficient to determine an exact histopathological diagnosis in most cases[30].

2. Endoscopic Stereotaxy

Since the beginning of this century endoscopy has been applied in neurosurgery[10,31]. The main indications for this technique were operative procedures on hydrocephalus[45].

For a long time no progress was made in the field of "endo-neurosurgery"[16].

Today the indications for endoscopic neurosurgery are enlarged. It is used for the evacuation of haematomas[2], for brain tumour diagnosis and – therapy especially in the cerebral midline[3] and for interventions on midline and intraventricular cysts[41,42].

In stereotactic neurosurgery application of endoscopes is rare. Endoscopes are used as a helpful tool for stereotactic evacuations of colloid cysts[17] and interventions on intra-axial solid and cystic brain tumours[37].

Common to most of these uses are endoscopes which are rigid and have diameters of more than 6 mm. These diameters are in contrast to the tissue-sparing stereotactic operation techniques especially in midline lesions.

Technical progress makes it now possible to use ultra-thin flexible, steerable endoscopes combined with ultralight microchipcameras in surgery. This development offers new perspectives even in stereotactic neurosurgery, particularly for biopsies of solid brain tumours under visual control.

We have combined these two methods in a new stereotactic operation technique which we term "endoscopic stereotaxy"[20].

Our results prove that stereotactic-endoscopic interventions on midline lesions have many advantages.

The stereotactic approach for these processes provides a less invasive, "sure-hitting" operation-technique. The endoscopic monitoring of the stereotactic procedure guarantees intra-operative visual control and offers the possibility of immediate intervention under direct view.

The indications for stereotactic-endoscopic interventions on processes of the cerebral midline are:

1. biopsy of undiagnosed solid and cystic tumours (Fig. 4 a),
2. evacuation of cystic processes,
3. installation of drainage-systems,
4. laser-therapy for small-sized lesions,
5. haemostatic procedures,
6. ventriculoscopy (Fig. 4 b).

3. Histopathological Diagnosis and Therapeutic Considerations

Squash and smear-preparations yield specimens in which the histological pattern is destroyed. Yet, by examination of material gained step by step through the lesion, a reconstruction of the histopathology is possible

Morphological diagnosis is absolutely necessary before further therapeutic interventions on cerebral midline tumours, to avoid gross errors of treatment, as the following statements will demonstrate.

Germinoma

Germinomas are the most common tumours of the pineal region[11]. These processes are extremely radiosensitive (Fig. 5 b).

There is no significant difference in survival-time between microsurgically treated and irradiated patients[25].

Tumour-resection with its high risk therefore is not required if diagnosis could be confirmed by stereotactic biopsy[39].

On the other hand some tumours of the pineal region, which have similar appearance in CT or MRI

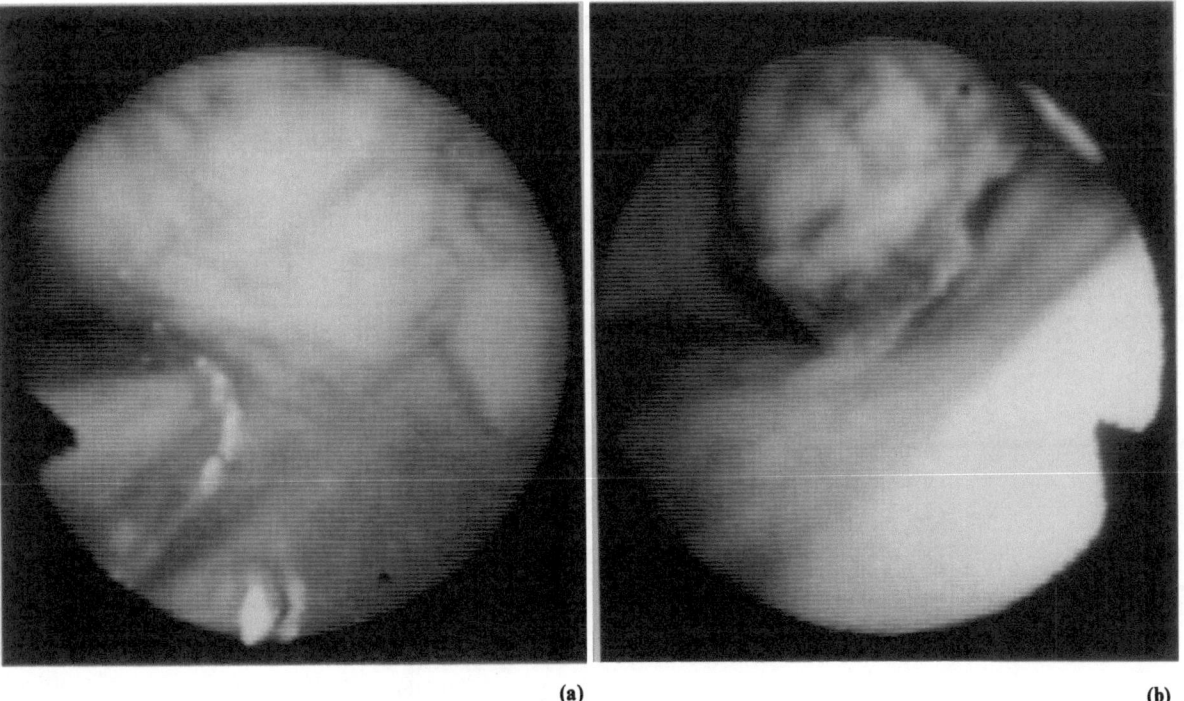

(a)   (b)

Fig. 4. Stereotactical application of ultra-thin endoscopes. a) Biopsy of a cystic midline tumour under direct view; see biopsy forceps and cyst wall. b) Ventriculoscopy: Small tumour in the lateral ventricle

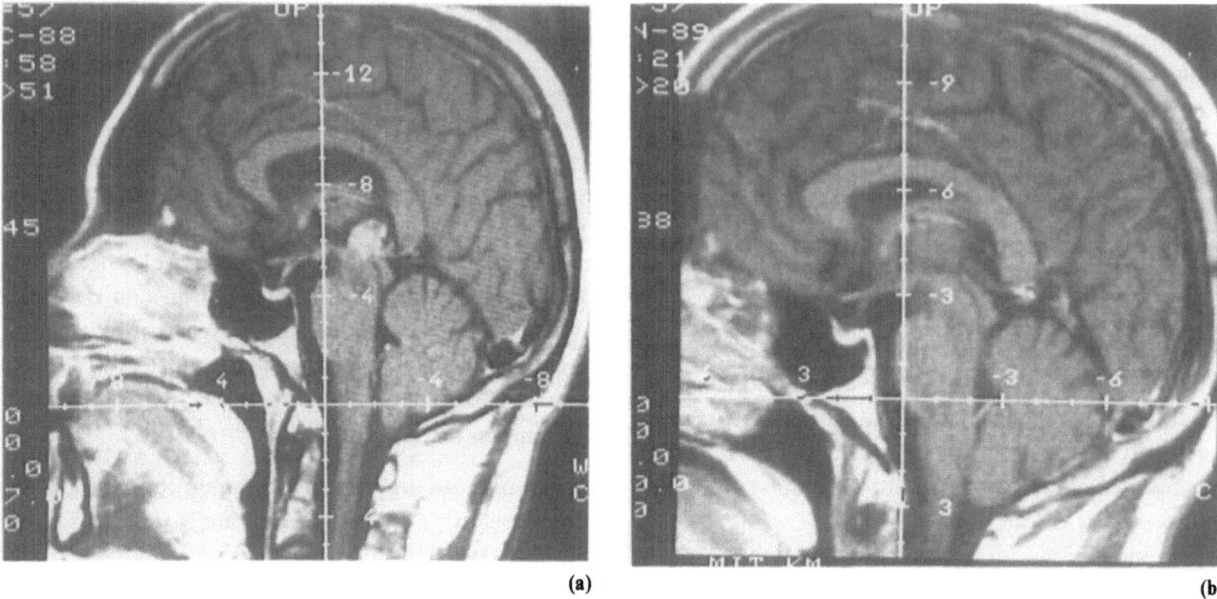

Fig. 5. a) MRI:contrast-enhancing tumour of the pineal, histo-pathological diagnosis: germinoma. b) Tumour after fractioned focal irradiation with 30Gy

as germinomas, are radioresistant. This fact implies that the formerly used "irradiation test" with application of one single dose of 2000 rad[43] should not be performed as a diagnostic method.

Because of the variety of tumour-types found in the pineal region treatment has to be differentiated. A biopsy should be obtained in all patients with pineal tumours[14].

Primary Cerebral Lymphoma

Two patients in our series of midline-tumours suffered from primary cerebral lymphomas, which could not be diagnosed with CT- or MRI-examination. The perifocal oedema was treated pre-operatively by the use of corticosteroids. Tumour-regression was the consequence (Fig. 6 b). This therapeutic effect is to be

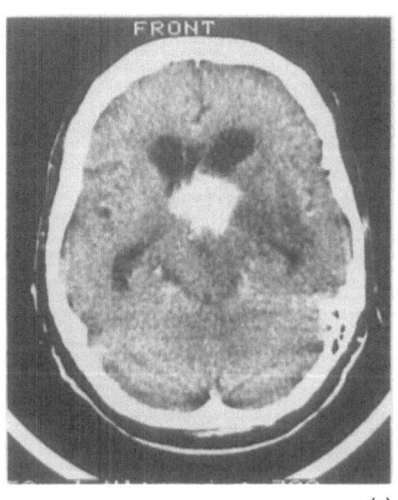 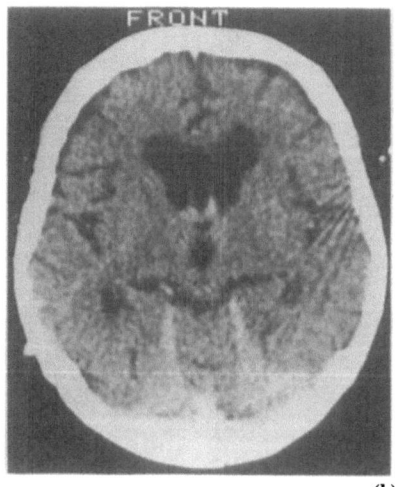

Fig. 6. a) CT:contrast-enhancing tumour of the cerebral mid-line, histopathological diagnosis: primary cerebral lymphoma. b) Tumour after one week with cortico-steroid-treatment

expected already after a short time[22] and could lead to the misfortune, that the tumour is missed during an explorative craniotomy[48].

Even if prognosis is very poor with a median survival time of less than one year[5] a post-biopsy therapy-regimen should include radiation-therapy[21] and chemotherapy[15].

The importance of stereotactic biopsy in the diagnosis of midline-lesions is underlined impressively by these comments.

Stereotactic procedures are safe[36] and reliable concerning smear-preparation diagnosis[29]. Empiric methods of treatment are no longer justified for treatment of these tumours[9].

4. Interstitial Curietherapy

Permanent stereotactic application of 125-Iodine-seeds is the treatment of choice for low-grade gliomas in the midline or other critical localizations in the brain, where a tumour resection has considerable risks.

This isotope is easy to handle and has excellent radiobiological properties for use in low-grade gliomas[33].

At the present time we have no long-term results on interstitial curietherapy with 125-Iodine for low-grade glioma, but we suggest from our data, that the outcome would be satisfactory.

This suggestion is in accordance with results which were presented with series with larger numbers of patients treated by intestitial low-dose curie-therapy[13,34].

Conclusion

As we have pointed out any therapeutic intervention on cerebral midline tumours requires an exact histopathological diagnosis.

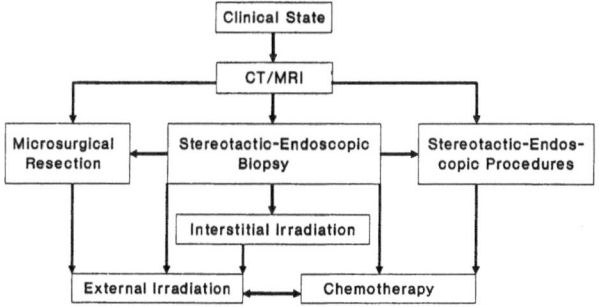

Fig. 7. Rational diagnosis and therapy of midline tumours

Radiological examinations like CT and MRI cannot solve this problem sufficiently accurately.

Stereotactic interventions are safe and accurate even in high-risk localizations as in pons[1] and brain stem[23].

Diagnostic errors relating to mistreatment are minimized with this method. As an important innovation endoscopy makes stereotactic interventions under direct vision possible.

The assembling of the neurological report, CT and MRI-findings together with the histopathological diagnosis of the stereotactic-endoscopic biopsy offers a useful concept for rational treatment of cerebral midline tumours[19] (Fig. 7).

References

1. Abernathey CO, Camacho A, Kelly PJ (1989) Stereotactic suboccipital transcerebellar biopsy of pontine mass lesions. J Neurosurg 70: 195–200
2. Auer LM (1985) Endoscopic evacuation of intracerebral haemorrhage. High-tec-surgical treatment – a new approach to the problem? Acta Neurochir (Wien) 74: 124–128
3. Auer LM, Holzer P, Ascher PW, Heppner F (1988) Endoscopic neurosurgery. Acta Neurochir (Wien) 90: 1–14
4. Baumgartner JE, Rachlin JR, Beckstead JH, et al (1990) Primary cerebral nervous system lymphomas: natural history and response to radiation therapy in 55 patients with acquired immunodeficiency syndrome. J Neurosurg 73: 206–211
5. Berry MP, Simpson WJ (1980) Radiation therapy in the management of primary malignant lymphoma of the brain. Int J Radiat Oncol Biol Phys 7: 55–59
6. Bogdahn U, Bogdahn S, Mertens HG, Dammasch D (1986) Primary non-Hodgkin lymphomas of the CNS. Acta Neurol Scand 73: 602–614
7. Bruce DA, Allen JC (1985) Tumor staging for pineal region tumor in childhood. Cancer 56: 1792–1794
8. Choksey MS, Valentine A, Shawdon H, et al (1989) Computed tomography in the diagnosis of malignant brain tumour: do all patients need biopsy? J Neurol Neurosurg Psychiatry 52: 821–825
9. Coffey, RJ, Lunsford, LD (1985) Stereotactic surgery for mass lesions of the midbrain and pons. Neurosurgery 17: 12–18
10. Dandy WE (1922) Cerebral ventriculoscopy. Bull Johns Hopkins Hosp 33:189
11. Edwards MS, Hudgins RJ, Wilson CB, et al (1988) Pineal region tumors in children. J Neurosurg 68: 689–697
12. Ferbert A, Gulotta F (1985) Remarks on the follow-up of cerebellar astrocytomas. J Neurol 232: 134–136
13. Frank F, Fabrizi AP, Gaist G, Frank-Ricci R, et al (1987) Late considerations on the treatment of low-grade malignancy cerebral tumors with Iodine-125-Brachytherapy. Appl Neurophysiol 50: 302–309
14. Futrell NN, Osborn AG, Cheson BD (1981) Pineal region tumors: computed tomographic-pathologic spectrum. AJR 137: 951–956
15. Gabbai AA, Hochberg FH, Linggood M, et al (1989) High-dose methotrexate for non-Aids primary central nervous system lymphoma. J Neurosurg 70: 190–194
16. Griffith HB (1986) Endoneurosurgery-endoscopic intracranial surgery. In: Symon L, et al (eds) Advances and technical standards in neurosurgery, Vol 14. Springer, Wien New York, pp 2–24

17. Heikkinen ER, Heikinnen MI (1987) New diagnostic and therapeutic tools in stereotaxy. Appl Neurophysiol 50: 136–142

18. Hellwig D, Rossberg C, Welcke, (1989) Die Bedeutung der stereotaktischen Biopsie für die Differentialdiagnose and Therapie intrazerebraler Raumforderungen. Zentralbl allg Pathol pathol Anat 135:84

19. Hellwig D, Mennel HD, List-Hellwig E, Rossberg C (1991) Der stereotaktische Eingriff als Beitrag zur Diagnose and Therapie mittelliniennaher Prozesse. Neurochirurgia 34: 62–68

20. Hellwig D, Bauer BL (1991) Endoscopic procedures in stereotactic neurosurgery. Acta Neurochir (Wien) [Suppl] 52: 30–32

21. Hochberg FH, Miller DC (1988) Primary central nervous system lymphoma. J Neurosurg 68: 835–853

22. Homo-Delarche F (1984) Glucocorticoid receptors in normal and neoplastic human lymphoid tissues: a review. Cancer Res 44: 431–437

23. Hood TW, McKeever PE (1989) Stereotactic management of cystic gliomas of the brain stem. Neurosurgery 24: 373–378

24. Jiddane M, Nicoli F, Diaz P, *et al* (1986) Intracranial malignant lymphoma. J Neurosurg 65: 592–599

25. Jooma R, Kendall BE (1983) Diagnosis and management of pineal tumours. J Neurosurg 58: 654–665

26. Kazner E, Wende S, Gumme Th, Stochdorph O (1988) Computer- und Kernspintomographie intrakranieller Tumoren aus klinischer Sicht, 2. Aufl. Springer, Berlin Heidelberg New York

27. Koos WT, Perneczky A, Horaczek A (1985) Problems in surgical technique for treatment of supratentorial midline tumours in children. Acta Neurochir (Wien) [Suppl] 35: 31–41

28. Mennel HD (1988) Geschwuelste des zentralen und peripheren Nervensystems. In: Doerr W, Seifert G (eds) Pathologie des Nervensystems, Band 13/III. Springer, Berlin Heidelberg New York

29. Mennel HD, Rossberg C, Lorenz H, Schneider H, Hellwig D (1989) Reliability of simple cytological methods in brain tumor biopsy diagnosis. Neurochirurgia 32: 129–134

30. Mills CM, Crooks LE, Kaufman L, Brant-Zawadzki M (1984) Cerebral abnormalities: use of calculated T1 and T2 magnetic resonance images for diagnosis. Radiology 150: 87–94

31. Mixter WJ (1923) Ventriculoscopy and puncture of the third ventricle. Bos Med Surg J 188: 277

32. Mundinger F, Birg W (1984) Stereotactic biopsy of intracranial processes. Acta Neurochir (Wien) [Suppl] 33:219–224

33. Mundinger F (1988) Stereotactic biopsy and technique of implantation (instillation) of radionuclids. In: Jellinger K (ed) Therapy of malignant brain tumours. Springer, Wien New York, pp 150 ff

34. Mundinger F (1988) Considerations in the usage and results of curietherapy. In: Lunsford LD (ed) Modern stereotactic neurosurgery. Martinus Nijhoff Publishing, Boston Dordrecht Lancaster, pp 245–258

35. Neuwelt EA Glasberg M, Frenkel E, Clark WK (1979) Malignant pineal region tumors. A clinico-pathological study. J Neurosurg 51: 597–607

36. Ostertag CB, Mennel HD, Kiessling MO (1980) Stereotactic biopsy of brain tumors. Surg Neurol 14: 275–283

37. Otsuki T, Jokura H, Yoshimoto T (1990) Stereotactic guiding tube for open-system-endoscopy. A new approach for the stereotactic endoscopic resection of intra-axial brain tumours. Neurosurgery 27: 326–330

38. Packer RJ, Batnitzki S, Cohens ME (1985) Magnetic resonance imaging in the evaluation of intracranial tumours of childhood. Cancer 56: 1767–1772

39. Pecker J, Scarabin JM, Vallee B, Brucher JM (1979) Treatment in tumours of the pineal region. Value of stereotactic biopsy. Surg Neurol 12: 341–348

40. Pedersen H, Gjerris F, Klinken L (1981) Computed tomography of benign supratentorial astrocytomas of infancy and childhood. Neuroradiology 21: 87–91

41. Powell MP, Torrens MJ, Thomson JLG, Horgan JG (1983) Isodense colloid cysts of the third ventricle: a diagnostic and therapeutic problem resolved by ventriculoscopy. Neurosurgery 13: 234–237

42. Powers SK (1986) Fenestration of intraventricular cysts using a flexible, steerable endoscope and the argon laser. Neurosurgery 18: 637–641

43. Rao YTR, Medini E, Haselow RE, *et al* (1981) Pineal and ectopic pineal tumours: the role of radiation therapy. Cancer 48: 708–713

44. Ramsey RG, Geremia GK (1988) CNS complications of AIDS: CT and MRI findings. AJR 151: 449–454

45. Scarf JE (1935) Third ventriculoscopy as the rational treatment of obstructive hydrocephalus. J Pediatr 6: 870

46. Segall H, Batnitzky S, Zee CH-S, *et al* (1985) Computed tomography on the diagnosis of intracranial neoplasms in children. Cancer 56: 1748–1755

47. Smith FW (1987) Magnetic resonance imaging of midline brain tumors using inversion recovery sequences of 0.08 T (3.4 MHz). Magn Reson Med 5: 118–128

48. Vaquero J, Martinez R, Rossi E, Lopez R (1984) Primary cerebral lymphoma: the "ghost tumor". Case report. J Neurosurg 60: 174–176

Correspondence: Dr. D. Hellwig, Neurochirurgische Klinik der Philipps-Universität Marburg, Baldingerstrasse, D-3550 Marburg, Federal Republic of Germany.

Acta Neurochirurgica, Suppl. 53, 33–36 (1991)
© by Springer-Verlag 1991

Diagnostic Potential of Stereotactic Biopsy of Midline Lesions

F. Alesch[1], K. Kitz[1], W. Th. Koos[1], and C. B. Ostertag[2]

Neurochirurgische Universitätsklinik [1]Wien, Austria, and [2]Freiburg, Federal Republic of Germany

Summary

The technique of CT-guided stereotactic biopsy is described and its reliability is discussed based on the experiences with a series of 1747 procedures. We could show that stereotactic biopsy has an overall diagnostic accuracy of 95% and therefore is a safe and reliable tool for planning the therapeutic strategy.

Keywords: Stereotactic biopsy; reliability; complications.

Introduction

Modern computer-assisted imaging techniques such as MRI or CT provide excellent topographic information and details about even the smallest lesions. They allow a tentative diagnosis, but cannot provide a histological one. The indication and the specific kind of surgical management, however, often depends on the histological nature of the lesion[1].

The histological diagnosis can only be made under the microscope. CT-guided stereotactic biopsy enables us to obtain samples of the lesion. However, the size and number of the stereotactic biopsy samples are limited and the questions, we are confronted with are: Is stereotactic biopsy a reliable method? How great is the diagnostic potential of the stereotactic biopsy? From a series of 1747 patients of the Department of Stereotactic Neurosurgery in Homburg/Saar in Germany and from the Department of Neurosurgery in Vienna, we studied the reliability, the diagnostic value, the limitations and the complications of stereotactic biopsy. This study in part updates previous reports[2,4,7].

Description of the Technique

In Vienna we mostly use the Riechert system and less often the Brown–Roberts–Wells system, in Homburg we exclusively used the Riechert system. Under mild sedation and local anesthesia the head ring of the stereotactic system is fixed to the patient's skull using four plastic posts, each one holding a Mayfield pin (Fig. 1). The patient is then brought to a CT-scanner. The ring is clamped to the CT-table with a specially designed ring holder. The latter holds the ring securely parallel to the scanning plan of the CT-gantry. Since the stereotactic apparatus uses rectilinear coordinates for indexing, we can directly transfer the coordinates from the CT-scanner without any modifications (Fig. 2).

After CT scanning, the patient is taken back to the operation theatre. If there is need for angiography, which is generally the case with midline lesions, it is then performed under stereotactic conditions. This allows the preservation of cerebral vessels or highly vascularised areas. The target point is then calculated using CT and angiographic data. Under local anesthesia a burrhole is made, generally in a right frontal site. Then, depending on the location and the size of the lesion, 2 to 12 (mean 6) tissue samples are taken stepwise at distances of 2 to 5 mm. The volume of each sample is approximately 1 mm³. For this we use a specially designed biopsy forceps. This technique, which is called serial biopsy, allows us to obtain a representative profile, even of heterogenous tumours. Moreover, it permits an estimation of the borders of a tumour when interstitial irradiation is planned.

Some samples are evaluated using an intraoperative smear technique. The probe is placed on glass slides and gently smeared or spread with needles, stained, and slightly pressed with a coverslip. The staining was done using Löffler's methylene blue, in Vienna we use May-Grünwald-Giemsa. When this procedure is employed a neuropathologist is present during the operation. The remaining samples are fixed for embedding and routine stains, including semi-thin sections and immunohistology.

In all cases the final neuropathological diagnosis is the result of the two diagnostic procedures described above. For this study clinical follow-up and the results of open surgery treatment or autopsy were also taken into account. For glial tumours we used a grading according to the World Health Organization (WHO)(10)*.

---

* **Acknowledgements:** The neuropathological evaluation was done by H. Budka, Neurological Institute, University of Vienna, M. Kiessling, Department of Neuropathology, University of Heidelberg, Germany and B. Volk, Department of Neuropathology, University of Freiburg, Germany.

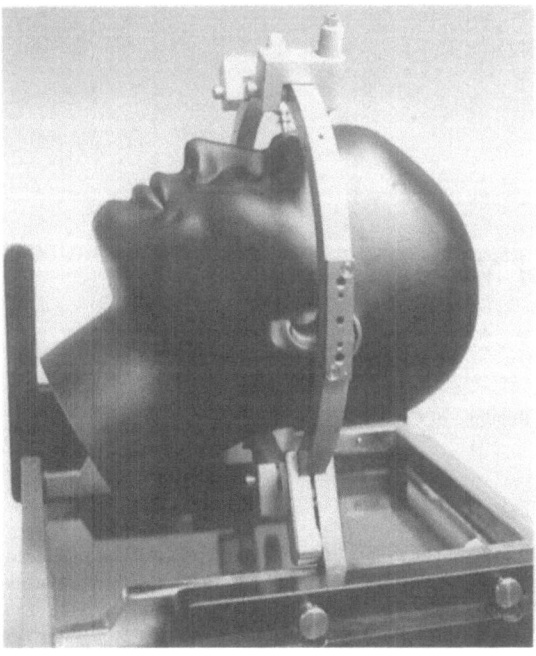

Fig. 1. The head ring of the Riechert stereotactic system is fixed on the patient's skull using four plastic posts, each one holding a Mayfield pin

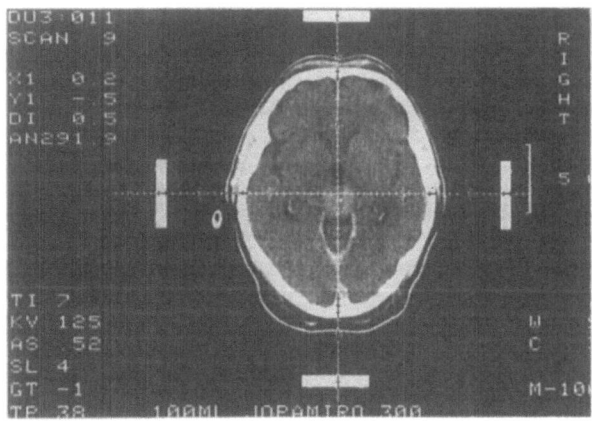

Fig. 2. The coordinates can be transferred directly from the CT-scanner's software without need of any modifications

Results

From April 1984 until March 1990 1564 stereotactic biopsies were performed in Homburg. In Vienna we performed 183 stereotactic biopsies from March 1986 until May 1990.

The distribution of location and diagnosis were very similar to those reported earlier[2,4,7]. The majority of the lesions were located in functionally critical areas. 32% of the lesions were in or near the midline (Table 1). 84% of the lesions were neoplastic, 11% were

Table 1. *Localization of Biopsied Lesions*

Frontal	20%	
Temporal	20%	944 cases (54%)
Parietal-occipital	14%	
Hypothalamus–chiasm	7%	
Basal ganglia–thalamus	11%	
Midbrain–pineal region	5%	559 cases (32%)
Pons–medulla	6%	
Ventricles	3%	
Cerebellum	3%	
Multilocular	8%	244 cases (14%)
Other	3%	

4/84–5/90 (n = 1747)

Table 2. *Diagnosis of Biopsied Lesions*

	N	%
Low grade glioma	526	30
High grade glioma	465	27
Colloid cyst	17	1
Pineozytoma/Pinealoblastoma	14	1
Germinoma	19	1
PNET	11	1
Craniopharyngeoma	28	2
Pituitary adenoma	18	1
Developmental tumour	20	1
Misc. tumour	42	2
Metastatic tumour	213	12
Meningioma	25	1
Lymphoma	67	4
Vascular lesion	100	6
Gliosis	92	5
Infection	32	2
Unclassified	58	3

4/84–5/90 (n = 1747)

of vascular origin, and 2% were infectious. 3% remain unclassified (Table 2). The tumours most frequently found were astrocytomas. These diagnoses are the synthesis of cytological as well as histological findings.

For the final pathological diagnosis other findings in addition to the histology were taken into account: patient data, including mainly follow-up, radiographic findings, consecutive intraoperative or autoptic findings. This allowed us to establish a correlation between the cytological and histological findings (Table 3).

In 60% tumour type and grade of the cytological evaluation could be confirmed, in 4.5% tumour type, and in 2.5% tumour presence. Absence of a tumour was confirmed in 10%. This yielded an overall confirmation of 77%. There was a discrepancy in

Table 3. *Correlation of Diagnosis Obtained from Smear Preparation and Paraffin Sections*

Confirmation	
Tumour type and grade confirmed	60.0%
Tumour type confirmed	4.5%
Tumour presence confirmed	2.5%
Absence of tumour confirmed	10.0%
Discrepancy	
Tumour type discrepancy	5.0%
Tumour grade discrepancy	4.0%
Tumour presence discrepancy	1.5%
No correlation possible	12.5%

4/84–5/90 (n = 1747)

Table 5. *Overall Diagnostic Potential of Cytological Diagnosis and Paraffin Sections*

Author	Year reported	Cases	Accuracy
Edner	(1981)	345	91%
Monsaingeon et al.	(1984)	268	92%
Sedan et al.	(1984)	309	91%
Kleihues et al.	(1984)	600	93%
Anagnostopoulos et al.	(1986)	1,236	95%
Own series	(1990)	1.747	95%

10.5%. No correlation was possible in 12.5%, in which cases the material was not representative either cytologically or histologically mainly as a result of sampling error. Further we studied 41 patients from the Vienna series who had been operated on after stereotactic biopsy. This gave us the possibility to study the correlation between the diagnoses from stereotactic biopsy and open surgery (Table 4).

In 38 cases (92.5%) we found an absolute correlation between biopsy and open surgery diagnoses, regarding both the nature of the tumour and its possible grading. In one patient (2.5%) we could confirm the nature of the tumour but not its grading. In two cases (5%) there was a discrepancy between the biopsy and open surgical diagnoses.

The overall complication rate was 2.3%. They occurred mostly in patients with an major mass lesion and were manifest as transient deterioration of the patient's neurological status due to peri- or intralesional haemorrhages. These haemorrhages disappeared in subsequent CT follow up scans corresponding to the clinical improvement. 16 patients (0.9%) died within 6 days after biopsy, mostly due to haemorrhage.

Table 4. *Accuracy of Stereotactic Biopsy: Correlation of Diagnosis – Stereotactic Biopsy versus Craniotomy/Autopsy (41 of 183 Cases)*

Confirmation		
Tumour type and grade confirmed	38	92.5%
Tumour type confirmed	1	2.5%
Total		95.0%
Discrepancy		
Tumour type discrepancy	1	2.5%
Tumour grade discrepancy	1	2.5%
Total		5.0%

Discussion

A review of the literature shows that the average overall diagnostic accuracy of stereotactic biopsy is about 90% (Table 5). In our series it was 95%. The main potential problem remains the sample size, especially in heterogenous tumours. This is also the reason why errors resulted in the sampling of anaplastic astrocytomas, metastatic tumours or mixed-cell tumours. The disadvantage of the small sample size can be compensated by careful targeting of the biopsy site, by taking serial biopsies and by the presence of the neuropathologist at the operation, so that an intraoperative cytological smear evaluation can be performed. Moreover, immunohistochemistry can help in the differential diagnosis in anaplastic tumours such as malignant gliomas and metastases.

Another error results from the failures to distinguish between infiltrative gliomas and reactive gliosis. This is mainly a neuropathological problem and is not unique to stereotactic biopsy. It also exists in open surgery. Unlike with open surgery, the stereotactic technique allows stepwise sampling, which facilitates arriving at the accurate tumour diagnosis and degree of infiltration.

In conclusion, we feel that stereotactic biopsy using modern imaging techniques together with the new neuropathological tools such as immunohistochemistry is a safe and reliable method of obtaining the information needed to plan the therapeutic strategy.

References

1. Alesch F, Moringlane JR, Ostertag CB (1988) Die stereotaktische Hirnbiopsie als Grundlage der Therapieplanung. Bull Soc Sci Méd 1: 5–13
2. Anagnostopoulos J, Kiessling M, Volk B (1988) Validität morphologischer Diagnostik an stereotaktischen Hirntumorbiopsien. In: Bamberg N, Sack H (eds) Therapie primärer Hirntumoren. W. Zuckschwerdt Verlag, pp 270–278
3. Edner G (1981) Stereotactic biopsy of intracranial space occupying lesions. Acta Neurochir (Wien) 57: 213–234

4. Kleihues P, Volk B, Anagnostopoulos J, Kiessling M (1984) Morphologic evaluation of stereotactic brain tumour biopsies. Acta Neurochir (Wien) [Suppl] 33: 171–181

5. Kleihues P, Kiessling M, Janzer RC (1987) Morphological markers in neuro-oncology. In: Seifert G (ed) Morphological tumor marker, current topics in pathology, Vol 77. Springer, Berlin Heidelberg New York, pp 307–338

6. Monsaingeon V, Daumas-Duport C, Mann M, Miyahara S, Szikla G (1984) Stereotactic sampling biopsies in a series of 268 consecutive cases – validity and technical aspects. Acta Neurochir (Wien) [Suppl] 33: 195–200

7. Ostertag CB (1988) Reliability of stereotactic brain tumor biopsy. In: Lundsford LD (ed) Modern stereotactic neurosurgery.

Martinus Nijhoff Publishing, Boston Dordrecht Lancaster, pp 129–136

8. Ostertag CB, Mennel HD, Kiessling M (1980) Stereotactic biopsy of brain tumors. Surg Neurol 14: 275–283

9. Sedan R, Peragut JC, Farnarier Ph, Hassoun J, Sethian M (1984) Intra-encephalic stereotactic biopsies. Acta Neurochir (Wien) [Suppl] 33: 207–210

10. Zülch KJ (1980) Principles of the new World Health Organization (WHO) classification of brain tumors. Neuroradiology 19: 59–66

Correspondence: Dr. F. Alesch, Neurochirurgische Universitäts-klinik, Währinger Gürtel 18–20, A-1090 Wien, Austria.

Acta Neurochirurgica, Suppl. 53, 37–41 (1991)

Pontine – Mesencephalic Cavernomas: Indications for Surgery and Operative Results

R. Fahlbusch, C. Strauss, and W. Huk

Department of Neurosurgery of the University of Erlangen-Nürnberg, Erlangen, Federal Republic of Germany

Summary

Cavernous haemangiomas cavernomas of the brainstem can be diagnosed by MRI and safely removed when elective surgery is performed in the subacute stage after haemorrhage. Recurrent haemorrhage and/or neurological deterioration are indications for surgery. In cases with additional venous malformation the cavernoma should be selectively removed.

The experiences with our own series of 18 cases are presented.

Keywords: Brainstem haematoma; cavernous haemangioma; cavernoma; brainstem surgery; magnetic resonance imaging.

Introduction

Cavernous haemangiomas of the brainstem are rare vascular lesions. They consist of large sinusoidal vessels without nerval tissue interposed[15,20,22]. Haemosiderin deposit within the lesion and the surrounding tissue gliosis suggest recurrent bleeding, which is not necessarily associated with clinical evidence of haemorrhage. The natural history of these lesions is unknown[22].

Before introduction of magnetic resonance imaging (MRI) diagnosis was made incidentally, when brainstem haematomas were evacuated[9,11,20,21]. MRI is the method of choice to identify cavernous haemangiomas, where as computed tomography (CT) and angiography failed to provide the diagnosis[11]. CT only demonstrates the haemorrhage, angiography possibly identifies an additional venous malformation, however not the cavernous haemangioma itself. This resulted in an increasing number of case reports of otherwise rare brainstem cavernomas[3,5,6,14] and to an increasing number of small series[1,2,4,7,8,18,19,21]. The management of these lesions, indications for surgical and non surgical treatment, timing of surgery and outcome is still being discussed[2,7,18,19,21] and so far has not been thoroughly evaluated[4].

Patients and Methods

Between 1986 and 1990 14 patients were admitted and treated in the department of Neurosurgery of the University of Erlangen-Nürnberg for brainstem haemorrhage. All cases presented with sudden onset of neurological deficit. Diagnostic work-up included CT scans and MRI with and without contrast and angiography. In all cases CT revealed a interamedullary haematoma and the MRI suggested presence of a cryptic vascular malformation. All cases underwent arterial digital subtraction angiography without evidence of vascular malformation, except a venous malformation in two cases.

Surgically Treated Cases

Surgery was performed in 9 patients with complete removal of the lesion in 8 cases (Table 1). The surgical approach varied according to the site of the lesion. In 2 patients surgery of pontomesencephalic lesions was achieved via subtemporal approach, in on case a supracerebellar midline approach was used. 6 pontine and pontomedullary lesions were approached using a suboccipital median approach. Somatosensory and auditory evoked potentials were monitored during surgery in all cases. Diagnosis of cavernous haemangioma was confirmed by histopathological examination. Postoperative follow-up included MRI 3 months after surgery.

Non Surgically Treated Cases

We have seen altogether 9 additional patients, 6 of them have been seen up to 6 months after haemorrhage. MRI was highly suggestive for cavernous haemangiomas in all patients with evidence of recurrent bleeding. Contrast enhancement revealed an additional venous malformation in one case. In 3 other cases incidental MRI revealed evidence of a cavernous haemangioma of the brainstem without clinical symptoms of haemorrhage. Surgery was advised to all of them in case of recurrent haemorrhage and/or deterioration of neurological symptoms, but in none of them till now surgery has been performed.

Table 1. *Summary of Surgically Treated Cavernous Haemangiomas*

Patients	Number of bleedings	Location	Surgery (weeks after bleeding)	Approach	Outcome	Follow up (months)
1. P R ♂, 17 yo	4	Pons	6	suboccipital	improved	39
2. T H ♂, 45 yo	2	Ponto-mesencephalic junction	12	subtemporal	improved	21
3. N G ♀, 43 yo	2	junction	4	supracerebellar	improved	18
4. W G ♂, 42 yo	2	Pons	17	suboccipital	additional morbidity	18
5. B K ♀, 2 yo	1	Pons	3	suboccipital	improved	10
6. S G ♂, 46 yo	3	Ponto-mesencephalic junction	3	subtemporal	improved	12
7. N E ♀, 39 yo	3	Ponto-medullary junction	2	suboccipital	improved	7
8. K G ♀, 32 yo	2	Pons	4	suboccipital	improved	6
9. T A ♂, 20 yo	2	Pons*	4	suboccipital	improved	5

* Additional venous malformation.

Case Reports

Case 1

A 17 year old male patient was admitted twice within two years with acute onset of double vision, tinnitus, vertigo and numbness of his right side. The neurological exam revealed a left sided VIth nerve palsy, tinnitus, nystagmus, and a right hemihypesthesia. The deficit resolved on both occasions. He was readmitted 4 weeks later with similar symptoms. His condition deteriorated and within 2 months he had developped a severe brainstem syndrome with a right hemiparesis, a left VIIth nerve paresis, a left $1\frac{1}{2}$ syndrome, tinnitus and nystagmus. Serial MRI revealed recurrent brainstem haemorrhage due to a suspected cavernous haemangioma within the brainstem below the floor of the 4th ventricle (Fig. 1). 6 weeks after the last bleeding the haemangioma was completely removed using a suboccipital median craniotomy. The fourth ventricle was exposed and a reddish bulging of the floor of the 4th ventricle slightly to the left slightly below the striae medullares was seen. Intramedullary haematoma was released through a longitudinal left paramedian incision and a cavernous angioma was removed. After surgery all symptoms continuously improved and resolved except for the VIth nerve palsy.

Case 3

A 43 year old woman was admitted for the second episode of acute diplopia. On exam a incomplete left oculomotor nerve paresis

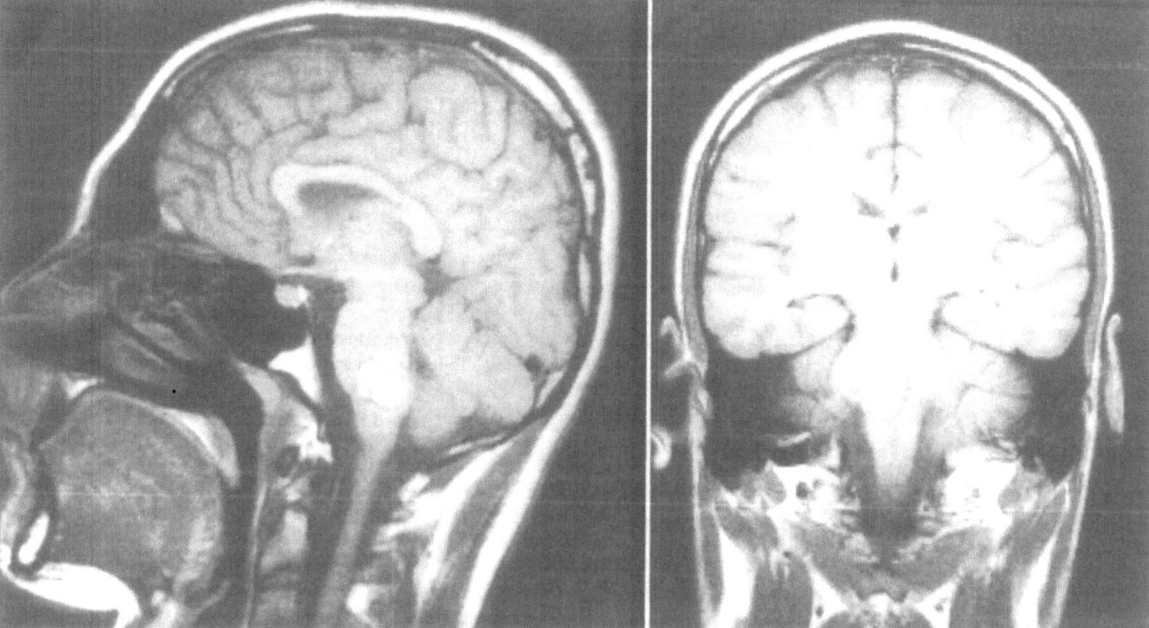

Fig. 1. Preoperative MRI in case 1, demonstrating recurrent bleeding due to a pontine cavernous haemangioma associated with deterioration of neurological function. Complete removal was achieved using a median suboccipital approach

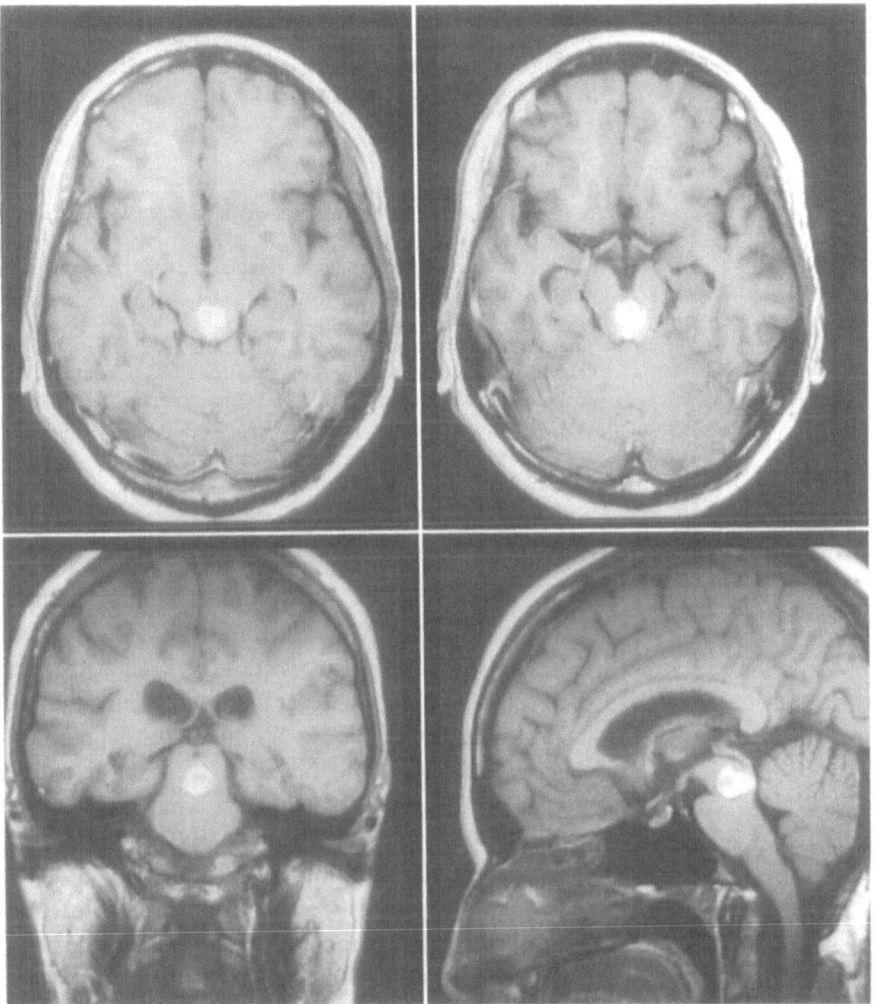

Fig. 2. Preoperative MRI in case 3 showing evidence of a pontine cavernoma. The lesion was removed via suboccipital supracerebellar approach

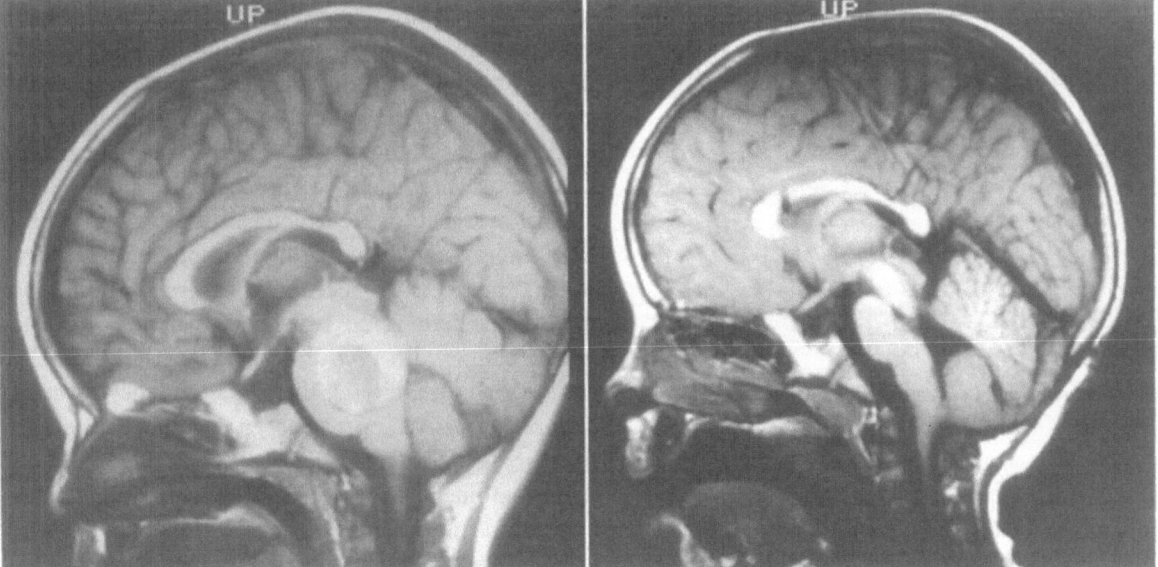

Fig. 3. Pre- and postoperative MRI in a 2 year old child (case 5) demonstrating a large pontine cavernous haemangioma, which was removed using a median suboccipital approach

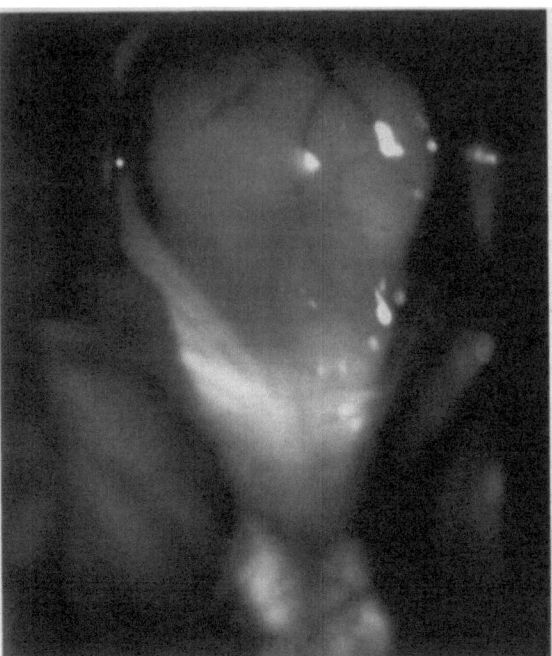

Fig. 4. Bulging of haematoma on the floor of the fourth ventricle in case 5

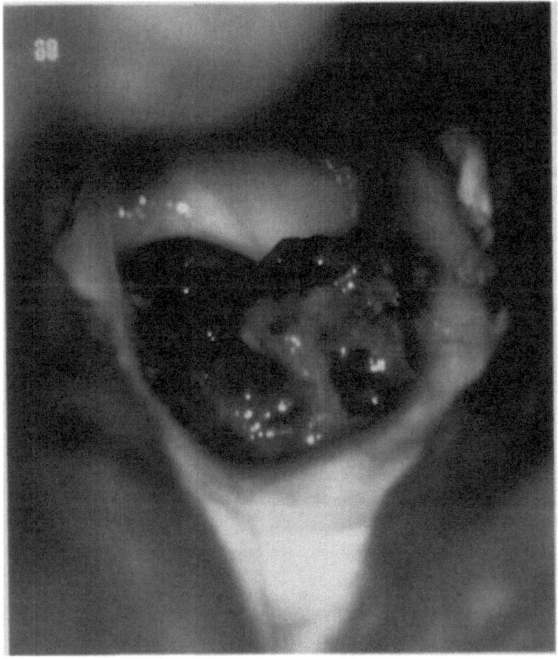

Fig. 5. Successful removal of cavernous haemangioma in case 5

was seen. MRI was suspicious for a cavernous haemangioma slightly below the level of the inferior colliculi with evidence of recurrent bleeding (Fig. 2). 4 weeks after onset of symptoms complete removal was achieved using a supracerebellar infratentorial approach with splitting of the medullary velum. The brainstem was entered below the inferior colliculus passing the aqueduct using a 10 mm longitudinal incision. After release of a haematoma the cavernous angioma could be removed. Directly after surgery the patient developed bilateral internuclear opthalmoplegia which already improved during the hospital course and resolved completely, as well as the oculomotor paresis after 3 months.

Case 5

A 2 year old girl presented with unsteady gait and diplopia after a single bleeding. The neurological exam revealed severe truncal ataxia and right $1\frac{1}{2}$ syndrome. On MRI evidence of a large pontine cavernous haemangioma of almost 2 cm size was found (Fig. 3). Because of the massive lesion and lack of neurological recovery surgery was performed using a suboccipital median approach. On the floor of the 4th ventricle a reddish paramedian bulging was encountered (Fig. 4). After release of a haematoma the incision was widened to 8 mm and the cavernoma was removed (Fig. 5). After surgery complete recovery of neurological deficit was observed within 3 months.

Discussion

The natural history of cavernous haemangiomas is unknown, bleeding within the brainstem however can be fatal[12, 21, 22]. The introduction of MRI helped to establish the diagnosis of cavernous haemangioma prior to surgery[4, 7, 11]. So far there have been few suggestions whether to operate cavernous haemangiomas at all and if to operate at what stage of the disease[1, 2, 4, 7, 18, 19, 20, 21].

We have analyzed a total of 18 patients with MRI suggestive for cavernous haemangiomas of the brainstem. In 9 patients surgery was performed and the diagnosis histologically verified. We have been following 6 other patients with suspected cavernous haemangiomas. Surgery was not performed because there was either only one haemorrhage in the history or the haemorrhage had occurred several months ago. In 3 patients the suspected cavernoma was an incidental finding. Analyzing the 9 successfully operated cases and comparing them with the 9 non-operated cases we feel confident with the following regimen: Cavernous brainstem angiomas presenting with clinical evidence of recurrent bleeding supported by MRI findings and negative angiography or associated with a progressive neurologic disorder should be removed. There is no experience whether a single haemorrhage with recovery should be followed by surgery or not, although there is a tendency towards a more aggressive approach even in single episodes of haemorrhage for fear of rebleed[7, 18, 21].

In combined lesions of cavernous haemangiomas and venous malformations we now feel confident that even in the brainstem the symptomatic cavernoma should be removed as done in case 9[4, 13].

The optimal timing for surgery remains difficult and

has not been addressed so far[4]. According to our experience surgery should be performed early after haemorrhage, as soon as the patient's condition has stabilized. Surgery in the subacute stage has the advantage of an incompletely organized haematoma and less reacting gliosis. The presence of haematoma facilitates dissection. The only case with additional postoperative neurologic deficit (case 4) was operated upon 4 months after haemorrhage. Removal at this stage is more difficult and may result in deterioration of neurological function[4].

The surgical approach to brainstem cavernomas varies according to the location. Pontomedullary cavernomas are removed via a posterior midline exposure of the 4th ventricle. Cavernous angiomas of the pontomesencephalic region are approached via subtemporal route. For pontomesencephalic midline lesions we recommend the supracerebellar infratentoriell approach.

The favorable results of operative removal of 9 symptomatic cavernous angiomas of the brainstem should encourage a more aggressive diagnostic and therapeutic approach in symptomatic cavernous haemangiomas of the brainstem. Early surgery within weeks after recurrent bleeding seems the treatment of choice in suspected cavernous angiomas of the brainstem.

References

1. Brühlmann Y, de Tribolet N, Berney J (1985) Les angiomes caverneux intracérébraux. Neurochirurgie 31: 271–279
2. Chyatte D (1989) Vascular malformations of the brainstem. J Neurosurg 70: 847–852
3. Durward QJ, Henry ChB, Barnett HJM, Barr HWK (1982) Presentation and management of mesencephalic hematoma. J Neurosurg 56: 123–127
4. Fahlbusch R, Strauss C, Huk W, Röckeleien G, Kömpf D, Ruprecht KW (1990) Surgical removal of pontomesencephalic cavernous hemangiomas. Neurosurgery 26: 449–457
5. Inoue Y, Sato O (1983) Successful removal of pontine hematoma due to rupture of cryptic arteriovenous malformation. Case report. Acta Neurochir (Wien) 69: 69–75
6. Kasai N, Fujiwara S, Yoshimoto T, Suzuki J (1981) "Cryptic" arteriovenous malformation of the brainstem. A successfully operated case. Neurol Surg 9: 1161–1165
7. Kashiwagi S, van Loveren HR, Tew jr JM, Wiot JG, Weil SM, Lukin RA (1990) Diagnosis and treatement of vascular brainstem malformations. J Neurosurg 72: 27–34
8. Konovalov AN, Spallone A, Makhmudov UB, Kukhlajeva JA, Ozerova VI (1990) Surgical management of hematomas of the brain stem. J Neurosurg 73: 181–186
9. Koos WT, Sunder-Plassman M, Salah S (1969) Successful removal of a large intrapontine hematoma. Case report. J Neurosurg 31: 690–694
10. Lemme-Plaghos L, Kucharcyzk W, Brant-Zawadzki M, Uske A, Edwards M, Norman D, Newton TH (1986) MR-imaging of angiographically occult vascular malformations. AJNR 7: 217–222
11. Pouyanne MH, Got M, Julien J, Riemesn V, Paoli M (1967) Deux cas d'hematomes intraprotubérantiels opérés. Etude critique. Neurochirurgie 13: 738–742
12. Pozzati E, Giuliani G, Nuzzo G, Poppi M (1989) The growth of cerebral cavernous angiomas. Neurosurgery 25: 92–97
13. Rigamonti D, Spetzler RF (1988) The association of venous and cavernous malformations. Report of four cases and discussion of the pathophysiological, diagnostic and therapeutic implications. Acta Neurochir (Wien) 92: 100–105
14. Russell B, Rengachary SS, McGregor D (1986) Primary pontine hematoma presenting as a cerebellopontine angle mass. Neurosurgery 19: 129–133
15. Russell DS, Rubinstein LJ (1977) Pathology of tumors of the nervous system. Baltimore, Williams & Wilkins, pp 127–141
16. Scott BB, Seeger JF, Schneider RC (1973) Successful evacuation of a pontine hematoma secondary to rupture of a pathologically diagnosed "cryptic" vascular malformation. J Neurosurg 39: 104–108
17. Steiger HJ, Markwalder TM, Reulen HJ (1987) Clinicopathological relations of cerebral cavernous angiomas: Observations in eleven cases. Neurosurgery 21: 879–884
18. Tung H, Gianotta SL, Chandrasoma PT, Zee C (1990) Recurrent intraparenchymal hemorrhages from angiographically occult vascular malformations. J Neurosurg 73: 174–180
19. Veerapen RJ, Sbeih IA, O'Laoire SA (1986) Surgical treatment of cryptic AVM's and associated hematoma in the brainstem and spinal cord. J Neurosurg 65: 188–193
20. Voigt K, Yasargil MG (1976) Cerebral cavernous hemangiomas or cavernomas. Incidence, pathology, localization, diagnosis, clinical features and treatment. Review of the literature and report of an unusual case. Neurochirurgia 19: 59–68
21. Weil SM, Tew Jr JM (1990) Surgical management of brainstem vascular malformations. Acta Neurochir (Wien) 105: 14–23
22. Wilkins RH (1985) Natural history of intracranial vascular malformations: A review. Neurosurgery 16: 421–430

Correspondence: Ch. Strauss, MD., Neurochirurgische Klinik der Universität Erlangen-Nürnberg, Schwabachanlage 6, D-W-8520 Erlangen, Federal Republic of Germany.

Acta Neurochirurgica, Suppl. 53, 42–47 (1991)
© by Springer-Verlag 1991

Unilateral Interhemispheric Keyhole Approach for Anterior Cerebral Artery Aneurysms

T. Fukushima, Sh. Miyazaki, Y. Takusagawa, and **M. Reichman**

Department of Neurosurgery, Mitsui Memorial Hospital, Tokyo, Japan

Summary

A special midline interhemispheric keyhole approach to the anterior communicating artery aneurysms is described. A small trephine opening of 3 cm in diameter is used in most cases. The detailed microsurgical technique of the unilateral interhemispheric exposure of the anterior cerebral artery complex is presented. For the past 10 years, a total of 138 patients, 112 with Acom AN and 26 with distal ACA AN, were operated upon through this approach. There were 16 cases with non-ruptured aneurysms and the postoperative results were excellent in all of them. The overall results in 122 cases with ruptured aneurysms were excellent and good (working) in 95 cases, fair in 10 cases, poor in 9 and death supervened in 8 cases. The mortality rate in 71 acute operation cases was 8% and 4% in 51 delayed cases. The advantages of this approach include simple and rapid craniotomy, minimum brain retraction, accurate midline exposure of all parent arteries and the aneurysm. This anterior interhemispheric approach is, in our experience, much superior to the conventional pterional approach.

Keywords: Anterior cerebral artery aneurysm; interhemispheric keyhole approach; results.

Introduction

Microsurgical management of aneurysms (AN) of the anterior cerebral artery complex remains one of the most exciting challenges in neurosurgery. The standard frontotemporal or pterional craniotomy, popularized and perfected by Yaşargil[6, 7], is the most common approach utilized in neurosurgical clinics around the world for repair of these anterior communicating (Acom) and anterior cerebral (ACA) artery aneurysms (AN). The interhemispheric approach for AN in this region was first described by Wilhelm Tönnis in 1936[5]. Lawrence Pool[4] suggested that Acom AN should be approached via a bifrontal craniotomy and midline subfrontal exposure. In 1967, Yaşargil[6] pioneered the currently accepted microsurgical

technique and subsequently has shown that most aneurysms can be adequately exposed microsurgically using the pterional trans-Sylvian exposure. Presently, very few centers utilize the microsurgical interhemispheric approach to Acom AN. During the period between 1980 and 1990, a total of 138 patients (112 with Acom AN, 26 with distal ACA AN) have been treated using this microsurgical unilateral interhemispheric keyhole approach at the Mitsui Memorial Hospital. The procedure, results and discussion are presented.

Clinical Material

Over a 10 year period (1980–1990), 138 cases of anterior cerebral artery aneurysms, 112 Acom AN and 26 distal ACA AN, were repaired via a unilateral interhemispheric keyhole approach. The ages ranged from 3 years to 80 years with a mean of 54 years. There were 76 males and 62 females in the series. Early surgery was performed in 71 cases (80% within 3 days, 20% in 4 to 7 days), and delayed surgery in 51 patients.

Operative Technique

The patient is placed in a supine position with the head elevated 15–20 degrees and with the neck moderately hyper-extended. The head is secured in a standard Mayfield 3 pin headholder (Fig. 1). In males and elderly patients, a straight transverse midforehead incision placed along a skin crease is used. A small coronal incision at the hairline can be used for younger female patients (Fig. 1). A 3 cm midline trephine craniotomy is made using a specially designed atraumatic thick blade trephine for routine Acom & ACA ANs (Fig. 2). A 3.5 cm or 4 cm trephine is used for

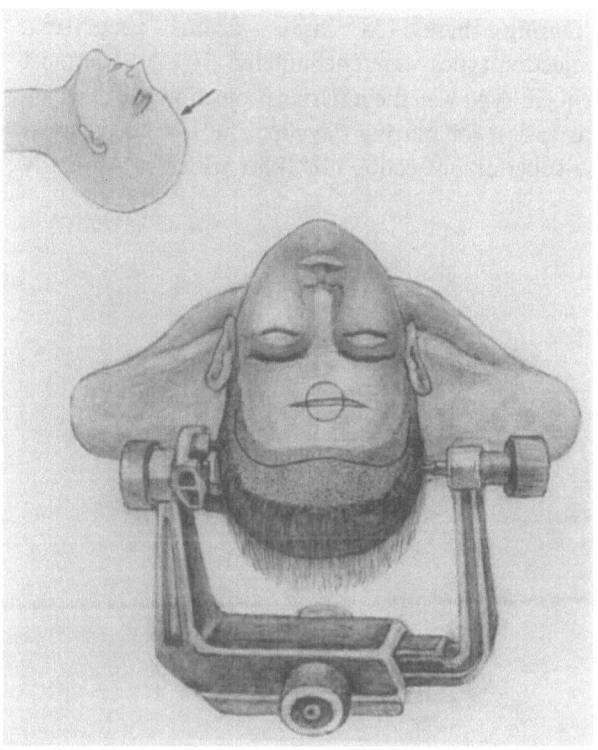

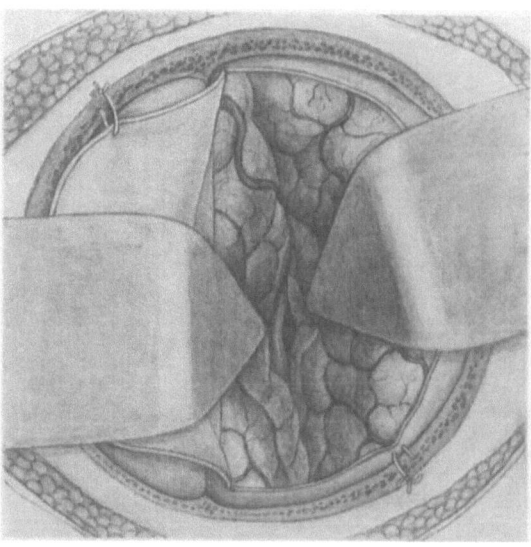

Fig. 3. The dura is incised only on the right side and the inter-hemispheric fissure is separated by microsurgical sharp dissection using a pair of non-reflecting black tapered spatulae

Fig. 1. Patient positioning, skin incision and location of a 3 cm trephine. The neck is moderately hyperextended to achieve the microscopic view angle at 45 degrees and to obtain comfortable access to Acom aneurysm. A straight midforehead incision is used for males and elderly patients and a coronal hairline incision for young ladies. For both procedures, strict cosmetic closure technique is required

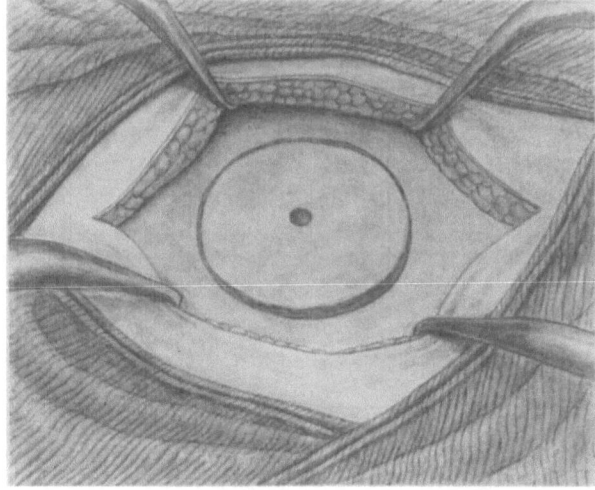

Fig. 2. A pair of Gelpi retractors are used to expose the midforehead skull surface. A specially designed Fukushima thick blade non-traumatic trephine (3 cm diameter) provides rapid bone opening

large and giant size ANs. The dura is incised on the right side of the superior sagittal sinus in a curvelinear fashion to provide an operative access of $1 \times 2 \, cm$ (Fig. 3). With this interhemispheric approach, only a very minimal amount of retraction of the medial frontal lobe is required. A 4 mm tapered black retractor is placed over the falx and a 2 mm tapered non-reflecting black retractor is gently placed on the mesial frontal surface (Fig. 3). Strict microsurgical technique must be mastered to safely utilize this approach, as the anterior communicating artery complex is at a significant distance from the craniotomy opening. By manoeuvering the operating microscope up and down or right to left, wide visualization of the corpus callosum, the genu and the anterior interhemispheric fissure can be achieved (Fig. 3). The arachnoid trabeculations and interdigitated gyri of the interhemispheric fissure are dissected sharply using microscissors and bipolar technique. The callosal bifurcation of the ACA–A2 segments are identified and the sharp dissection is continued proximally along the A2 arteries toward the Acom complex to visualize the Acom AN (Fig. 4). The A1 segments can be exposed by continuing the dissection along the proximal A2 vessels laterally and inferiorly, leaving the area of AN rupture untouched till the last moment. In some cases, only the dominant A1 artery can be controlled prior to placing an initial preliminary clip on the AN neck. The aneurysmal dome can then be dissected completely and the neck is defined accurately with

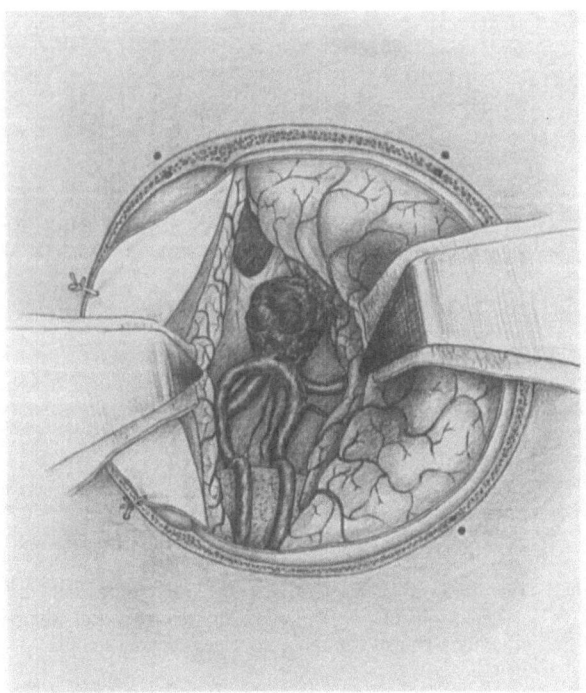

Fig. 4. From the callosal bifurcation, the A2 segments of ACA are followed proximally to expose the Acom complex. The dissection should be performed sharply in a non-traumatic fashion from the non-ruptured area. The dissection of the rupture point must be done at the last moment before clipping. The anatomical identification of the location of the A1 vessels and perforators is the most crucial issue for a successful result

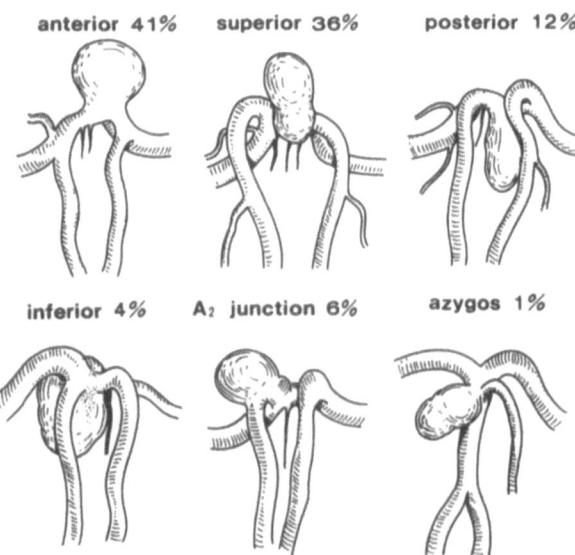

Fig. 5. Dome projection types and frequency of Acom aneurysms

identification of all parent vessels and hypothalamic-septal perforating branches (Fig. 4). After confirming all vascular anatomy, the final clipping is made with particular care to obliterate the AN neck completely and to preserve perforators.

During these 138 cases, various aneurysmal projection types were encountered (Fig. 5). The most frequent type was the anterior projection (41%) which was easiest for placing the clip. The second type was the superior projection (36%) for which it was fairly

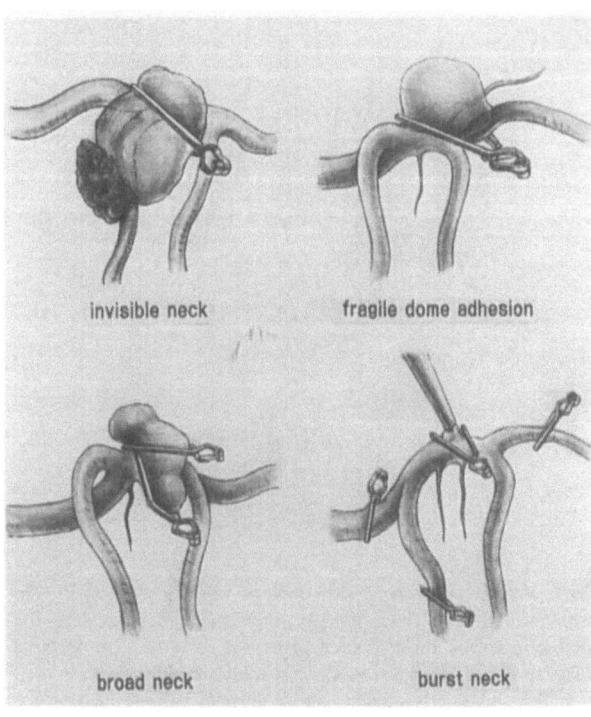

Fig. 6. Various clipping techniques for difficult Acom aneurysms

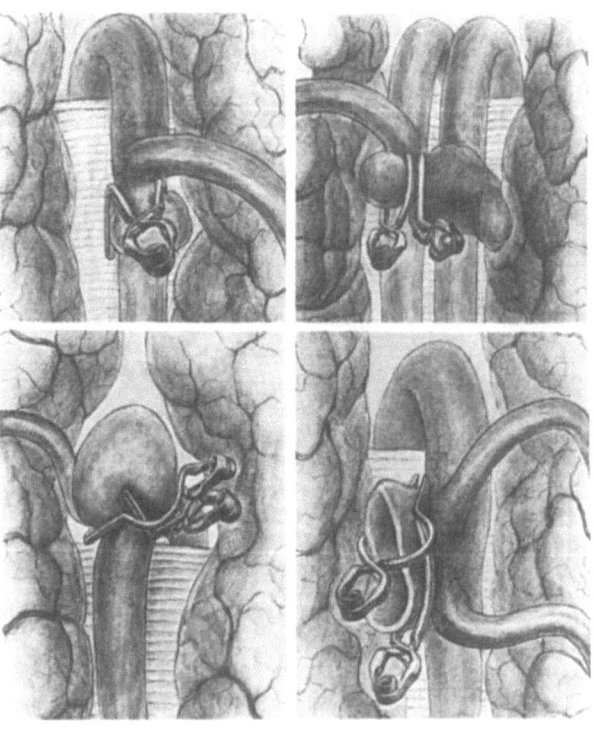

Fig. 7. Multiple clipping techniques for distal ACA aneurysms

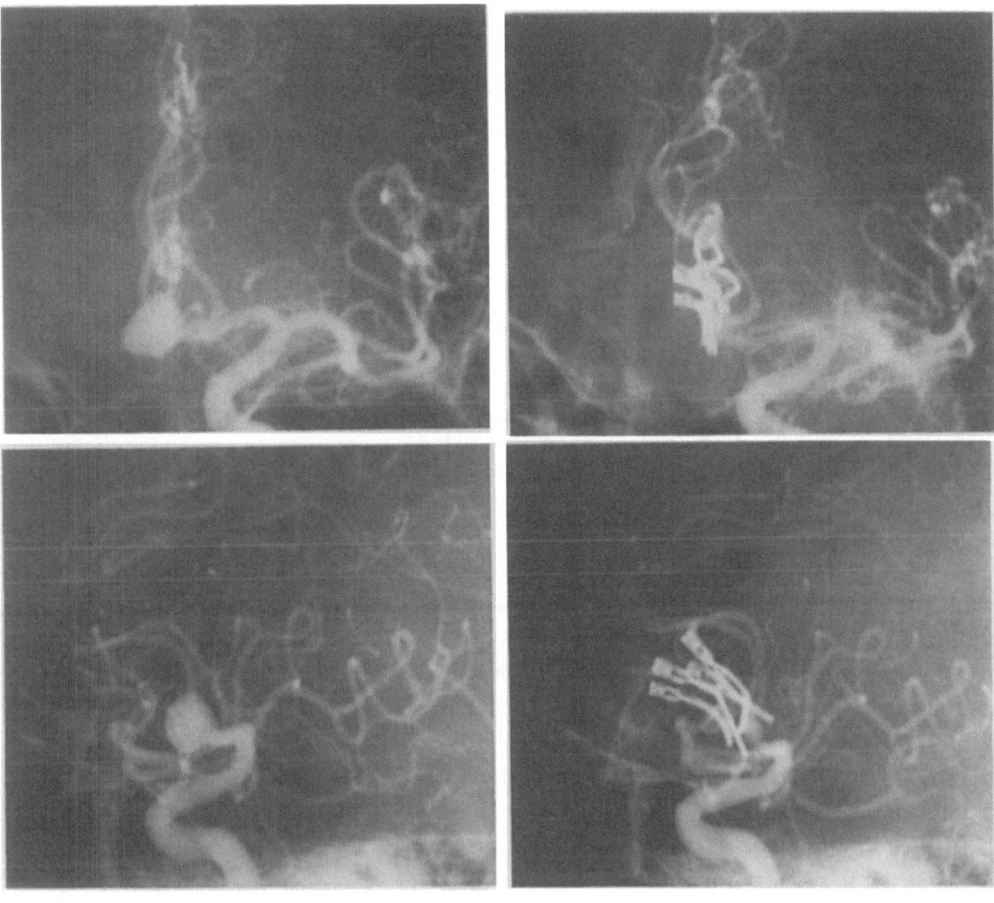

Fig. 8. An example of thick wall and broad neck Acom aneurysm in a 65 year-old female. Four clips of various shapes were necessary to repair this aneurysm. Surgery on day 1 at grade II

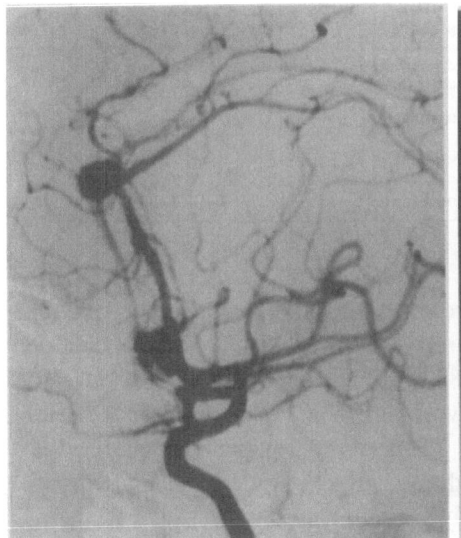
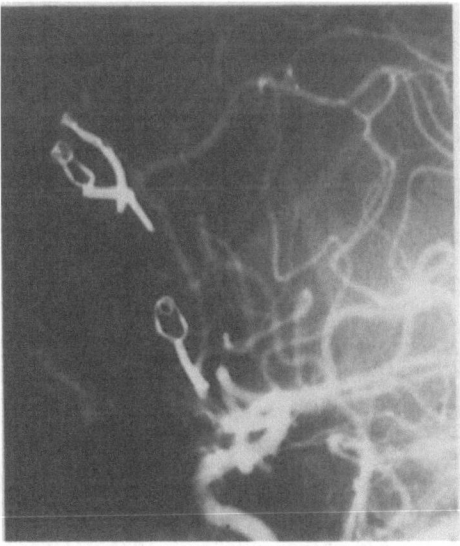

Fig. 9. An example of tandem aneurysms with Acom plus ACA callosal bifurcation aneurysms in a 56 year-old woman. Clipping was performed through a single tunnel operative field on the day of bleed at Grade II

difficult to make an exposure because the dome appears first before dissection of proximal vessels can be undertaken. The posterior and inferior projection types were rather infrequent, but these types were also to be handled carefully due to adhesion of the perforators to the AN dome.

Figure 6 illustrates various clipping techniques for difficult ANs. When the neck is invisibly covered by a large dome, a preliminary clip is placed over the dome and the neck together. Then, the rest of the dome and the rupture point are dissected from the surrounding tissues and the AN dome is reflected anteriorly to separate the perforators and to visualize the neck. When the very thin fragile AN wall is adherent to the parent vessels, a preliminary clipping should be made before its dissection, to prevent premature bleeding. When the neck is damaged or burst ruptured, 2 or 3 temporary clips are necessary for the control of bleeding and a final clipping is made while sucking the residual neck. To accomplish a precise clean microsurgical dissection and accurate suction, various sizes of pressure adjustable malleable tapered suckers with a tear-drop shaped side hole are indispensable. Also, to apply a clip in such a narrow operative space, various types of thin key-hole clip appliers with vari-angle groove cutting are required (Fujita Corporation, Tokyo, designed by Fukushima). Most ANs were successfully obliterated with a single clip, however, in some cases with a broader neck, a multiple clipping technique was required (Fig. 6). Figure 7 demonstrates various multiple clipping methods for distal ACA aneurysms. A couple of clinical examples of complicated clipping procedures are shown in Figs. 8 and 9. Needless to say, the angiogram, CT and MRI studies should be all carefully evaluated to ascertain the dome projection and the neck configuration. The surgeon will then be adequately prepared should he encounter the aneurysm dome early during dissection.

Operative Results

Of 138 patients, acute surgery was performed in 71 cases (57 cases, 80% within 3 days after the bleed and 14 cases, 20% in 4 to 7 days). Delayed surgery was done in 51 cases. There were 16 cases (Acom 9, A2–3 7 cases) operated on for non-ruptured AN. The patient's outcome based on surgical timing is summarized in Table 1. In 71 patients operated on in the acute stage, excellent and good results (working) were obtained in 72%, fair results (independent) in 13%, poor results (wheel chair or bed-ridden) in 7% and death occurred in 8%. In delayed cases, excellent and good results were obtained in 86%, fair results in 2%, poor results in 8% and death in 4%. All of 16 cases operated on for non-ruptured AN had excellent results. Overall, 111 patients (80%) were working at 3 months evaluation after surgery, 10 patients (7%) were walking independently with some neurological deficits, 9 patients (7%) were disabled and there was an overall mortality rate of 6% (Table 1).

The patients' preoperative status in 122 ruptured cases and their postoperative outcome are shown in

Table 1. *Surgical Timing and Operative Outcome in 138 Cases of Acom and A2–3 Aneurysms*

INTERHEMISPHERIC APPROACH: 138 cases

ACUTE vs DELAYED

				Working	Independent	Disabled	†
Acute 0-7 day	**71**	Acom	64	45	9	5	5
		A2-3	7	6			1
				72 %	13 %	7 %	8 %
Delayed >1 w	**51**	Acom	39	34	1	3	1
		A2-3	12	10		1	1
				86 %	2 %	8 %	4 %
Non-rup	**16**	Acom	9	9			0
		A2-3	7	7			0
total	**138**			111 (80%)	10 (7%)	9 (7%)	8 (6%)

Table 2. *Pre-operative Neurological Status and Postoperative Outcome in 122 Patients with Ruptured Aneurysm.* The patients immediate pre-operative clinical condition is classified into 3 categories. "Good Condition" includes patients in Grade I and II as well as early Grade III (slightly lethargic cases). "Fair Conditio" includes cases in definite drowsiness and stupor. "Poor Conditions" means the patients are in semicoma and coma

INTERHEMISPHERIC APPROACH: 122 ruptured cases

GRADES & OUTCOME

	Grading		Working	Independent	Disabled	†
83	GOOD COND.	I awake II ⟨ IIIa sleepy	76	4	2	1
25	FAIR COND.	IIIb definite drowsy IVa ⟨ stupor	16	4	2	3
14	POOR COND.	IVb semicoma ⟨ V coma	3	2	5	4

Table 2. There were 83 patients categorized in the "Good Condition" group (Grade I, II and early Grade III). Of these 83 patients, 76 (92%) had excellent and good results (working), 4 had a fair result and 2 cases were disabled. There were 25 patients categorized in the "Fair Condition" group (Grade III, definite drowsiness and early Grade IV stupor). Of these 25 cases, 16 (64%) were working, 4 independent and 2 disabled. There were 14 patients categorized in the "Poor Condition" group (semicoma and coma). Of these, only 3 patients (21%) were working and 2 were walking independently. An overall mortality rate of 5.8% (8 cases) resulted from these 138 patients. Of these 8 patients, 4 were in the poor condition as a result of the initial subarachnoid haemorrhage. The three

patients initially in fair condition died; 2 due to severe vasospasm and one due to hypothalamic injury from massive intraoperative rupture. The single death among the good condition patients occurred secondary to bilateral occipital infarctions and subsequent herniations on the second postoperative day (third post-haemorrhage day). This may have been a complication of the initial angiography.

Discussion

The interhemispheric approach to Acom AN was first described by Tönnis in 1936[5]. He performed a large craniotomy with a transcallosal approach for muscle wrapping of an Acom AN. In 1961, Lawrence Pool[4] advocated a large bifrontal craniotomy for midline subfrontal exposure of Acom AN. Subsequently, Lyle French[1], in 1966, reported a unilateral frontal craniotomy with antero-medial wedge resection of the frontal lobe to expose the Acom complex. Microsurgical bilateral interhemispheric approach was first described by Lougheed in 1969[3]. However, after introduction of the standard Yaşargil's pterional craniotomy[6, 7], few surgeons have subsequently pursued this interhemispheric approach. Ito revived Lougheed's bifrontal interhemispheric exposure of Acom An with some modification in Japan in 1974 achieving excellent results[2]. He is the person who motivated the author (T. F.) to pursue further the microsurgical interhemispheric approach to Acom AN. The approach has been subsequently modified and refined to a small trephine craniotomy and with a unilateral keyhole "target" exposure. Since 1980, this midline unilateral interhemispheric keyhole technique has been utilized exclusively by the authors for the microsurgical management of Acom and distal ACA ANs. The advantages of this approach include simple and rapid craniotomy, minimum brain retraction, avoidance of frontal lobe base elevation and gyrus rectus resection, preservation of the olfactory

nerves and direct exposure of all parent arteries and perforating vessels. The disadvantage may be that the exposure is deeper and the operative field is narrow and occasionally the AN dome is encountered prior to gaining proximal control. These disadvantages can be minimized with a sound knowledge of microsurgical anatomy and microsurgical expertise and experience. The clinical results of the present series are very comparable to other large series of Acom AN surgery in which a standard pterional approach was utilized[6, 7].

In this paper, the authors stress that a microsurgical interhemispheric approach can be accurately and safely utilized with satisfactory operative results to treat Acom and ACA ANs. Re-emphasis of strict and meticulous microsurgical technique and skills are warranted as a very small keyhole approach is utilized for exposure of ANs located deep at the midline skull base.

References

1. French LA, Chou SN, Story JL, Schultz EA (1966) Aneurysms of the anterior communicating artery. J Neurosurg 24: 1058–1062
2. Ito Z (1982) The microsurgical anterior interhemispheric approach suitably applied to ruptured aneurysms of the anterior communicating artery in the acute stage. Acta Neurochir (Wien) 63: 85–99
3. Lougheed WM (1969) Selection, timing, and technique of aneurysm surgery of the anterior circle of Willis. Clin Neurosurg 16: 95–113
4. Pool JL (1961) Aneurysms of the anterior communicating artery. J Neurosurg 18: 98–101
5. Tönnis W (1936) Erfolgreiche Behandlung eines Aneurysma der Art commun ant cerebri. Zbl Neurochir 1: 39–42
6. Yaşargil MG, Fox JL (1975) The microsurgical approach to intracranial aneurysms. Surg Neurol 3: 7–14
7. Yaşargil MG, Fox JL, Ray MW (1975) The operative approach to aneurysms of the anterior communicating artery. In: Krayenbühl H, et al (eds) Advances and technical standards in neurosurgery, Vol 2. Springer, Wien New York, pp 113–170

Correspondence: T. Fukushima, M. D., D. M. Sc., Department of Neurosurgery, University of Southern California Medical Center, Los Angles, CA 90033, U.S.A

Acta Neurochirurgica, Suppl. 53, 48–49 (1991)

Endovascular Treatment of Berry Aneurysms by Endosaccular Occlusion

J. Moret

Department of Interventional Neuroradiology, Fondation Rothschild Hospital, Paris, France

Summary

In 90 cases with 93 berry aneurysms endovascular occlusion of the aneurysms was attempted, in 73 of them successfully. There has been a 12% complication rate, including 4% mortality and 8% of cases with neurological deficit, and 9 recurrences.

The indications for endovascular treatment of berry aneurysms are discussed. This method seems to be an alternative especially for carotiophthalmic and basilar artery aneurysms.

Keywords: Berry aneurysm; endovascular occlusion; indications; results; complications.

Although the surgical experience of treatment of aneurysms is tremendously large in comparison with the endovascular one, it becomes possible to have a good idea of what the future will be as far as we have a better approach of the endovascular treatment possibilities and results. In order to avoid to comparison of apples and potatoes, this study will take into account only what are commonly called "Berry aneurysms", that is to say typical surgical aneurysms whose sizes are equal or smaller than 1.5 cm, and which extend intracranially and in almost all the cases totally in the subarachnoid space (see Table 1).

Table 1. *Berry Aneurysms*. Location of 93 Aneurysms Treated by Endosaccular Occlusion

Intracavernous (partially)	4
Carotido-ophthalmic	23
Post. communicating artery	7
Carotid bifurcation	8
Basilar artery (tip or trunk)	27
Middle cerebral artery	7
Ant. communicating or cer. art.	10
Post. cerebral art.	3
P.I.C.A.	2
Subarach. vert. art.	2
	93

Material and Methods

The specificity of our study is double: First it is indeed strictly comparable to the neurosurgical series regarding the material as it has been described above, second all the aneurysms have been treated by the same team, using the same endovascular technique and the same rules of follow up (first control angiogram four or six months after the endosaccular occlusion, second control angigram one year after the first one). Only 20% of the patients have had the second control angiogram since our technique has only been used for two and a half years.

All the aneurysms underwent an endosaccular occlusion using a latex balloon filled with (100% of) polymerizing substance (POLYMERAN from BALT Company). Navigation, positioning and detachment of the balloon have been performed using a catheter specially designed for that use (Magic BD 2L from BALT Company). Endosaccular occlusion is achieved according to three different methods: "Endosaccular clipping, endosaccular packing and endosaccular valving" (Fig. 1).

At the time of paper 93 aneurysms in 90 patients have had an attempt at treatment. 16 cases were acute patients (bleeding within 48 hours before treatment), 34 cases were non-acute patients (bleeding 10 days to some weeks before treatment), 43 patients had never bled. Because of arteriosclerosis or the impossibility of occluding the aneurysmal sac or impossibility of entering the aneurysmal neck, the endosaccular treatment failed in 24 cases (7 of those failures could be treated by parent vessel occlusion). In three cases although the balloon was perfectly occluding the aneurysm, we decided to quit because the anchorage of the balloon was suspected to be weak and we did not want to take any risk in asymptomatic patients. Finally 73 of the 93 cases have been successfully occluded.

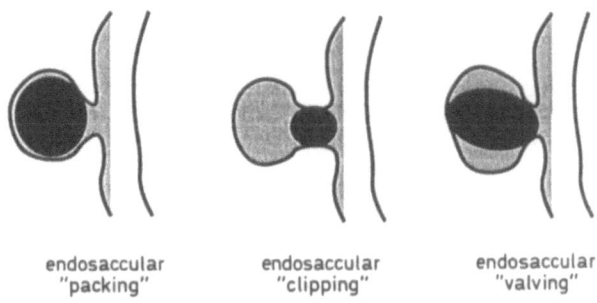

endosaccular "packing"   endosaccular "clipping"   endosaccular "valving"

Fig. 1. Methods of endovascular occlusion

Results

The long term follow-up shows 9 recurrences. A retrospective analysis of those recurrences demonstrates in all of them a small remaining neck at the base of the aneurysm on the immediate control angiogram. 5 of the 9 recurrences underwent a second endovascular treatment (3 of the retreated cases were successfully occluded). 2 of the 9 recurrences underwent surgical treatment. 1 of the 9 recurrences occurred very early after an "endosaccular clipping" (displacement of the balloon two days after its placement leading to a secondary haemorrhage). 1 of the 9 recurrences is scheduled for another endovascular treatment.

We have had to accept 12 complications in 93 cases which represent in fact 98 different attempts of treatment because of the 5 retreated cases after recurrence. Analysis of these complications reveales 4 deaths and 8 patients with neurological deficit. All the deaths occurred in the posterior fossa, 2 because of brainstem ischaemia and 2 because of aneurysmal rupture (1 during the procedure, 1 two days after treatment because of early recurrence). 5 of the 8 neurological deficit case are related to clotting phenomena despite the fact that all the treatments have been performed under full heparinization. 2 of the 8 neurological deficits are related to a secondary migration of the balloon. (1 lack of repositioning, 1 failure of repositioning). 1 of these 8 occurred after migration of the polymerizing substance because of rupture of the balloon before total solidification of that substance (this was related to the use of a wrong! HEMA which had degraded the latex balloon at the beginning of our experience).

Discussion

Analysis of complications we have avoided is also very important as it shows that eventhough we are working remote from the aneurysms itself, we have the possibility of escaping from dangerous situations. Repositioning of the balloon after detachment is one of the major technical tricks that makes the technique safer. In 11 cases a secondary migration of the balloon occurred (it was always a few minutes after detachment), leading to the occlusion of the parent vessel. In 1 case (the first one in our experience) we did not reposition the balloon and we witnessed an ischaemic complication. In all of the 10 other cases we repositioned the balloon using a second non-detachable balloon catheter. In 9 of those 10 cases repositioning was successfull and complications were avoided.

Looking at the complications and their percentage of occurence one must take into account all the attempts of treatment that is to say 98 procedures (93 cases + 5 retreatments). The risk of complications is therefore 12%, including 4% mortality and 8% with neurological deficits, independently of the localization of the aneuryms. If we want to compare our results with the neurosurgical results, the anatomical localization is very important as far as it is the only strictly identical parameter between both techniques of treatment. Carotid-ophthalmic and basilar aneurysms are known to be difficult or dangerous or both with regard to the neurosurgical approach. We must consider that those two later localizations represent respectively 25% and 29% of the aneurysms we have treated, this means that the neurosurgical treatment might have been tricky and/or dangerous in 54% of our cases for open skull surgery.

At this stage of our experience the timing of treatment regarding the onset of the haemorrhage versus the clinical results cannot be reliably taken into account because 16 cases treated by endosaccular occlusion as emergencies are too small a series. Nevertheless the therapeutic trauma of endovascular treatment is without doubt much less than the neurosurgical trauma.

Finally behind the statistical numbers which are absolutely necessary to evaluate the performance of a given technique, it is the philosophy of treatment of Berry Aneurysms which has changed. Endosaccular occlusion is definitely an alternative treatment the indications of which must be discussed as a priority for carotid-ophthalmic and basilar aneurysms whatever the circumstances of diagnosis are. In asymptomatic aneurysms a carefull attempt of endovascular treatment carries few risks and seems to be also the first choice of treatment, especially because its failure can be immediately followed by a surgical procedure. In emergency cases except for the carotid-ophthalmic and basilar localizations, our experience of endosaccular treatment needs to be greater for a more appropriate analysis.

Correspondence: J. Moret, M. D., Department of Interventional Neuroradiology, Fondation Rothschild Hospital, 25–29, rue Manin, F-75940 Paris Cedex 19, France.

Acta Neurochirurgica, Suppl. 53, 50–59 (1991)

Arterio-Venous Malformations of the Basal Ganglia.
Surgical versus Endovascular Treatment

B. Richling and **G. Bavinzski**

Department of Neurosurgery, University of Vienna Medical School, Vienna, Austria

Summary

Technique, indications and results of endovascular occlusion by superselective embolization of basal ganglia arterio-venous malformations (AVM's) are discussed, based on personal experiences with 21 cases and 41 embolizations.

Follow-up was available in 17 cases. Total occlusion could be achieved in 4 cases, partial occlusion in 12, and one was extirpated microsurgically.

Further haemorrhages after partial occlusion occurred in two cases. Neurological symptoms improved in 6 cases and remained unchanged in 11.

Keywords: Arterio-venous malformation; basal ganglia; embolization; extirpation; indications; results.

Introduction

From the very beginning of AVM surgery, arterio-venous malformations of the basal ganglia have posed a special challenge to the surgeon. Described as principally inoperable by the first authors on this topic[9,10] it was in the sixties that the first reports on the successful surgical removal of basal ganglia angiomas, predominantly angiomas of the head of the caudate nucleus, were published[2,4,5,6,18].

The development of endovascular techniques for the preoperative or final treatment of cerebral vascular malformations[12] introduced a new approach to the treatment of lesions of this type. However, in the early days of embolization, with the then common purely flow-dependent systems, the selective endovascular accessibility of basal ganglia AVMs was dependent on sufficiently large vascular lumina and high flow rates. An embolization of most basal ganglia AVMs, with the perforating branches of striolenticular or choroidal vessels branching off at right or acute angles and usually being of low to middle diameters, resulted in great problems before flow independent catheter systems were devise[14].

The development of guide-wire supported micro-catheters with progressive softness[3,11] has recently made possible the advancement along vessels of both low diameter and low flow and, in addition, the advancing through such vessels to beyond the "physiological zone" into the nidus of the AVM. With these technical advances embolization techniques have matured to constitute a therapeutic alternative to the treatment of basal ganglia AVMs.

The chances but also the risks involved with the two therapeutic approaches will be discussed on the basis of our case histories and the presentation of three typical cases.

Case Reports

Twenty-one of all cerebral angiomas treated between 1985 and 1990 were basal ganglia angiomas. See Table 1 for a breakdown of sites and sizes of these malformations.

The main sign in 12 patients was a ventricular haemorrhage; 3 of them suffered from progressive neurological deficit that was not caused by the haemorrhage. Two further patients suffered from a cerebral haemorrhage without detailed definition. In 4 patients a pure progressive neurological deficit appeared as a steal phenomenon, 4 patients suffered from epilepsy (2 grand mal epilepsies, 2 temporal lobe epilepsies); 1 of them died from a ventricular haemorrhage before commencement of the treatment. One patient suffered from exophthalmus due to marked dural involvement. Five patients suffered from internal

Table 1. *AVM's of the Basal Ganglia*

Localization

Thalamus ant. + head of caudate nucleus	5
– middle	1
– post	3
– post + Trigonum	5
– ant + post	4
– complex	3

Size

Giant	> 6 cm	3
Large	4–6 cm	4
Moderate	2–4 cm	12
Small	1–2 cm	2
Micro	0.5–1 cm	0

Table 2. *Clinical Presentation*

Ventricular haemorrhoges	12
SAH	2
Epilepsy	4
Progred. neurol. deficit	7
Headache	11
Hydrocephalus	5
Exophthalmus	1

Table 3. *Forms of Treatment*

n = 21	
Embolized	15
Operation	1
Embolized + operation	1
Untreated	4
(No. of embolization	41)

Clinical Results:

n = 17	
Further haemorrhage (after part. emb.)	2
Neurol. deficit – improved	2
– unchanged	3
– worse	2
Epilepsy (with med. therapy) – improved	1
– unchanged	2
– died before treatment	1
Headache – improved	3
– unchanged	6
– died before treatment	2

Technical Results:

n = 17	
Total occlusion	4
Total exstirpation	1
Part. occlusion	11
Part. occl. + part. surg. fistula isolation	1

hydrocephalus (not caused by the haemorrhage), while 11 patients complained about chronic headache (Table 2).

Pre-operatively all patients were at least examined angiographically once; with all patients all main cerebral vessels were demonstrated. In addition, CT examinations and, in most cases, MRI examinations were carried out. Out of the 21 patients, 1 only was operated on, 15 were embolized and 1 patient was subject to multiple embolizations followed by an operation. Four patients were not treated at all (2 died before the planned treatment could be started, 2 suffered from AVMs that proved to be inoperable and not accessible by endovascular techniques). Table 3 sets out a summary of the technical and clinical results obtained. Of the 17 angiomas which were treated 1 was completely removed and 4 permanently occluded. In 5 out of 11 angioma patients who were subject to partial embolization the nidi could be reduced by more than 50 percent. Two patients suffered from bleeding after partial embolization (i.e., between the endovascular sessions). The pre-operative neurological deficit could be improved in 2 cases and remained unchanged in 3 cases. Two patients suffered from transient deterioration of their neurological condition due to the intervention (1 hemianopia, 1 hemiparesis).

Three typical cases from the above case histories are described.

Case 1

A 54-year old female patient suffered from a ventricular mass bleeding, with unconsciousness and hemiparesis. After a ventricular drainage and intensive care in another hospital the patient fully recovered and was transferred to our hospital in a condition without neurological findings. A further examination showed an AVM at the head of the left caudate nucleus (Fig. 1). While it was possible to advance the microcatheter into the feeding artery (perforating branch arising from M1) on the occasion of an endovascular session (Fig. 2), a sufficiently distal catheter position peripheral to the physiological zone could not be reached. Therefore, surgical intervention was necessary: via a left transventricular approach to the lateral ventricle the head of the left caudate nucleus was approached. There in the ventricular wall the discolored red AVM draining vein could be located; following this vein the angioma was discovered and dissected (Fig. 3 B). After shrinking the nidus through coagulation finally the feeding perforating branch could be located in the depth and severed after coagulation. Postoperatively the patient did not show any deficit; a follow-up angiogram performed 1 month after the intervention did not show any cerebral vascular abnormalities (Fig. 4).

Case 2

A 32-year old female patient was admitted to another hospital on account of severe ventricular bleeding. Her case history showed that she had suffered from a similar bleed three years before. The patient recovered after ventricular drainage and finally did not show any clinical abnormalities and no neurological deficit. A follow-up angiogram showed an anterior thalamic AVM which typically drained via the deep venous system. The panoramic angiogram (Fig. 5) pictures the anterior choroid artery as the main feeder with possible contributions from perforating branches of the M1 segment on the right. A particularly fine guide-wire controlled microcatheter

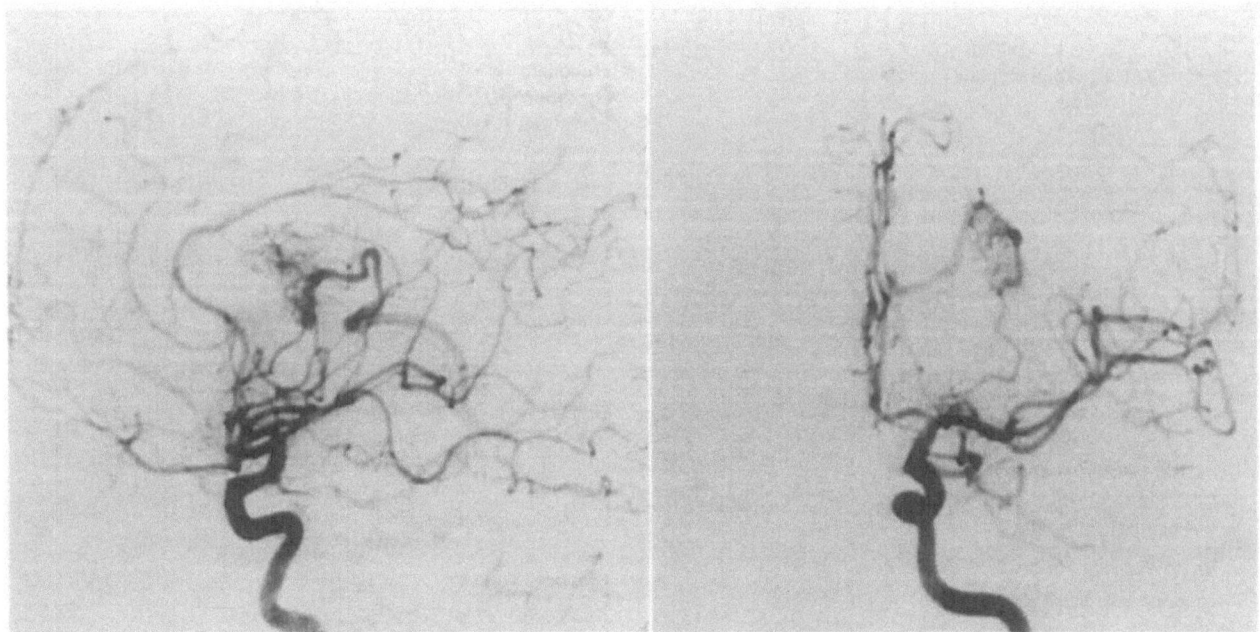

Fig. 1. AVM at the head of the caudate nucleus. Case report 1

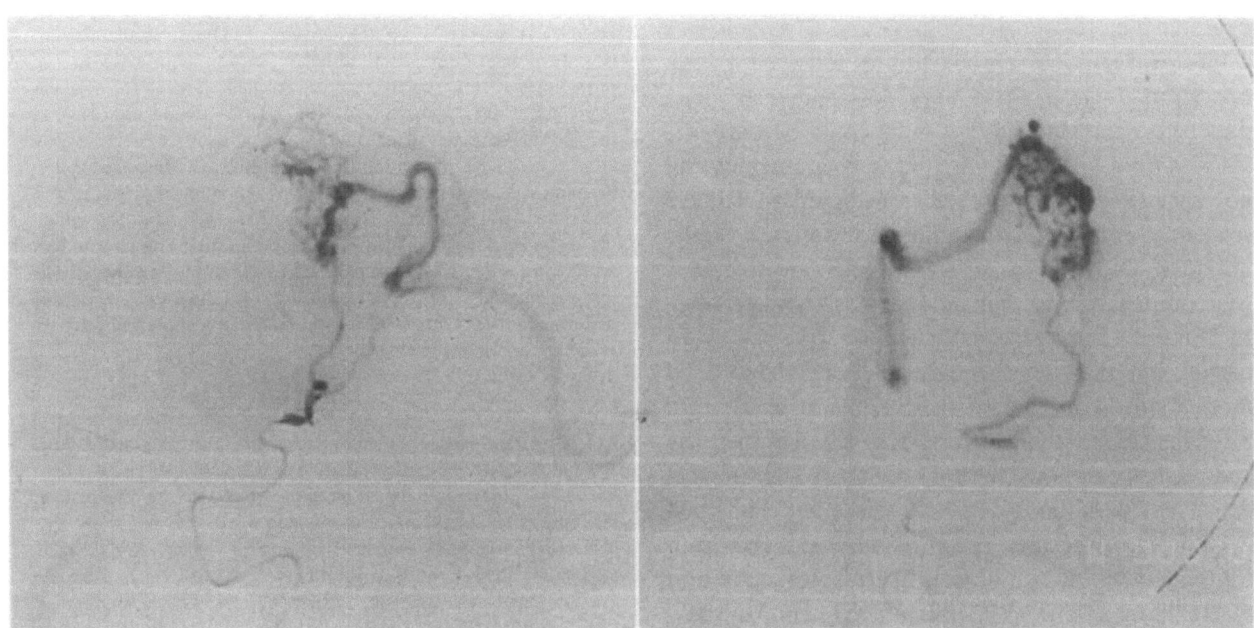

Fig. 2. Microcatheter entering the performating artery (M1) feeding the AVM. A more distal position of the catheter tip could not be reached

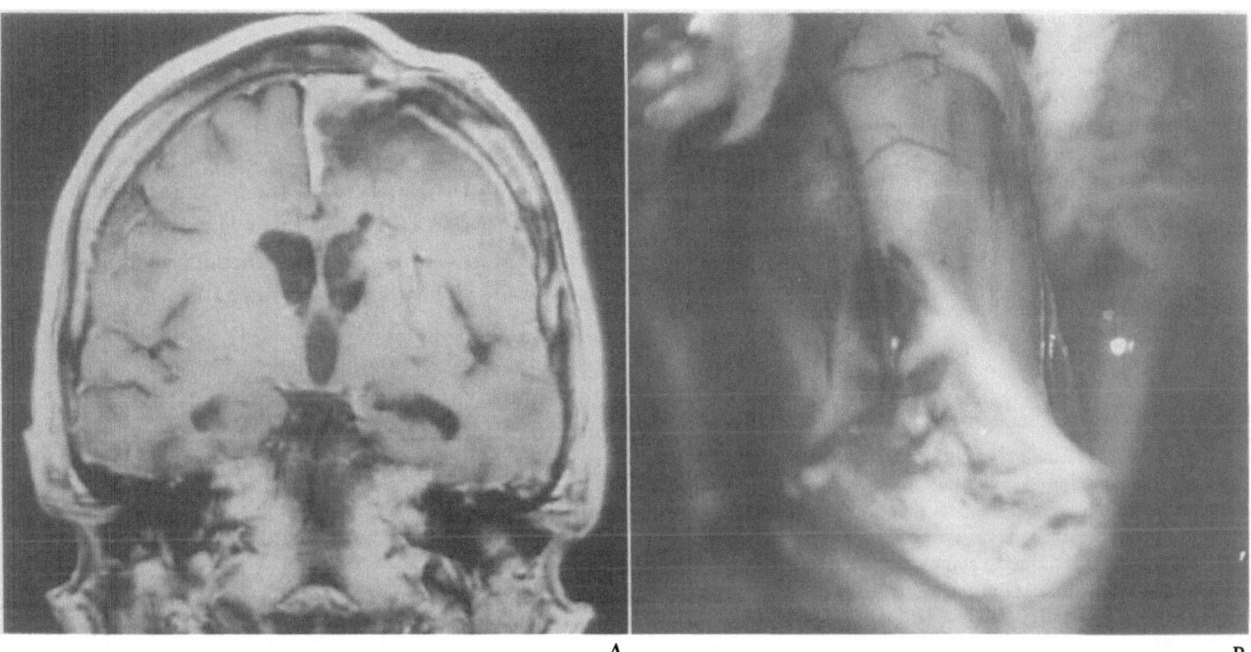

Fig. 3. A) MRI showing the AVM with in the head of the caudate nucleus. B) AVM-draining vein in the ventricular wall leading to the AVM nidus

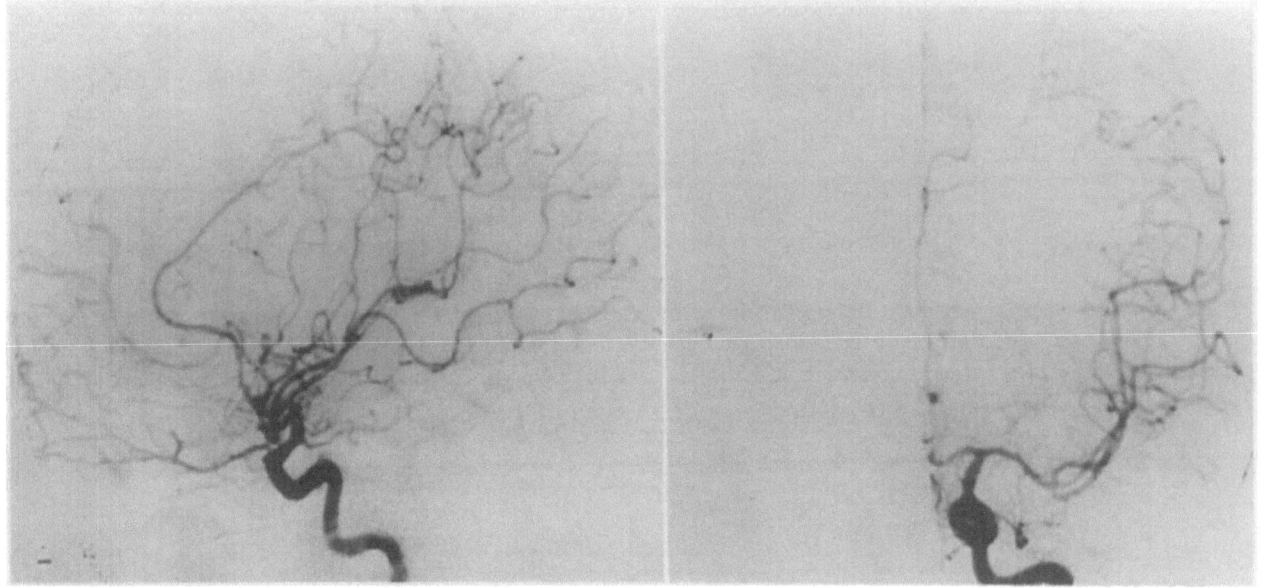

Fig. 4. Postoperative angiogram of case report 1

(Tracker 10) was used in an endovascular session to advance along the possibly contributing perforating branch. However, the selective angiographic representation from this artery showed that it did not contribute (Fig. 6). A Tracker 18 catheter was used to advance along the feeding artery (anterior choroidal artery) to arrive at a selective catheter position close to the nidus (Fig. 7). An Amytal test (75 mg) was performed; the result was negative. Then the nidus was embolized with 0.25 ml of a mixture of histoacryl blue/Lipiodol ultrafluid (ratio 1:2). Fig. 9 shows the casting of the nidus of the angioma by the embolizing mixture. After the intervention, and for two years now, the patient has not shown any neurological abnormalities. A follow-up angiogram one year after the embolization showed that the vascular malformation did not reappear (Fig. 8).

Case 3

A 14-year old female patient had developed a progressive right-side hemiparesis over the past three years and, in addition, suffered from aphasia over the past months. CT and MRI showed the widespread presence of an angioma of the basal ganglia on the left. The angiograms showed a complex AVM of the entire left basal ganglia, fed via perforating branches from the M1 segment of the anterior choroidal artery and via perforating branches from the posterior communicating artery and the P1 segment as well as from the posterior choroidal arteries (Fig. 10).

Two endovascular sessions were held over a period of 4 months; part of the contributory vessels could be catheterised along selectively, positioning the wire-controlled, flow-independent microcatheter at selective positions close to the nidus in this vessel (Fig. 11). While after the first embolization, at which three compartments were embolized, the neurological condition of the patient at first remained unchanged, the hemiparesis and aphasia markedly improved over the following weeks. The second endovascular session was held 4 months after the first. Again selective compartments were occluded; however, there was no comparable improvement of the patient's condition after this intervention. Figure 12 shows the angiogram of the complex AVM

after two endovascular sessions. A third session is planned for the near future.

Discussion

The aim of the any treatment of cerebral AVMs is either the total extirpation by surgical means or the permanent and total occlusion through endovascular intervention. The third possibility, the total obliteration by stereotactic radiosurgery, will not be discussed here. In every individual case, however, the risk inherent in surgical intervention and that involved with one or several endovascular sessions must be assessed and compared against that of the natural course of the illness.

An assessment of the risks involved must take into account that basal ganglia AVMs show a higher disposition to bleed than cerebral malformation in general. Basal ganglia AVMs are reported to bleed at a rate of 100 percent[13,14]. In our case histories the rate was 70 percent. Major studies of the general bleeding frequency of cerebral angiomas quote figures of between 40 percent[7,8] and 60 percent[9]. Hence the bleeding risk of basal ganglia angiomas is close to the bleeding risk of cerebral aneurysms, constituting an absolute indication for an invasive surgical intervention or an endovascular approach. It is in particular the smaller basal ganglia angiomas that involve a higher bleeding risk; a phenomenon that is by some

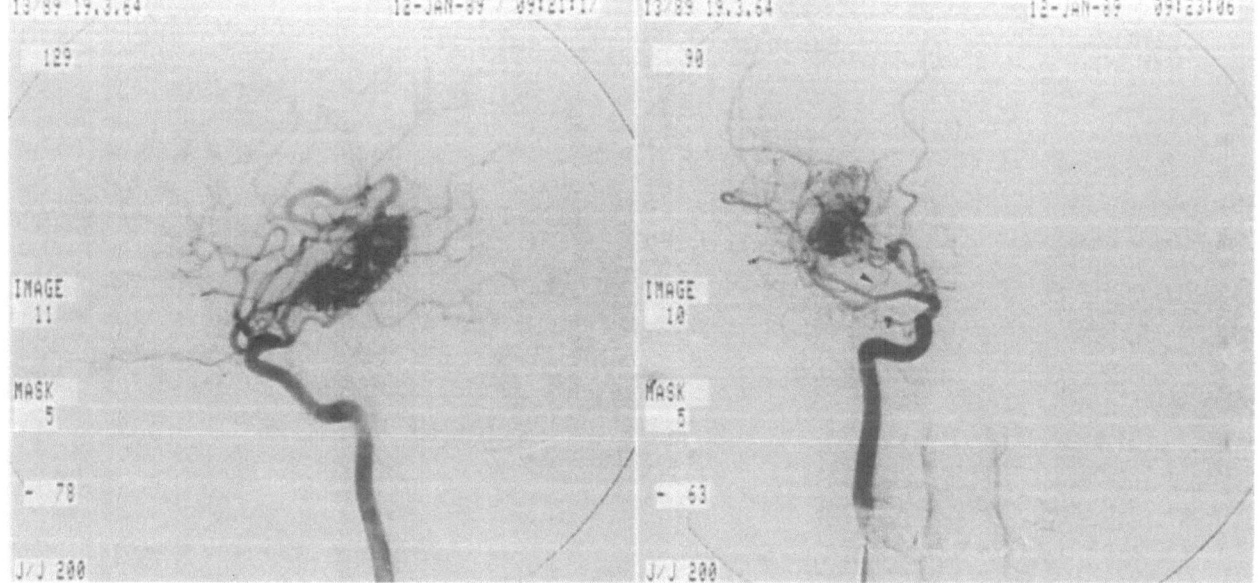

Fig. 5. Pre-embolization angiogram showing the thalamic AVM of case 2. Arrow indicates the perforating branch demonstrated selectively in Fig. 2

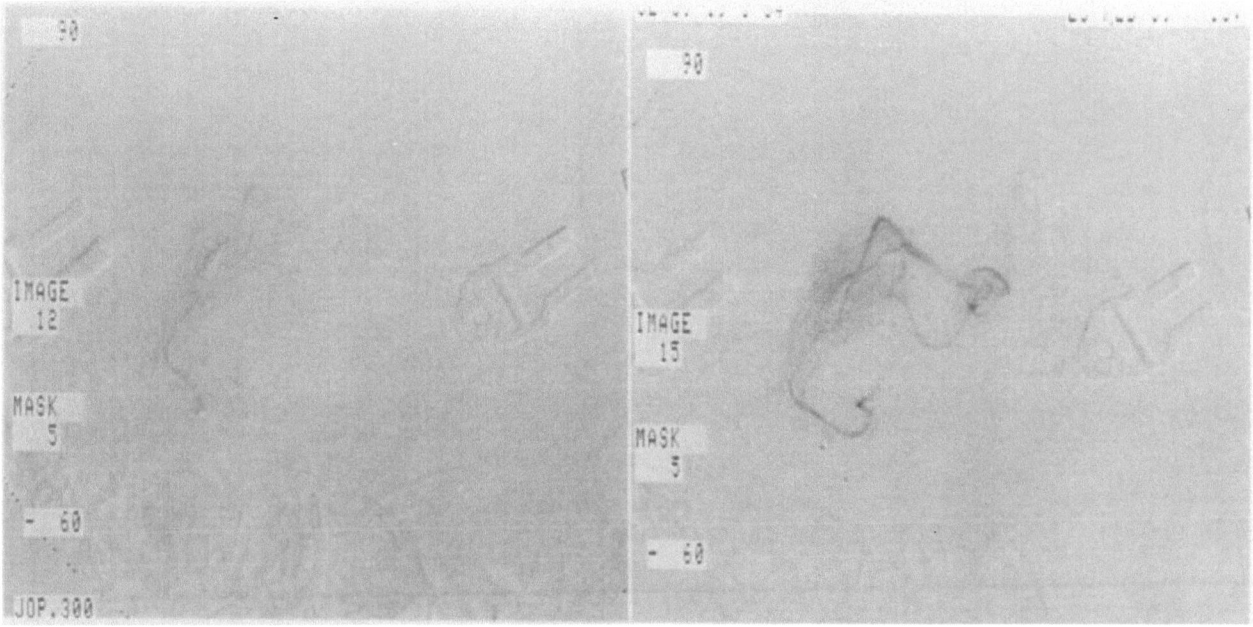

Fig. 6. Selective injection into the perforating branch (Tracker 10, ap view). Early (*left*) and late (*right*) phase. No contribution to the AVM by this artery

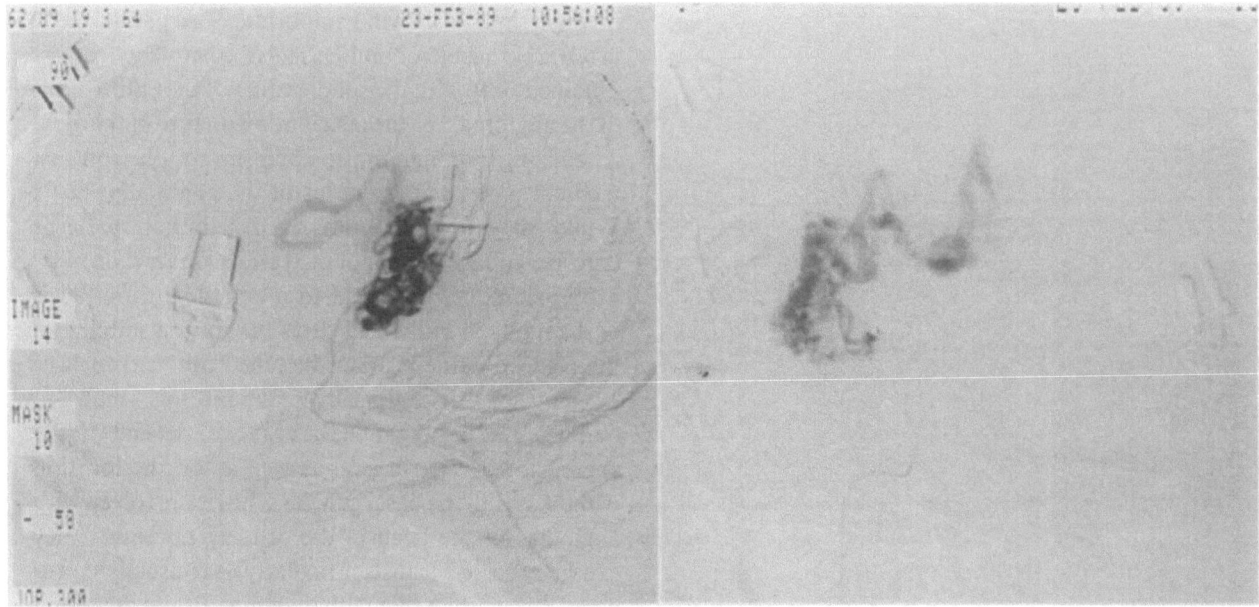

Fig. 7. Selective approach of the microcatheter (Tracker 18) to the thalamic AVM-nidus before embolization. (Note the EEG electrodes for intraoperative monitoring)

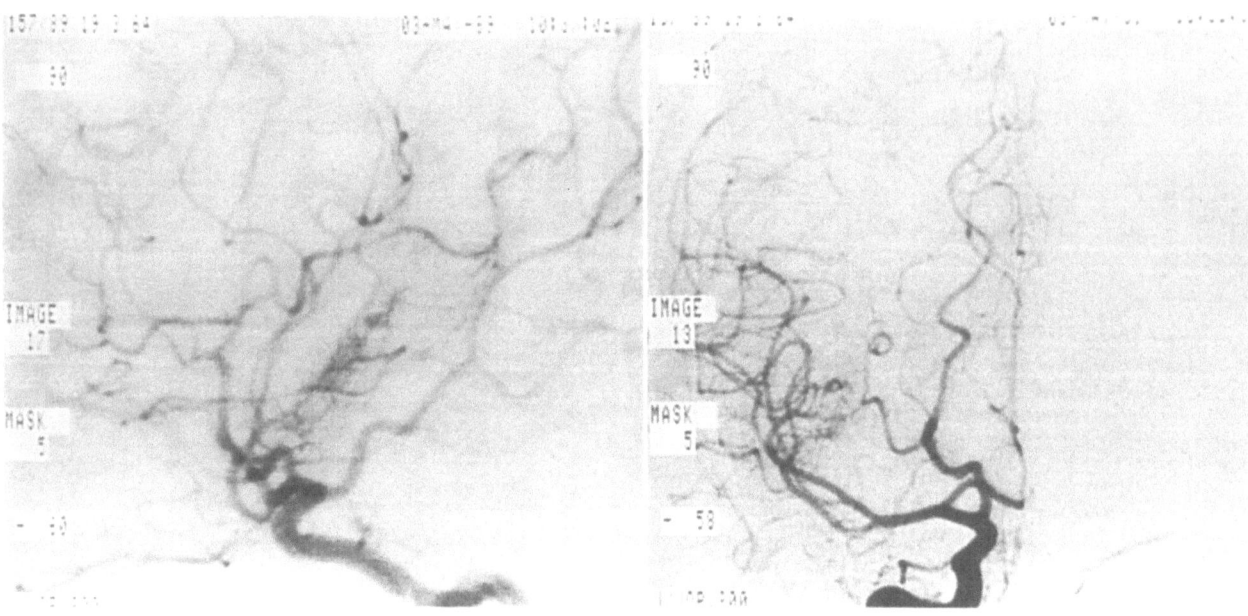

Fig. 8. Follow-up angiogram 1 year after the embolization of the thalamic AVM of case 2

authors[1] linked to the reduced number of draining veins and their position in the ventricular system. Thus the small basal ganglia angiomas with their readiness to bleed constitute the high-risk group that invariably requires definitive treatment.

The decision whether surgical intervention or an endovascular approach is indicated will generally be based on the ruling local circumstances and the personal capabilities of the medical staff. Modern

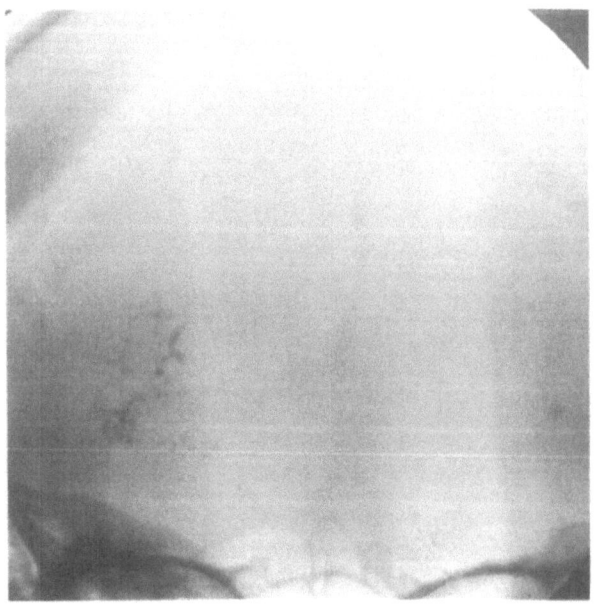

Fig. 9. Solid casting using Histoacryl/Lipiodol in the nidus of the AVM presented in case 2

flow-independent microcatheters, in particular the state-of-the-art miniatures, in many cases make possible a direct access into the nidus of the angioma, even along striate and choroidal vessels. The risk inherent in such endovascular approaches is low, if embolization is performed meeting the need of an absolutely selective catheter position at the nidus of the angioma. However, it is not only the position of the catheter when embolization is performed, but also the type, quantity and distribution of the embolizing medium that is of vital importance. A permanently favourable result of endovascular treatments can be obtained only with the solid casting of the entire nidus of the angioma, i.e., the distribution picture of the acryl embolizing medium must conform to the contrast medium picture of the nidus of the angioma (Fig. 9). While all other materials or distribution patterns (particle collagen, alcohol mixture, histoacryl drop by drop technique) may lead to a complete thrombosis of the nidus in individual cases the certain stability of the result obtained cannot be relied on.

The risk of surgical treatment of small to middle-sized basal ganglia AVMs will depend on the experience of the surgeon as well as on the location of the AVM in the basal ganglia. The risk involved with angiomas at the head of the caudate nucleus – (they can be accessed transventricularly) – is usually considered lower[5] than that with thalamo-striatal locations. It is true that most of the small to middle-sized basal ganglia AVMs have become operable using the

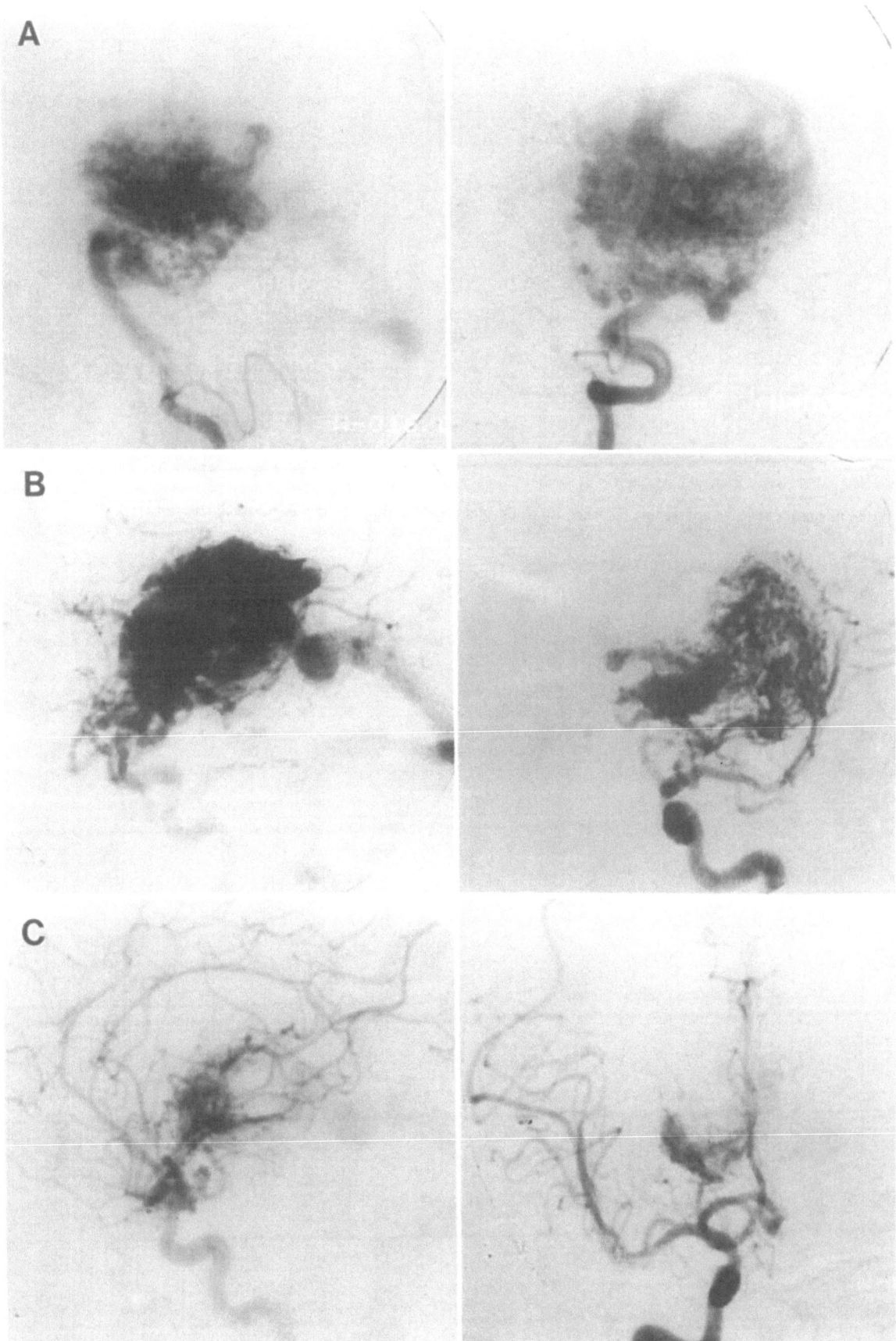

Fig. 10. Giant, complex AVM of the basal ganglia (case 3), fed by both carotid and vertebral arteries. A) Vertebral A., B) left Carotid A., C) right Carotid A

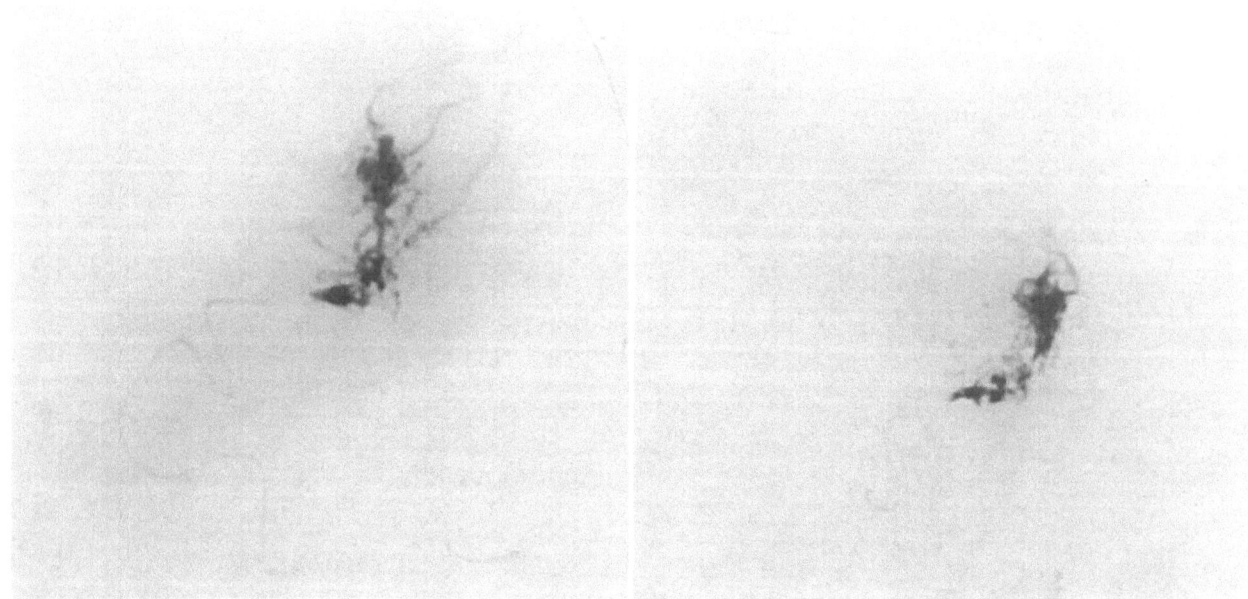

Fig. 11. One of the numerous selective approaches (Tracker 10) to the giant AVM during the two endovascular sessions

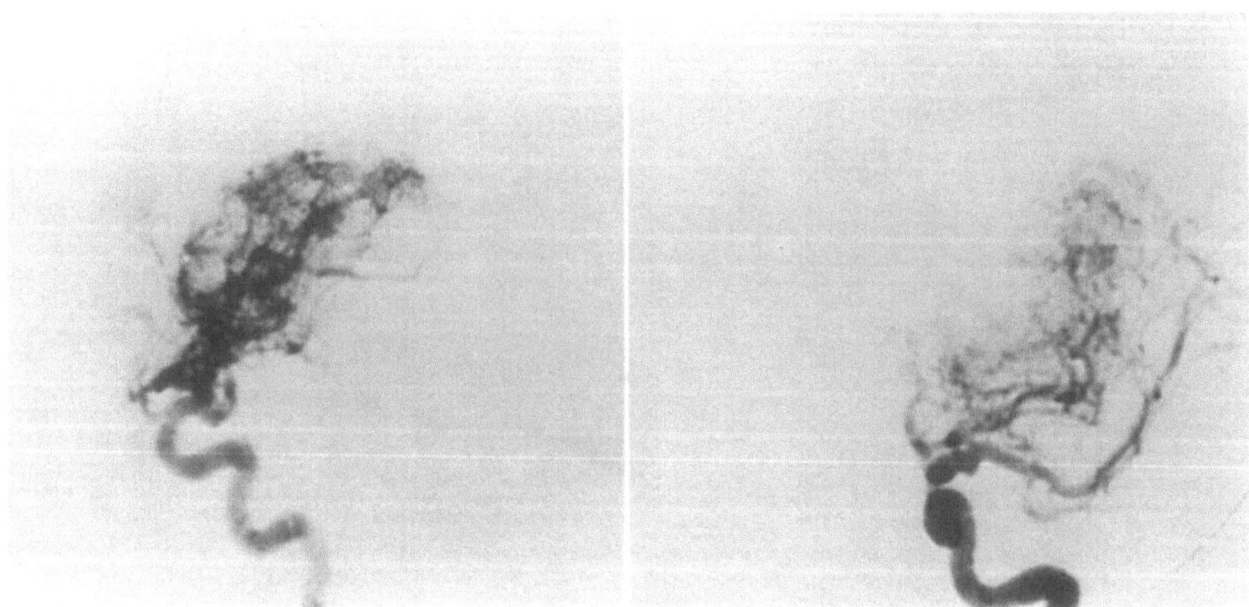

Fig. 12. Angiographic result after two endovascular sessions (case 3). Partial reduction of shunt-activity, increased flow to the functional cerebral territories (left Carotid)

operating microscope and modern radiodiagnostic techniques (MRI); zero-mortality and morbidity below 30 percent, however, will be achieved by centers specializing in angioma surgery (14, 17).

Assessing the risks inherent in endovascular and surgical techniques we at first attach priority to embolization. During the session (under local anaesthesia, with neurophysiological monitoring) it will become evident whether a sufficiently selective catheter position for embolization can be reached. Only if this ideal catheter position for embolization is reached, is embolization performed, aiming at a solid casting of the nidus. If this result cannot be obtained due to vascular or haemodynamic characteristics, total resection by surgical means has to be performed.

Giant basal ganglia AVMs more often than not comprise several vascular territories and pose a complex venous draining system. In most cases the symptoms and signs are neurological deficits and cerebral "fits" rather than bleeding. While their spontaneous risk consequently is low, the risk of treatment is higher. By employing all modern diagnostic and microsurgical techniques and performing staged operations the total resection even of giant basal ganglia angiomas[15] is possible, the complex giant basal ganglia angiomas, however, in particular in the light of their mostly undermatic symptomatology, do not constitute a primary indication for operation[16]. In these cases endovascular techniques and staged approaches may not lead to a total elimination of AVMs, a percent reduction of the AV shunt, however, will in most cases be possible. As shown in case report 3, symptoms and signs like neurological deficits, headache, epileptic fits and hydrocephalus (caused by venous stasis) may, however, be reduced. The disadvantage involved with staged endovascular approaches is that after each session the feeders are left that are more problematic to reach and hence pose a higher risk, increasing the intervention risk from session to session. In addition, the effects of a volume reduction of below 30 percent do not become clinically manifest or are compensated by the angioma's haemodynamic mechanisms within a short time. Despite all these drawbacks a staged endovascular approach to the limit of what is currently feasible from a technical point of view may lead to a reduction of the AV shunts, improving the clinical condition and the patient's quality of life.

References

1. Albert P (1982) personal experience in the treatment of 178 cases of arteriovenous malformation of the brain. Acta Neurochir (Wien) 61: 207–226
2. Andreussi L, Cama A, Grossi G, Marino C, Servato R (1979) Microsurgical excision of a strio-insular arteriovenous malformaation. Surg Neurol 12: 499–502
3. Chuang VP (1986) Superselective catheterization and embolization with tracker 18 infusion catheter. Cardiovascular and interventional radiology and new imaging modalities. Congress proceedings porto cervo
4. Dany A, Vallat JN, Gaudin H, Valegeas A (1968) Les anevrismes cirsoides du cops calleux. Neurochirurgie 14: 489–498
5. Juhasz J (1978) Surgical treatment of Arteriovenous angiomas localised in the corpus callosum, basal ganglia and near the brain stem. Acta Neurochir (Wien) 40: 83–101
6. Lapras C, Bochu M, Russel F, Sindou M (1972) Les angiomes de la tete du noyau caude (a propos de 8 cas opérés). Neurochirurgie 18: 471–483
7. Moody RA, Poppen JL (1970) Arteriovenous malformations. J Neurosurg 32:503–511
8. Parkinson D, Bachers G (1980) Arteriovenous malformations. Summary of 100 consecutive supratentorial cases. J Neurosurg 53: 285–299
9. Perret G, Nishioka H (1966) Arteriovenous malformations. An analysis of 545 cases of cranio-cerebral arteriovenous malformations and fistulae reported to the cooperative study. J. Neurosurg 25: 467–490
10. Pool JL, Potts DG (1965) Aneurysms and arteriovenous anomalies of the brain. Diagnosis and treatment. Harper and Row, New York, 463 pp
11. Richling B (1991) Embolization techniques in the treatment of cerebral arteriovenous malformations. Advances in Neurosurgery 19: 41–45
12. Serbinenko FA (1974) Balloon catheterization and occlusion of major cerebral vessels. J Neurosurg 41: 125–145
13. Shi Y-Q, Chen X-C (1987) Surgical treatment of arteriovenous malformations of the striatothalamocapsular region. J Neurosurg 66: 345–356
14. Solomon RA, Stein BM (1987) Interhemispheric approach for the surgical removal of thalamocaudate arteriovenous malformations. J Neurosurg 66: 345–351
15. Tsutsumi K, Shiokawa Y, Kubota M, Avoki N, Mizutani H (1990) A case of large basal ganglia AVM totally removed by staged operation. No-Shinkei-Geka 18: 871–876
16. Viale GL, Turtas S, Pau A (1980) Surgical removal of striate arteriovenous malformations. Surg Neurol 14: 321–324
17. Wilson CB, Martin NA (1984) Deep supratentorial arteriovenous malformations. In: Wilson, Stein (eds) Intracranial arterio-venous malformation. Williams & Wilkins, Baltimore London, pp 184–208
18. Yaşargil MG, Jain KK, Antic J, Laciga R (1976) Arteriovenous malformations of the splenium of the corpus callosum: microsurgical treatment. Surg Neurol 5: 5–14

Correspondence: Prof. Dr. B. Richling, Department of Neurosurgery, University of Vienna Medical School, Währinger Gürtel 18–20, A-1090 Wien, Austria.

Acta Neurochirurgica, Suppl. 53, 60–64 (1991)

Proliferation in Pituitary Adenomas: Measurement by MAb KI 67

K. Kitz, E. Knosp, W. Th. Koos, and **A. Korn**

Department of Neurosurgery, Vienna Medical School, Wien, Austria

Summary

The monoclonal antibody MAb KI 67 reacts with a nuclear antigen throughout the entire cell cycle and allows easy evaluation of proliferating tumour cells on routinely prepared smear and frozen sections. 120 pituitary adenomas were investigated by use of the monoclonal antibody KI 67 in a two-step avidin-biotin-peroxidase complex (ABC) technique. The KI 67 labelling index (LI) ranged in all adenomas from 0.2 to 4.6%. In 90 cases of transphenoidally operated adenomas the dura of the sella floor was investigated histologically. Adenomas with histologically proven dural infiltration showed a statistically significant higher KI 67 LI (p < 0.001) compared to non-invasive adenomas.

Keywords: Dural invasiveness; monoclonal antibody KI 67; pituitary adenoma.

Introduction

Neurosurgical treatment of pituitary adenomas aims at improving or preventing visual disturbances and at curing hormonal hypersecretion. Pre-operative serum hormone levels[11,16,24,25,33,37,38] tumour size[10,11,25,38] and distinct immunohistological and ultrastructural patterns[20] were related to the chance of surgical cure. Although pituitary adenomas in general are benign and slowly growing tumours invasive growth into dura and surrounding bony sturctures has been demonstrated radiologically, surgically and histologically[19,21,35,36,39].

Except for rare cases of pituitary carcinomas, histological patterns of malignancy are seldom found in pituitary adenomas. Nuclear and cellular pleomorphism without an increase of mitotic activity in histological specimens have proven to be no reliable criteria for rapid regrowth of pituitary adenomas[19,34].

Immunocytochemical detection of a proliferation associated nuclear antigen by the monoclonal antibody KI 67 allows easy and rapid determination of

the cellular growth rate in biopsy samples of human cell populations[5,6,19,22,23].

In the study MAb KI 67 was used to determine the proliferative activity of 120 pituitary adenomas, comprising 64 hormonally active and 56 hormonally inactive adenomas.

Material and Methods

Fresh tissue samples of pituitary adenomas were smeared on glass slides and stained immunohistochemically using the ABC method as described[19] (Fig. 1). Small biopsies of the dura of the sella floor were embedded in Tissue-Tek O.C.T. compound, frozen and stored at − 70°C. Frozen sections were incubated for MAb KI 67 as described[5,6,19]. Larger specimens were further embedded in epoxy resin and semi-thin sections were stained with toluidine blue (Fig. 2). Proliferative activity was determined in highly positive areas. More than 2000 adenoma cells in at least 4 areas were counted and the ratio of KI 67 labelled cells and the total number of adenoma cells was expressed as a percentage (KI 67 Labelling Index, KI 67 LI).

Results

This enlarged series of 120 cases of pituitary adenomas[19] comprises all immunohistological types of pituitary adenomas and represents nearly all pituitary adenomas operated on in our department since 1987. We investigated 56 non functioning and 64 hormonally active adenomas.

The mean value of KI 67 LI (Labelling Index) of all investigated pituitary adenomas was 1.59% (SD ± 0.84) within a range of 0.2 to 4.6% (Table 1).

The group of the non functioning adenomas (NE) represented the largest group in our series (46.6%) and the measured KI 67 LI was 1.42% (SD ± 0.64) mean value, ranging from 0.2 to 3.29% of all nuclei.

In the group of 64 hormonally active adenomas we investigated 27 cases (22.5%) of adenomas secreting

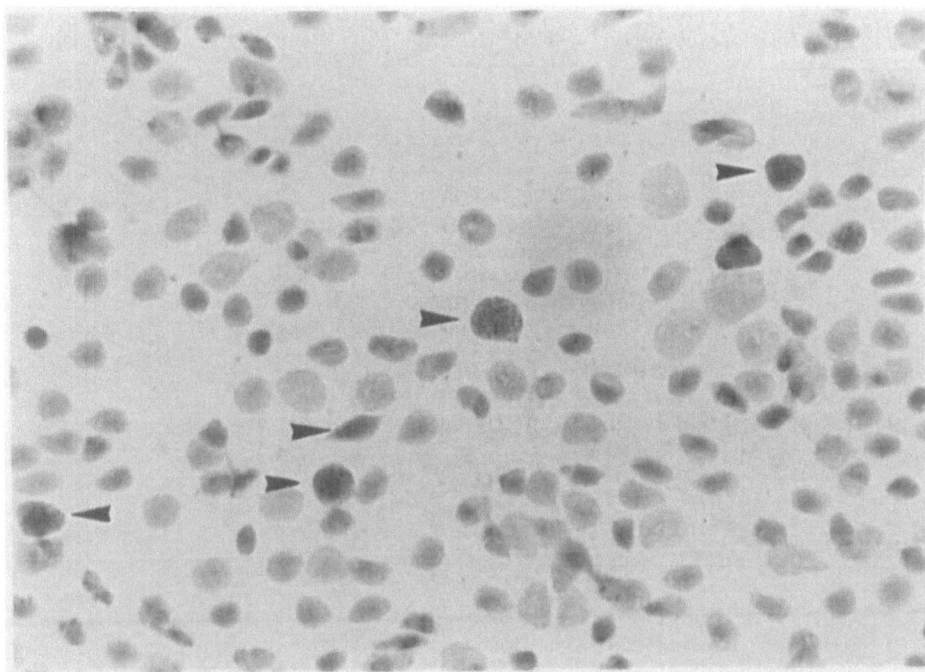

Fig. 1. Several nuclei positively stained for KI 67 in ABC technique (arrows), smear preparation of pituitary adenoma, Hematoxilin counter-stain, x 640

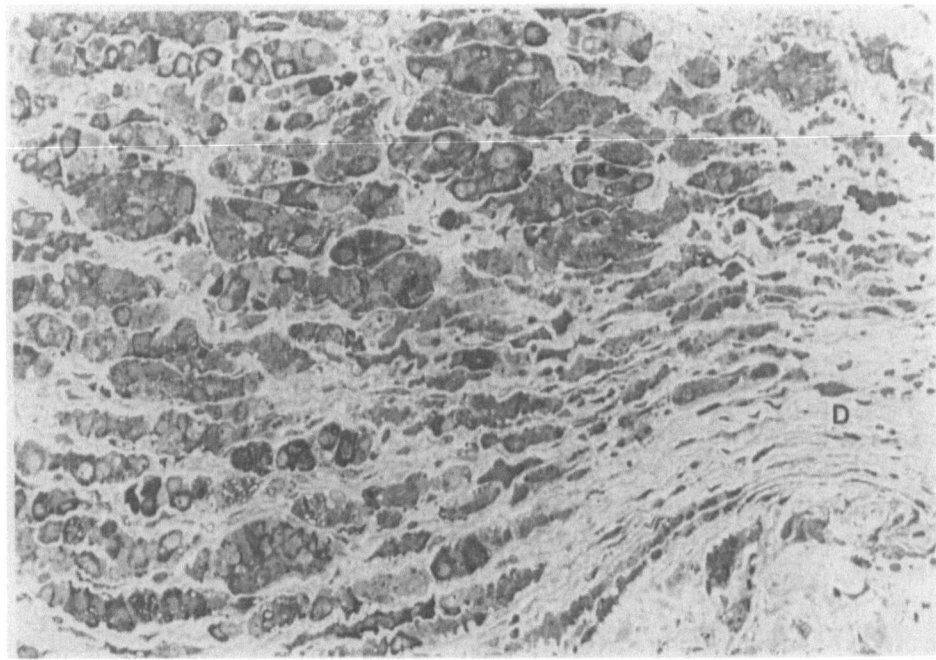

Fig. 2. Clusters of adenoma cells infiltrating the dura of the sella floor (D = dura). Semi-thin section, Toluidine blue, x 320

prolactin, 24 cases (20%) of adenomas secreting growth hormone, 6 cases (5%) of adenomas secreting adrenocorticotropic hormone, 5 cases of Nelson tumours and 2 cases of adenomas secreting luteinizing hormone.

In Prolactinomas (PRL) the proliferation activity (KI 67 LI) was 1.71%, within a range from 0.3 to 3.31%.

In 24 cases of growth hormone secreting adenomas (GH) the mean value of the KI 67 LI (Labelling Index) was 1.21% (SD ± 0.66), ranging from 0.2 to 2.42%.

5 cases of adenomas secreting adrenocorticotropic hormone (ACTH) showed an average proliferative activity (KI 67 LI) of 1.82% (SD ± 0.98) within a range from 0.44% to 3.02%.

Outstanding high mean values of KI 67 LI 3.34%

Table 1. *Proliferation Rate in 120 Pituitary Adenomas: Measurement by MAb Ki-67*

Number of cases	Immuno-histology	Sex (M/F)	Mean age (year)	Ki-67 LI mean in %	Range (%)
56	NF	27/29	53	1.42 (SD ± 0.64)	(0.20–3.29)
27	PRL	10/17	38	1.71 (SD ± 0.75)	(0.43–3.31)
24	GH	11/13	46	1.21 (SD ± 0.66)	(0.20–2.42)
6	ACTH	3/3	39	1.82 (SD ± 0.98)	0.44–3.02)
5	NELSON	2/3	41	3.34 (SD ± 0.90)	(2.36–4.60)
2	LH	0/2	54	1.04 (SD ± 0.08)	(0.98–1.10)
120		**53/67**	**45**	**1.59 (SD ± 0.84)**	**(0.20–4.60)**

NF, non functioning adenoma; PRL, prolactin; GH, growth hormone; ACTH, adrenocorticotropic hormone; LH, luteining hormone; NELSON, Nelson tumour.

Table 2. *Histological Examination of 89 Dural Biopsies*

Number of cases	Immuno-histology	Sex (M/F)	Age (years)	Ki-67 LI (mean in %)	Range (%)	Dural infiltration
13	NF	5/8	50	0.89 (SD ± 0.43)	(0.20–1.44)	−
8	PRL	0/8	29	1.35 (SD ± 0.57)	(0.43–2.90)	−
8	GH	3/5	55	0.82 (SD ± 0.40)	(0.46–1.47)	−
1	ACTH	1/0	55	0.67		−
2	LH	0/2	54	1.04 (SD ± 0.08)	(0.98–1.09)	−
32		**9/23**	**48**	**0.98 (SD ± 0.47)**	**(0.20–2.90)**	**−**
26	NF	8/18	55	1.60 (SD ± 0.75)	(0.31–3.29)	+
12	PRL	5/7	40	1.85 (SD ± 0.88)	(0.51–3.31)	+
12	GH	5/7	42	1.46 (SD ± 0.64)	(0.20–2.42)	+
4	ACTH	2/2	36	1.87 (SD ± 0.87)	(0.90–3.02)	+
3	NELSON	2/1	46	3.50 (SD ± 1.24)	(2.60–4.60)	+
57		**22/35**	**44**	**1.81 (SD ± 0.92)**	**(0.31–4.60)**	**+**

NF, nonfunctioning adenoma; PRL, prolactin; GH, growth hormone; ACTH, adrenocorticotropic hormone; LH, luteining hormone; NELSON, Nelson tumour.

(SD ± 0.90) were found in 5 cases of Nelson tumour. In two cases of an adenoma secreting luteinizing hormone we found KI 67 LI's of 0.98 and 1.10%.

With exception of the group of Nelson tumours, no further statistically significant difference in the KI 67 LI could be found. Neither between different groups of hormonally active adenomas, nor in the inactive tumour group. A comparison of KI 67 Labelling Index with tumour size, hormonal secretion, sex, and age of the patients did not show any significant correlation[19,22,23].

Histological Examination of Dural Infiltration

89 cases of pituitary adenomas (74%) were operated on transsphenoidally. In all cases the dura of the sella floor was subjected to histological examination on frozen and semi-thin sections. In 32 cases (36%) no evidence of dural infiltration was found (Table 2). In 57 cases (64%), however, different patterns of individual cell penetration into the dura or invasion by clusters of adenoma cells were found (34) (Fig. 2).

The KI 67 LI in the noninvasive group ranged from 0.20 to 2.90% (0.98, ± 0.49; mean, ± SD). A nearly two-fold increase in the KI 67 LI from 0.31 to 4.6% (1.81, ± 0.92; mean, ± SD) was found in the group of invasive adenomas, indicating a statistically significant higher growth rate ($p < 0.001$, Student's t test).

Even in smaller subgroups, such as non functioning adenomas and adenomas secreting growth hormone, correlation between invasive to noninvasive groups revealed statistically significant differences (NF, $p < 0.01$; GH, $p < 0.05$; Student's t test).

Discussion

The results obtained with the MAb KI 67 correspond well with the proliferative activity measured by [H³]thymidine uptake[2,6,17], or the incorporation of 5-bromodeoxyuridine (BrdU) into the DNA[8,14,29]. In contrast to the above-mentioned methods, MAb KI 67 can be applied routinely on untreated, fresh biopsy material prepared by smear preparation or frozen section technique. Both techniques provide the investigator with nearly indentical results[22].

In this series of 120 investigated adenomas we found the KI 67 LI ranging from 0.2 to 4.6% with a mean value of 1.59% (SD ± 0.84). In comparison to our published series[19] we found higher mean values of KI 67 LIs in all adenoma types, probably due to the fact that 12 cases of recurrent adenomas were added to our series. In nearly all reoperated adenomas we measured higher values of KI LI than in specimens of prior operations (unpublished data).

In 66% of 90 dura specimens tumour invasion was demonstrated histologically. These findings correspond with the results of other authors[3,4,21,22,26,34,36] and with our published measurements[19]. In our series, a statistically significantly higher KI 67 LI was found not only in the group of all invasive adenomas 1.81, ± 0.92 (mean, SD; p < 0.001, Student's t test), but also in invasive adenomas secreting growth hormone and in invasive adenomas of the nonfunctioning type (GH, p < 0.05; NF, p < 0.01; Student's t test) (Table 2).

Aggressive growth has been correlated with certain immunohistological and ultrastructural findings[12,13,20]. Our material does not encompass rare immunohistological types of acidophilic stem cell adenoma or the silent corticotropic adenoma, whereas in our 5 cases of Nelson tumour outstanding high KI 67 LI's were found.

By use of KI 67, it is possible to demonstrate different proliferative activities ranging from 0.2 to 4.6%, which indicates that there exists no biological uniform group of adenomas. In cases of lack of hormone secretion, cure rates and regrowth of residual tumour can only be demonstrated by repeated postoperative computed tomography and magnetic resonance imaging scans. The decision of whether or not radiation therapy should be given is far more difficult than in secreting pituitary adenomas. Therefore, the measurement of the proliferative activity (KI 67 LI) on routinely prepared smear and frozen sections might become a useful tool in postoperative decision making.

Acknowledgement

The authors thank Mrs. Schmiedel Brigitte, Department of Neurosurgery, University of Vienna, for her skillful technical assistance.

References

1. Ciric I, Mikhael M, Stanford T, Lawson L (1983) Transsphenoidal microsurgery of pituitary macroadenomas with long term follow up results. J Neurosurg 59: 395–402
2. Cooper EH, Frank GL, Wright DH (1966) Cell proliferation in Burkitt tumors. Europ J Cancer 2: 377–384
3. Ebershold MJ, Quast LM, Laws ER, Scheithauer B, Randall RV (1986) Long term results in transsphenoidal removal of non functioning pituitary adenomas. J Neurosurg 64: 713–719
4. Fahlbusch R, Buchfelder M, Schreu K (1987) Short time preoperative treatment of macroprolactinomas by dopamine agonists. J Neurosurg 67: 807–815
5. Gerdes J, Schwab U, Lemke H, Stein H (1983) Production of a mouse monoclonal antibody reactive with a human nuclear antigen associated with cell proliferation. Int J Cancer 31: 13–20
6. Gerdes J, Lemke H, Baisch H, Wacker HH, Schwab U, Stein H (1984) Cell cycle analysis of a cell proliferation-associated human nuclear antigen defined by monoclonal antibody KI 67. J Immunol 113: 1710–1715
7. Goz B (1977) The effects of incorporation of 5 halogenated deoxyuridines into the DNA of eukaryotic cells. Pharmakol Rev 29: 247–272
8. Gratzner HG (1982) Monoclonal antibody to 5-bromo and 5-iododeoxyuridine: A new reagent for detection of DNA replication. Science 218: 474–475
9. Guesdon JL, Ternynck T, Avrameas S (1979) The use of avidinbiotin interaction in immunoenzymatic techniques. J Histochem Cytochem 27: 1131–1139
10. Hardy J (1969) Transsphenoidal microsurgery of the normal and pathological pituitary. Clin Neurosurg 16: 185–217
11. Hardy J (1983) Transsphenoidal microsurgery of prolactinomas: Report of 355 cases. In: Tolis G, Stefanis C, Mountokalakis T (eds) Prolactin and prolactinomas. Raven Press, New York, pp 431–440
12. Horvath E, Kovacs K, Killinger DW, Smyth HS, Platts ME, Singer W (1980) Silent corticotropic adenomas of the human pituitary gland: A histopathologic immunocytologic and ultrastructural study. Am J Pathol 98: 617–638
13. Horvath E, Kovacs K, Singer W, Ezrin C, Kerenyi A (1977) Acidophil stemcell adenoma of the human pituitary. Arch Pathol Lab Med 101: 594–599
14. Hoshino T, Nagashima T, Murovic JA (1986) In situ cell kinetics studies on human neuroectodermal tumors with bromodeoxyuridine labeling. J Neurosurg 64: 453–459
15. Hsu SM, Raine L, Fanger H (1981) Use of Avidine-Biotin-Peroxidase Complex (ABC) in immunoperoxidase techniques. A comparison between ABC and unlabelled antibody (PAP) procedures. J Histochem Cytochem 29: 577–580
16. Hubbard JL, Scheithauer BW, Abboud CHF, Laws ER (1967) Prolactin secreting adenomas: The preoperative response to bromocriptine treatment and surgical outcome. J Neurosurg 67: 816–821
17. Johnson HA, Haymaker WE, Rubini JR (1960) A radioautographic study of a human brain and glioblastoma multiforme after in vivo uptake of tritiated thymidine. Cancer 13: 636–642
18. Knosp E, Krisch K, Schmidbauer M, Budka H (1988) Immunologischer Hormonnachweis bei Hypophysenadenomen:

Korrelation von Serumhormonbefunden mit immunzytochemischem Hormonbefund am Tumorschnitt. Wien Klin Wochenschr 100: 322–325

19. Knosp E, Kitz K, Perneczky A (1989) Proliferation activity in pituitary adenomas: Measurement by monoclonal antibody KI 67. Neurosurg 25: 927–930

20. Kovacs K (1984) Light and electron microscopic pathology of pituitary tumors: Immunohistochemistry. In: Black McL, Zervas NT, Ridgeway EC, Martin JB (eds) Secretory tumors of the pituitary gland. Raven Press, New York, pp 365–375

21. Landolt AM (1980) Biology of pituitary microadenomas. In: Faglia G, Giovanelli MA, Mac Leod RM (eds) Pituitary microadenomas. Academic Press, London, pp 107–122

22. Landolt AM, Shibata T, Kleihues P (1987) Growth rate of human pituitary adenomas. J Neurosurg 67: 803–806

23. Landolt AM, Shibata T, Kleihues P, Tuncdogan E (1988) Growth of pituitary adenomas: Facts and speculations. Adv Biosciences 69: 53–62

24. Laws ER, Piepgras DG, Rendall RV (1979) Neurosurgical management of acromegaly: Results in 82 patients treated between 1972–1977. J Neurosurg 50: 454–461

25. Laws ER (1984) The Neurosurgical management of acromegaly. In: Black McL, Zervas NT, Ridgeway EC, Martin JB (eds) Secretory tumors of the pituitary gland. Raven Press, New York, pp 169–173

26. Martins AN, Hayes GJ, Kempe LG (1985) Invasive pituitary adenomas. J Neurosurg 22: 268–276

27. Morimura T, Kitz K, Budka H (1989) In situ analysis of cell kinetics in human brain tumors. A comparative immunocytochemical study of S-phase cells by a new in vitro BrdU labeling technique and of proliferating pool cells by monoclonal antibody KI 67. Acta Neuropathol (Berl) 77: 276–282

28. Nagashima T, Murovic JA, Hoshino T, Wilson CB, Dearmond SJ (1986) The proliferative potential of human pituitary tumours in situ. J Neurosurg 64: 588–594

29. Nagashima T, Hoshino T, Cho KG, Senegor M, Waldman F, Nomura K (1988) Comparison of bromodesoxyuridine labeling indices obtained from tissue sections and flow cytometry of brain tumours. J Neurosurg 68: 388–392

30. Naritoku WY, Taylor CR (1982) A comparative study of the use of monoclonal antibodies using three different immunohistochemical methods: An evaluation of monoclonal and polyclonal antibodies against human prostatic acid phosphatase. J Histochem Cytochem 30: 253–260

31. Nishizaki T, Orita T, Saiki M, Furutani Y, Aoki H (1988) Cell kinetic studies of human brain tumors by in vitro labeling using anti BrdU monoclonal antibody. J Neurosurg 69: 371–374

32. Ross DA, Wilson CB (1988) Results of transsphenoidal microsurgery for growth hormone secreting pituitary adenomas in a series of 214 patients. J Neurosurg 68: 854–867

33. Seager W (1977) Die Hypophysentumore: Zytologische und ultrastrukturelle Klassifikation, Pathogenese, endokrine Funktionen und Tierexperiment. Fischer G, Stuttgart New York, pp 39–42

34. Selman WR, Laws ER, Scheithauer BW, Carpenter SM (1986) The occurrence of dural invasion in pituitary adenomas. J Neurosurg 64: 402–408

35. Scheithauer BW, Kovacs KT, Laws ER, Randall RV (1986) Pathology in invasive pituitary tumors with special reference to functional classification. J Neurosurg 65: 733–745

36. Tindall GT, Tindall SC (1984) Transsphenoidal surgery for acromegaly; Long term results in 50 patients. In: Black McL, Zervas NT, Ridgeway EC, Martin JB (eds) Secretory tumors of the pituitary gland. Raven Press, New York, pp 175–178

Correspondence: K. Kitz, M.D., Department of Neurosurgery, Vienna Medical School, Währinger Gürtel 18–20, A-1090 Wien, Austria.

Acta Neurochirurgica, Suppl. 53, 65–71 (1991)
© by Springer-Verlag 1991

Pituitary Adenomas with Parasellar Invasion

E. Knosp[1], **K. Kitz**[1], **E. Steiner**[2], and **Ch. Matula**[1]

Departments of [1]Neurosurgery and [2]Radiology, Vienna Medical School, Wien, Austria

Summary

Pituitary adenomas with extension into the parasellar space, the so called "cavernous sinus" can be demonstrated best using MRI. To improve the delineation from the venous compartments the use of unenhanced and enhanced MRI scans is essential. In 25 pituitary adenomas with surgically proven infiltration into the space of the cavernous sinus we correlated the MRI findings with our surgical observations. When the adenoma encases the intracavernous internal carotid artery or reaches as far as to the lateral aspect of the artery, invasion was present in all cases. The critical area where invasion could not be predicted from MRI is the distance between the medial and the lateral aspect of the intracavernous internal carotid artery. By measurement with the monoclonal antibody KI-67 it could be shown, that pituitary adenomas infiltrating the parasellar space have a statistically significant higher growth rate ($p < 0.001$), compared to non-invasive adenomas. This is of special interest, because surgical cure becomes unlikely, when invasion into the space of the cavernous sinus is present.

Keywords: Pituitary adenomas; cavernous sinus; MRI; growth rate; invasiveness.

Introduction

Since we use MRI in the diagnosis of pituitary adenomas routinely, the parasellar anatomy for the first time becomes visible before operation. The challenge of MRI is not only to confirm the diagnosis of an adenoma but also to give a clear picture of the parasellar pathology. To improve the delineation of the adenoma from the surrounding structures, the application of Gd-DTPA is mandatory. We could demonstrate that this improves delineation of the adenoma from the normal gland as well as from the suprasellar structures and especially from the parasellar space up to 91% compared to unenhanced MRI scans[21].

Although pituitary adenomas are benign in their histological appearance, invasiveness can be demonstrated radiologically[1], surgically and histolo-gically[19,20,23]. When looking grossly at the dura of the sella floor a invasiveness was found in 40%[18] and in 94% when looking histologically[20].

In adenomas with histologically proven dura invasion, we could demonstrate a significantly higher proliferation rate[13] as did other authors[14].

It is possible to excise dura specimens for histological examination from the sellar floor without risk, whereas biopsies from the medial wall of the cavernous sinus carry a high risk for routine investigation. Therefore parasellar invasiveness remains a surgical observation which needs much experience[4,19,20,18] but represents a great surgical challenge.

With the advent of MRI the demonstration of parasellar anatomy and pathology, it is possible to see gross infiltration of the space of the "cavernous sinus"[2].

In order to distinguish between infiltration and compression of the 'cavernous sinus" we investigated all pituitary adenomas which had suspected involvement of the medial wall of the cavernous sinus. In these 25 cases with surgically proven infiltration, we correlated the MRI findings with our surgical observations. We also measured the proliferation rate with the monoclonal antibody KI-67 in order to determine the growth rates of these invasive adenomas.

Material and Methods

All patients undergoing surgery for pituitary adenomas had MRI investigation on a 1.5 T superconducting MR imaging system (Magneton 63 tm SIEMENS). Sagittal and coronal sections were obtained before and after intravenous administration of Gadolineum-DTPA (Magnevist R Schering) using 0.02 mmol/kg body weight.

Surgery was performed in all cases using different approaches according to the size and shape of their suprasellar extension. Most cases, however, had transsphenoidal surgery as the only or as the initial surgical treatment. In cases of the transsphenoidal approach, dura of the sella floor was excised and examined histologically.

Tumour specimens were taken for routine histological investigations (Haemallaun) and immunhistological staining) as well as for smear and frozen sections. All specimens were stained immunohistochemically with the monoclonal antibody (Mab) KI-67 in the ABC technique as described previously[13].

During tumour removal special attention was paid to the appearance of the medial wall of the "cavernous sinus" with regard to signs of invasiveness.

The observation of so called trabeculae or the uncovered wall of the intracavernous ICA were regarded as a clear sign of invasiveness.

In cases in which we found a hole in the medial wall of the cavernous sinus and venous bleeding after gentle tumour removal we also classified this as invasion of the cavernous sinus. In some cases, however, we were not able to exclude invasiveness unequivocally (these cases are excluded from the present study).

Surgical Results

All 25 patients underwent surgery and the histological confirmation of a pituitary adenoma. 18 patients had the transsphenoidal approach and 7 patients underwent craniotomy due to large and polycyclic extra-axial supraseller extensions. In all but two cases of the transsphenoidally treated cases the dura, overlying the sella floor, was investigated histologically for signs of invasiveness. In 11 of these patients infiltration of the basal dura was found. In two cases of tumour recurrence dura biopsy could not be performed. There were only 3 out of 15 cases with parasellar extension which had no invasion of the dura of the sella floor.

In all cases of subfrontally approached patients the tumour grew through the lateral wall or the roof of the cavernous sinus or had encased the intracavernous carotid artery totally, as demonstrated by MRI. In both circumstances, invasion of the parasellar space was evident.

In all cases operated upon transsphenoidally infiltration of the medial wall of the "cavernous sinus" was observed directly. In only a few cases, however, we were able to take biopsies from the medial wall of the cavernous sinus for histological examination (see Fig. 4). Within the space of the cavernous sinus we only used suction and blunt curettes for tumour removal. Usually venous bleeding occurs when the tumour is removed. In those cases with a large tumour mass within the space of the cavernous sinus we could see ligaments of the parasellar space which we know from our anatomical studies[11,12] (and unpublished data). In general, tumour removal becomes increasingly difficult with extension laterally. Tumour parts lateral to the internal carotid artery usually become inaccessible.

Although most cases had significant parasellar extensions, we had no additional morbidity or mortality in this series. The only fatality occurred in the largest tumour of this group (see Table 1) after transcranial removal which resulted in hypothalamic failure. In one case with a cavernous sinus syndrome the oculomotor palsy and trigeminal hypaesthesia resolved completely within five weeks after transsphenoidal operation. There were two patients with cavernous sinus syndrome in our 25 cases although in 9 cases (10 sides) the intracavernous carotid artery was completely surrounded by tumour.

13 patients had hormonal hypersecretion with elevation of prolactin (PRL) in 7 cases, growth hormone (GH) in 5 cases and adrenocorticotropic hormone (ACTH) in one case, which was a Nelson tumour developing 9 years after adrenalectomy. Cure from hormonal hypersecretion was unlikely and was found in 2 cases only (one PRL and one GH secreting adenoma).

Radiological Results

With increase in tumour size the medial compartment of the cavernous venous plexus did not enhance in MRI (Fig. 1). Depending on the direction of parasellar growth in relation to the internal carotid artery the superior and/or inferior compartment of the cavernous venous plexus did not enhance (Fig. 2). Finally the ICA became totally enclosed by the adenoma (Fig. 3). In most of these cases the lateral wall of the "cavernous sinus" was displaced with a convex contour (Fig. 3). When compared with CT, this was the most certain sign of "cavernous sinus" invasion. In all cases with tumour growth around the ICA, we found invasion of the 'cavernous sinus' during surgery.

The same holds true for all cases in which the adenoma grew as far as to the lateral border of the intracavernous ICA. If the tumour reaches the wall of the ICA or slightly progressed into the superior or inferior compartment of the "cavernous sinus", invasion was not seen in every case. In our experience the critical distance where tumour invasion of the space of the "cavernous sinus" becomes very likely is between the medial and the lateral aspects of the intracavernous ICA.

Beside parasellar extension of the adenoma, suprasellar growth was present in 16 cases. In 4 cases into the suprasellar cistern (SS 1) in 7 cases with displacement of the optic chiasm (SS 2) and in 6 cases with

Table 1. *Pituitary Adenomas with Invasion into the Parasellar Space.* Summary of 25 cases

NN	Age	Sex	App	DM	SU	Extension			Immuno-histol.	KI67 LI%	Invasiveness Dura
						SS	RCS	LCS			
E.	35	f	S	45	+	1	+	+	NF	1.25	+
A.	70	f	T	25		2	+	−	NF	1.37	+
R.	54	m	T	25	+	2	+	−	NF	1.44	+
K.	66	f	T	40	+	3	+	+	NF	2.27	+
H.	52	f	T	20		0	+	−	NF	2.94	+
T.	53	f	T	40	+	2	−	+	NF	3.29	+
K.	46	m	T	10		0	−	+	PRL	0.95	+
D.	22	f	T	20		0	+	−	PRL	1.50	+
M.	37	m	T	15		0	−	+	PRL	2.50	+
S.	23	f	T	25		0	+	−	PRL	2.90	+
W.	39	m	T	15		2	+	−	GH	2.42	+
F.	20	f ʟ	T	18		0	+	−	GH/PRL	2.27	+
P.	48	m	T	25		0	+	−	NF	1.12	−
H.	53	f	T	35		3	−	+	NF	2.30	−
M.	25	f	T	15		0	−	+	PRL	0.78	−
S.	37	f	T	25		1	−	+	ACTH*	3.80	nd
E.	52	f	S	35		1	+	−	GH	1.64	nd
T.	23	m	T	15		1	+	−	GH	1.87	nd
C.	39	m	S	40	+	3	+	+	GH	2.19	nd
A.	45	m	S	40	+	3	−	+	GH	3.50	nd
K.	57	m	S	70		3	+	+	NF	1.27	nd
P.	38	f	T	25		2	−	+	NF	1.27	nd
M.	53	f	S	40		3	+	+	NF	2.93	nd
J.	48	m	S	40		2	+	+	PRL	1.33	nd
B.	27	f	T	15		2	−	+	PRL	0.80	nd
25				28.7 (±13.3; mean, SD)						1.95 (±0.85; mean, SD)	

Summary of 25 cases with invasion into the parasellar space: Approach (App); trans-sphenoidal (T); subfrontal (S). Diameter (DM) in mm. Extension: subsellar (SU); suprasellar (SS); into the suprasellar cistern (1), with displacement of the optic chiasm (2), with displacement of the third ventricle (3). LCS (left cavernous sinus), RCS (right cavernous sinus) surgically observed infiltration of the cavernous sinus (+); no infiltration (−). Immunohistology: non functioning (NF); prolactin (PRL); growth hormone (GH); adrenocorticotropic hormone (ACTH*) – in this case a Nelson tumour was present. Proliferation rate: KI-67 labelling index (LI) expressed as percentage (%). Dura: histologically proven infiltration (+) of the dura of the sella floor; not invasive (−) ; not done (nd).

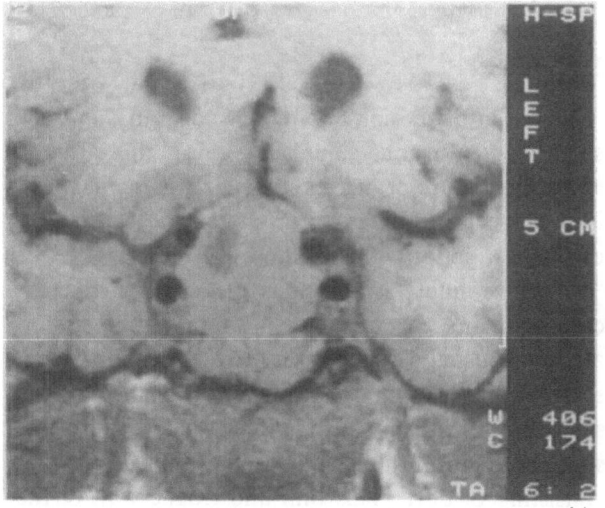
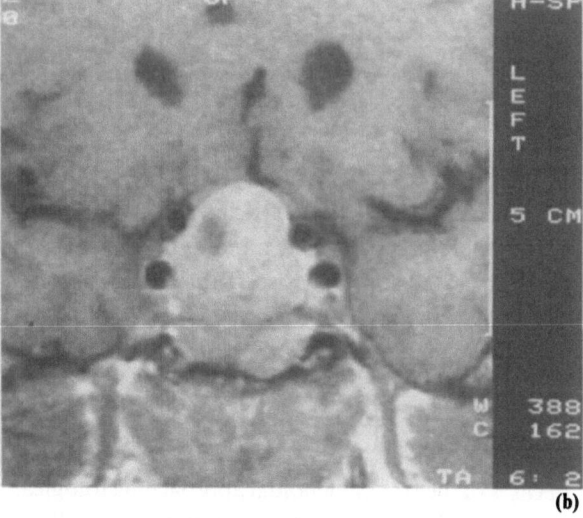

(a) **(b)**

Fig. 1. Coronal MRI scan before (a) and after (b) application of Gd-DTPA. The medial compartments of the cavernous sinus are compressed by the adenoma whereas the compartments lateral, superior and inferior to the intracavernous carotid artery are enhanced in (b). During surgery no invasion of the cavernous sinus was found. Invasion of the sphenoid sinus was present

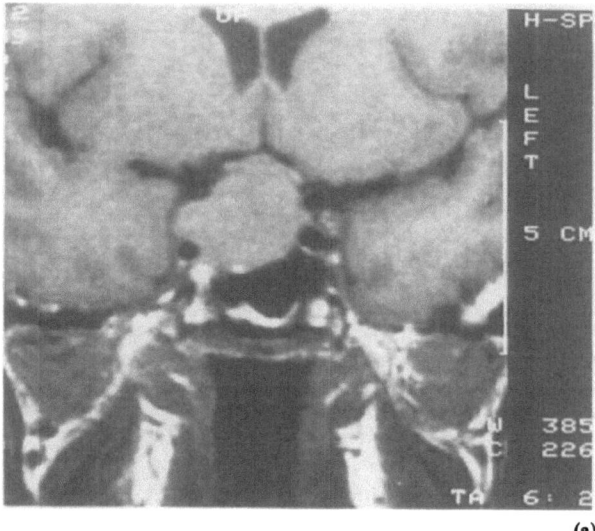 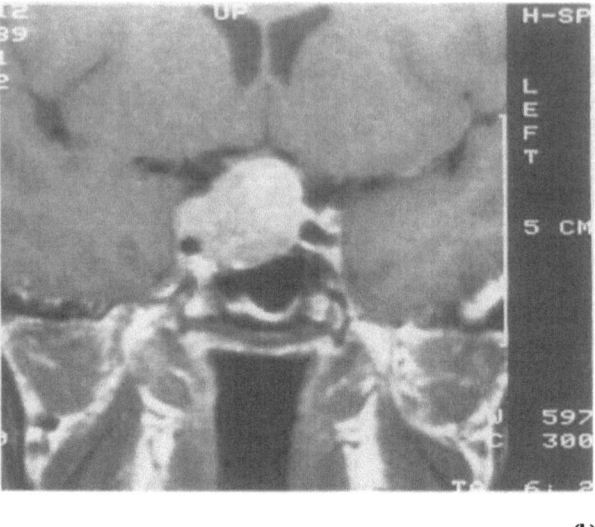

(a)   (b)

Fig. 2. Invasion of the right cavernous sinus with the tumour reaching the lateral wall of the cavernous sinus. On the left side no parasellar extension is present with all compartments of the cavernous venous plexus enhancing

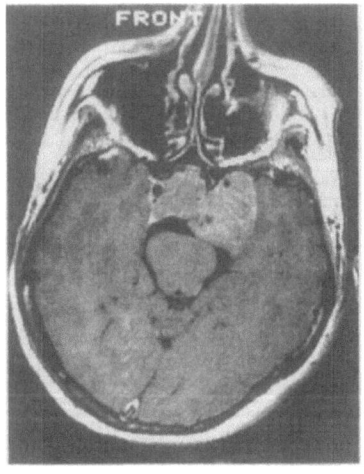

Fig. 3. Recurrent adenoma with total encasement of the left internal carotid artery and pronounced bulging of the lateral cavernous sinus wall, producing a cavernous sinus syndrome

displacement of the third ventricle (SS 3). In 8 cases, however, there was parasellar tumour growth without suprasellar extension (see also Table 1). In 6 cases tumour perforated the sella floor and appeared within the sphenoid sinus (Figs. 1 and 3).

Biological Results

In cases of the transsphenoidal approach histological investigation included immunohistology as well as investigation of dura biopsies taken from the sellar floor (Table 1). Growth rate of adenoma cells was measured by the monoclonal antibody KI-67 using the smear and frozen section technique as described previously[13].

The proliferation rate (KI 67 Labelling Index in %) in this group of 25 pituitary adenomas with parasellar extension ranged from 0.8% to 3.5% with a mean proliferation rate of 1.95% ($+/-0.85$; SD). When compared to non-invasive adenomas from our total series of 120 cases[10], pituitary adenomas infiltrating the space of the "cavernous sinus" showed a statistically significant higher proliferation rate ($p < 0,001$) as did those with histologically proven invasion of the dura of the sella floor-regardless of parasellar invasion.

Discussion

Parasellar extension of pituitary adenomas into the so called "cavernous sinus" first raises the question about the nature of the "cavernous sinus", which still is a subject of discussion[22,6,16,12,3]. According to our investigations[12] and those of others[22,16] the "cavernous sinus" is a venous plexus with different compartments. In relation to the internal carotid artery we usually can demonstrate a medial, lateral, superior and inferior compartment of veins within the space of the cavernous sinus. The medial wall of the space of the cavernous sinus is the only border not consisting of dura. This thin and fragile wall of the venous plexus is beyond the detection in MRI, so infiltration can not be demonstrated directly. Administration of Gd-DTPA can demonstrate the different compartments of the venous plexus, and is essential

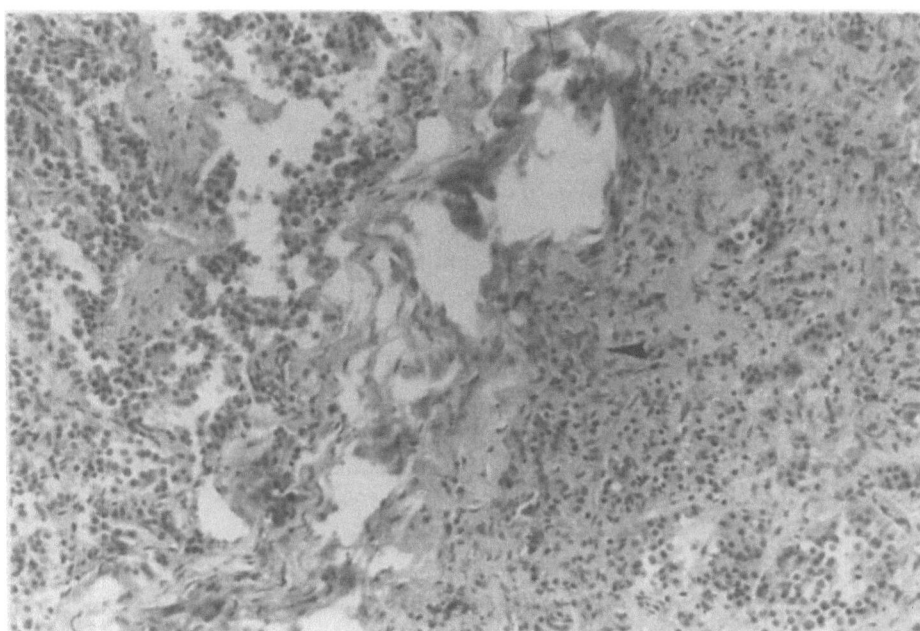

Fig. 4. Specimen of cavernous sinus (medial wall) infiltrated by pituitary adenoma. Groups of adenoma cells invading collagenous bundles (arrow). H&E, X 320 magnification

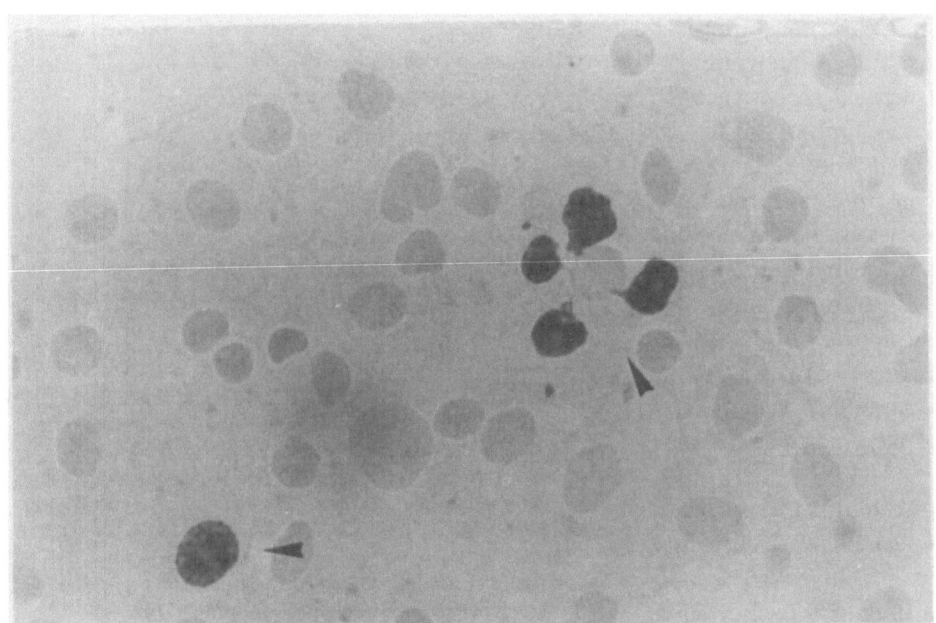

Fig. 5. MAb KI-67 positive cells (arrow) of a pituitary adenoma, smear preparation, X 730 magnification

for the demonstration of parasellar growth of pituitary adenomas. We could show that the use of unenhanced and enhanced MRI scans improves the delineation of the adenoma from the parasellar structures from 47% up to 91%[21]. Only encasement of the internal carotid artery has been regarded as a definitive sign of infiltration of the cavernous sinus when using unenhanced MRI alone[19].

Failing enhancement of different compartments of the cavernous venous plexus – in the absence of thrombosis – may speak for compression as well as for

invasion of the "cavernous sinus". Absent enhancement of the medial compartment alone, did not correlate with surgically observed infiltration. Whereas in all cases in which the adenoma surrounded the internal carotid artery completely or the adenoma reaches the lateral aspect of the artery, invasion was present. In our experience the critical area where cavernous sinus invasion becomes very likely, is the distance between the medial and the lateral aspects of the internal carotid artery. As the surgical observation is the criterion for proving invasion of the medial wall of the "cavernous sinus", the interpretation is dependent upon experience[18]. To be able to compare results between different groups a radiological criterion, which correlates with invasion, would be desireable.

Increasing surgical difficulties and increasing risk of damage to the internal carotid artery are encountered with adenomas which surround the artery in part or totally. This fact makes surgical cure unlikely[4]. We could achieve cure from hormonal hypersecretion in only 2 cases out of 15 hormonally active adenomas.

The transsphenoidal approach provides a safe and appropriate procedure even for adenomas with para-sellar extension[4,15,7]. We used this approach as the primary or only approach for 18 cases of adenomas with parasellar invasion with no mortality and with no additional morbidity.

The only death in this series was related to hypothalamic damage after transcranial resection of the largest tumour in this series.

If the adenoma bulges the lateral wall of the "cavernous sinus" a transcranial transcavernous approach provides as alternative route although rarely used for pituitary adenomas. Despite increasing experience[3,17], this approach through the lateral wall of the "cavernous sinus" carries the risk of cranial nerves damage.

Development of a cavernous sinus syndrome is a rare finding in pituitary adenomas even when reaching huge size. In most cases it is attributed to tumour apoplexy or haemorrhage. A cavernous sinus syndrome developed in 6% of adenomas with parasellar growth[4] and was present in two of our cases. In one case this was due to intra-tumourous haemorrhage and this was the case where the symptoms resolved completely.

Although benign in their histological appearance, pituitary adenomas can show signs of invasiveness into surrounding structures[23,19,20,8,9]. Invasiveness into the dura of the sella floor has been observed in up to 94% when this was investigated histologically[20]. Infiltration of the dura has been related to the immuno-histological findings[18] as well as to the size of the adenoma[20]. We found histological invasion of the sella floor in 66% of our cases without relation to tumour size or to immunhistology[13].

In contrast to conventional histological staining techniques, the monoclonal antibody KI-67 is capable of recognizing proliferating cell populations and can therefore be used to identify the proliferating cell pool of human tumours[5,14,13]. A statistically significant increase in the proliferation rate was found in invasive adenomas[13] but we could not find different growth rates with regard to hormone secretion, as did other authors[14].

In this group of 25 pituitary adenomas with surgically observed invasion of the "cavernous sinus" we found statistically significant higher proliferation rates ($p < 0.001$), when compared to our whole series[10]. This indicates a higher growth rate not only in adenomas infiltrating the dura but also when infiltration of the parasellar space was present. Invasion of the "cavernous sinus" without invasion of the dura of the sella floor was a rare finding in our series, present in 3 cases only.

Information of the biological behaviour of adenomas with invasive parasellar growth is of paramount importance, because surgical cure is far less likely compared to non-invasive adenomas and additional treatment is necessary to control the disease. Immuno-histological staining with the monoclonal antibody KI-67 for measuring the proliferation rate has been shown to be a reliable method to obtain this information.

References

1. Ahmadi J, North CM, Segall HD, Zee CS, Weiss MH (1985) Cavernous sinus invasion by pituitary adenomas. AJNR 6: 893–898
2. Daniels DL, Pech P, Mark L, Pojunas K, Williams AL, Haughton VM (1985) Magnetic resonance imaging of the cavernous sinus. AJNR 6: 186–192
3. Dolenc VV (1983) Direct microsurgical repair of intracavernous vascular lesions. J Neurosurg 58: 824–831
4. Fahlbusch R, Buchfelder M (1988) Transsphenoidal surgery of parasellar pituitary adenomas. Acta Neurochir (Wien) 92: 93–99
5. Gerdes J, Schwab U, Lemke H, Stein H (1983) Production of a mouse monoclonal antibody reactive with a human nuclear antigen associated with cell proliferation. Int J Cancer 31: 13–20
6. Harris FS, Rhoton AL (1976) Anatomy of the cavernous sinus, a microsurgical study. J Neurosurg 45: 169–180
7. Hashimoto N, Kikuchi H (1990) Transsphenoidal approach to infrasellar tumors involving the cavernous sinus. J Neurosurg 73: 513–517
8. Horvath E, Kovacs K, Killinger DW, Smyth HS, Platts ME, Singer W (1980) Silent corticotropic adenomas of the human pituitary gland. A histopathologic immunocytologic and ultrastructural study. Am J Pathol 98: 617–638
9. Horvath E, Kovacs K, Singer W, Ezrin C, Kerenyi A (1977) Acidophil stemcell adenoma of the human pituitary. Arch Pathol Lab Med 101: 594–599
10. Kitz K, Knosp E, Korn A, Koos WTH (1991) Proliferation-rate in 120 pituitary adenomas: Measurement by MAb Ki-67. Acta Neurochir (Wien) [Suppl] (this volume)
11. Knosp E, Mueller G, Perneczky A (1987 A) The blood supply of the cranial nerves in the lateral wall of the cavernous sinus. In: Dolenc VV (ed) The cavernous sinus. Springer, Wien New York, pp 67–80

12. Knosp E, Mueller G, Perneczky A (1987 B) Anatomical remarks on the fetal cavernous sinus and on the veins of the middle cranial fossa. In: Dolenc VV (ed) The cavernous sinus. Springer, Wien New York, pp 104–116

13. Knosp E, Kitz K, Perneczky A (1989) Proliferation activity in pituitary adenomas: Measurement by monoclonal antibody Ki-67. Neurosurgery 25: 927–930

14. Landolt AM, Shibata T, Kleihues P (1987) Growth rate of human pituitary adenomas. J Neurosurg 67: 803–806

15. Laws ER, Kern EB (1976) Complications of transsphenoidal surgery. Clin Neurosurg 23: 401–416

16. Parkinson D (1965) A surgical approach to the cavernous portion of the carotid artery: Anatomical studies and case report. J Neurosurg 23: 474–483

17. Perneczky A, Knosp E, Matula CH (1988) Cavernous sinus surgery. Approach through the lateral wall. Acta Neurochir (Wien) 92: 76–82

18. Scheithauer BW, Kovacs KT, Laws ER, Randall RV (1986) Pathology of invasive pituitary tumors with special reference to functional classification. J Neurosurg 65: 733–754

19. Scotti G, Yu CY, Dillon WP, Norman D, Colombo N, Newton TH, De Groot J, Wilson CB (1988) MR Imaging of cavernous sinus involvement by pituitary adenomas. AJNR 9: 657–664

20. Selman WR, Laws ER, Scheithauer BW, Carpenter SM (1986) The occurrence of dural invasion in pituitary adenoma. J Neurosurg 64: 402–408

21. Steiner E, Imhof H, Knosp E (1989) Gd-DTPA enhanced high resolution MR imaging of pituitary adenomas. Radiographics 4: 587–598

22. Taptas NJ (1982) The so called cavernous sinus: A review of the controversy and its implications for neurosurgeons. Neurosurg 11: 712–717

23. Wrightson PH (1978) Conservative removal of small pituitary tumours. Is it justified by the pathological findings? J Neurol Neurosurg Psychiatry 41: 283–289

Correspondence: E. Knosp, M.D., Department of Neurosurgery, Vienna Medical School, Währinger Gürtel 18–20, A-1090 Wien, Austria.

Acta Neurochirurgica, Suppl. 53, 72–76 (1991)
© by Springer-Verlag 1991

Long-term Follow-up Results in Hormonally Active Pituitary Adenomas After Primary Successful Transsphenoidal Surgery

M. Buchfelder, R. Fahlbusch, W. Schott, and J. Honegger

Neurochirurgische Klinik mit Poliklinik der Universität Erlangen-Nürnberg, Erlangen, Federal Republic of Germany

Summary

The long-term results of transsphenoidal surgery for hormonally active pituitary adenomas were assessed in 3 follow-up studies. Eight out of 50 patients with microprolactinomas developed a persisting postoperative re-increase of prolactin levels during an average follow-up period of 4.1 years. None of the 43 acromegalic patients who had achieved a suppression of growth hormone to below 2 ng/ml during an oral glucose load shortly after surgery relapsed. However, when the remission criterion was only based on basal growth hormone below 5 ng/ml 4 out of 61 patients showed a re-increase of growth hormone levels to persistently elevated values during an average follow-up period of 6.1 years. 14 out of 66 patients followed-up for an average of 8.2 years after successful primary microadenomectomy for Cushing's disease developed recurrent hypercortisolism as documented by an abnormal suppression of cortisol after oral low dose dexamethasone.

Keywords: Acromegaly; Cushing's disease; pituitary adenoma; prolactinoma; transsphenoidal surgery; long-term results.

Introduction

It is well established that transsphenoidal selective adenomectomy of hormone secreting pituitary adenomas is an efficient and safe method to rapidly correct the respective oversecretion. Since most of the follow-up studies reported to date were either performed on a limited number of patients or cover only a short observation period, we have reviewed our own data on prolactin- (PRL), growth hormone- (GH) and ACTH-secreting adenomas in a retrospective study. However, since there is variable terminology used in describing the outcome after therapy of a hormonally active adenoma, it is necessary to define a few terms which we have used[10]. We consider it essential that for the evaluation of long-term results after treatment of patients with hormonally active pituitary disease a differentiation is made between an immediate (acute) postoperative normalisation of elevated hormone levels

and a persistent hormonal oversecretion (Fig. 1). Even cases with amelioration of the hormone oversecretion should be regarded as patients still suffering from active disease, as long as the levels of the oversecreted hormone are not completely normalized. Spontaneous remissions, sometimes refered to as spontaneous "cures", may very rarely occur as a result of tumour infarction or haemorrhage. As opposed to a persistent normalisation of the hormone excess for years, real recurrences are defined as a relapse of the hormone excess following initial normalisation.

Patients and Methods

A non-consecutive series of patients with microprolactinomas, acromegaly or Cushing's disease has been chosen for this retrospective study. For every patient examined, the relevant hormone hyper-secretion (PRL, GH, ACTH) was acutely normalized following transsphenoidal microsurgical selective adenomectomy. Follow-up periods for patients with microprolactinomas (n = 50), acromegaly (n = 61) and Cushing's disease (n = 66) were 3.5–13 years (mean: 4.1 years), 3–14 years (mean: 6.1 years) and 5–14 years (mean: 8.2 years), respectively. The operations were carried out between 1971 and 1986. Postoperative activity of the disease was assessed clinically and biochemically. Prolactin (normal < 500 µU/ml;

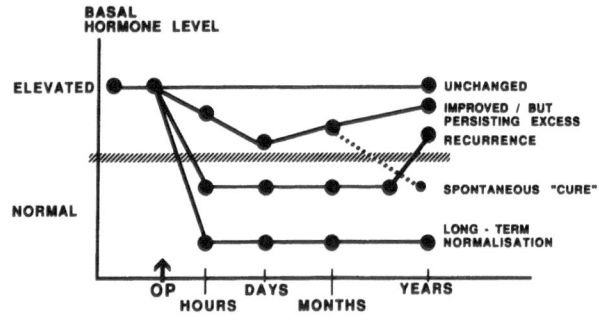

Fig. 1. Basic principles and definitions of operative results in hormonally active pituitary adenomas

kit: Behringwerke, Marburg, Germany), growth hormone (normal < 5 ng/ml; kit: Cis-Sorin, Saluggia, Italy) and cortisol levels (normal 10–25 µg/dl; kit: Abbott, Wiesbaden, Germany) were measured by commercially available radioimmunoassay kits. In addition, GH levels in acromegaly were measured during an oral glucose tolerance test (OGTT) after an overnight fast. A suppression to below 2 ng/ml at 60 minutes was regarded as normal. For Cushing's disease, cortisol levels before and after low dose dexamethasone were determined. For these latter studies, blood samples were drawn at 9 a.m. after the ingestion of 2 mg dexamethasone at 10 p.m. on the previous evening. A suppression of cortisol levels to below 2 µg/dl was regarded as a normal response.

Results

Prolactinomas

Out of 50 patients with microprolactinomas who achieved an acute normalisation of basal prolactin-levels one week after surgery, 8 developed recurrent hyperprolactinaemia. The rapid normalisation observed in these 8 patients was followed by a later re-increase of the hormone to persistently abnormal levels which occurred between 2 months and three years after surgery. Clinically, only 3 out of the 8 patients had a recurrence of galactorrhea and 2 were found to have anovulatory cycles. There was no neuroradiological evidence of recurrent tumour in any of these patients. Two patients became pregnant after the re-occurrence of hyperprolactinaemia. Their prolactin levels remained unchanged after delivery as compared to the pre-pregnancy levels. The course of prolactin levels and details of patient management are described in detail in another publication[4].

Acromegaly

Out of the 61 patients who had shown an acute normalisation of GH one week after surgery and who also had normal basal GH-levels three months after adenomectomy, basal GH-levels were found to be elevated above 5 ng/ml in four patients at the last follow-up visit (Fig. 2). The reincreases of GH occurred one to three years after surgery. These patients also had an abnormal GH response during OGTT and abnormal somatomedin C levels. However, when the normalisation criteria after surgery were based on a normal suppression of growth hormone to below 2 ng/ml during oral glucose tolerance testing, 60 minutes after glucose intake, none of the 43 patients in whom GH could readily be suppressed developed a repeatedly abnormal secretion dynamics of growth hormone (Fig. 3). None of the patients had clinical signs of active acromegaly at the last follow-up visit.

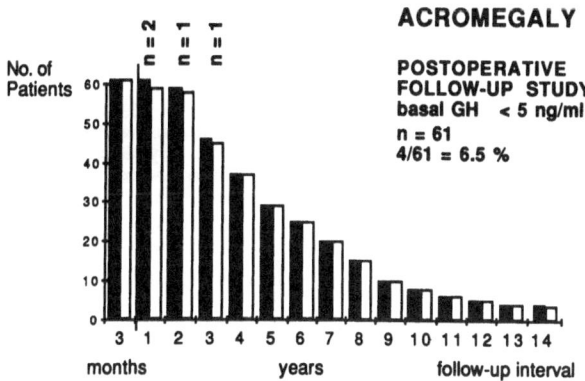

Fig. 2. Follow-up study of 61 acromegalic patients with basal GH-levels < 5 ng/ml 3 months after surgery

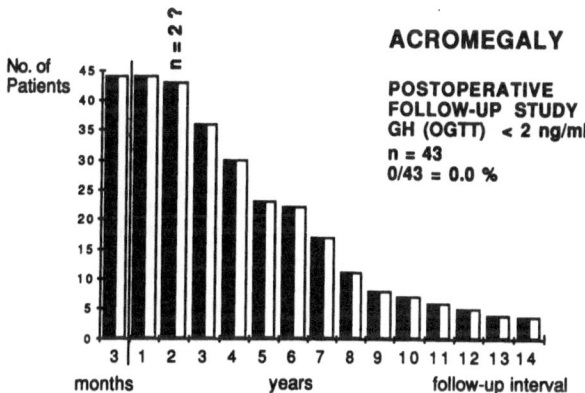

Fig. 3. Follow-up study of 43 acromegalic patients with suppressed GH-levels < 2 ng/ml during an OGTT 3 months after surgery

Two of the patients were, however, found to have a temporarily abnormal secretion pattern of GH during an OGTT and also abnormal somatomedin C levels, which remitted spontaneously and were not found to recur in later follow-up visits. Of the 23 patients who had a suppression of GH to below 1 ng/ml one week after surgery, all retained a similar suppression throughout the observation period. None of the patients had neuroradiological evidence of recurrent tumour.

Cushing's Disease

The figures in this report basically represent the follow-up data of our initial series of patients with Cushing's disease operated on between 1971 and 1984[9]. The initial remission rate was 76%. Only one patient was lost to follow-up. 4 patients died of other diseases or conditions associated with Cushing's disease within 5 years after surgery, but had no signs

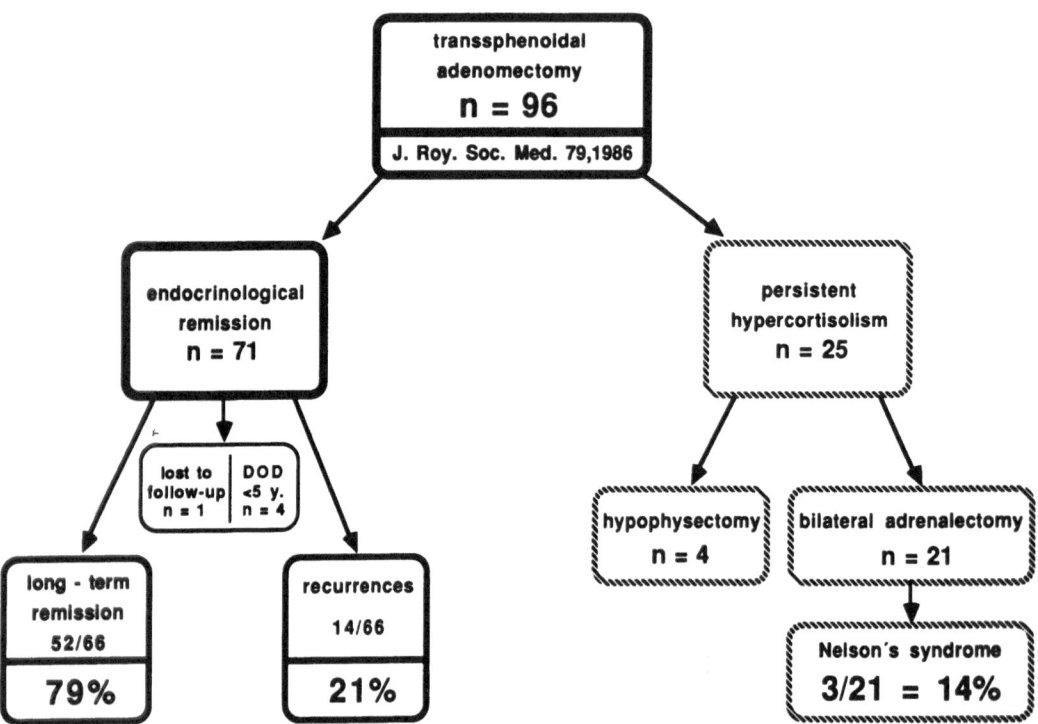

Fig. 4. Follow-up study of 71 patients with Cushing's disease who initially underwent a remission after transsphenoidal selective adenomectomy (long-term results of[9])

of recurrent hypercortisolism. Out of the remaining 66 patients followed-up after initially successful resection of an ACTH-secreting microadenoma, causing Cushing's disease (Fig. 4), 14 (21%) developed recurrent hypercortisolism. 52 of the 66 patients still do not exhibit clinical or biochemical signs of recurrent disease. 10 of them have now been followed-up for more than 10 years. The recurrences occurred as early as 1 year and at the latest 6.5 years after primary surgery. However, most of them were detected between 2 and 4 years after the operation. The clinical and endocrinological characteristics and management problems in the cases with recurrent hypercortisolism have been reported extensively elsewhere[5].

Discussion

An overview on the literature dealing with long term follow-up results of patients who underwent initially successful transsphenoidal surgery for *micro-prolactinomas* is shown in Table 1.

Whereas other authors report a similar recurrence rate as indicated by our results over a similar observation time, Serri *et al.*[24] have followed-up the patients operated on by Hardy for 6.2 years on average and found relapses in 12 out of 24 patients. Recurrent

hyperprolactinaemia frequently constitutes a laboratory diagnosis without any major clinical significance[4, 23]. By the time a relapse of prolactin levels to above the normal range occurs years after surgery, many patients would have already solved their problems of family planning. Furthermore, apart from promoting osteoporosis, mild hyperprolactinaemia itself usually does not seem to cause serious symptoms or morbidity.

An overview on the literature about long term follow-up of *acromegalic patients* (Table 2) shows that the oral glucose tolerance test seems to be one of the most reliable parameters. The present and other studies confirm that this test is a simple and cheap method to assess the activity of acromegaly in the long-term run, particularly when the suppressed GH level is measured at a single time point after a large dose of glucose. The authors have followed the suggestion of Quabbe *et al.*[20] and others and arbitrarily defined the upper limit of a normal suppressed level as 2 ng/ml. Recurrences are extremely rare once growth hormone levels can be suppressed to below this limit two to three months after surgery. Somatomedin-C- (Insulin-like growth factor I) levels seem to be almost as reliable[1, 14].

In long-term follow-up studies of patients operated

Table 1. *Recurrences After Transsphenoidal Surgery for Prolactinomas – a Survey of the Recent Literature*

Authors	Number of patients followed-up	Follow-up period mean (range) in years	Recurrence rate absolute (%)	Tumour type
Faglia et al. 1983[8]	39	3.5 (?–?)	6/39 (15%)	microadenomas
Serri et al.1983[24]	24	6.2 (5–10)	12/24 (50%)	microadenomas
Rodman et al. 1984[21]	29	4.2 (0.9–6.7)	5/29 (17%)	microadenomas
	5	3.4 (?–?)	1/5 (20%)	macroadenomas
Schlechte et al. 1986[23]	31	5.0 (5–5)	12/31 (39%)	micro- and macroadenomas
Maira et al. 1989[16]	73	? (1–8)	10/73 (14%)	micro- and macroadenomas
Ciccarelli et al. 1990[6]	22	6.5 (4–9)	8/22 (36%)	micro- and macroadenomas
This series	50	4.1 (3.3–13)	8/50 (16%)	microadenomas

Table 2. *Recurrences After Transsphenoidal Surgery for Acromegaly – a Survey of the Recent Literature*

Authors	Number of patients followed-up	Follow-up period mean (range) in years	Recurrence rate absolute (%)	Criteria of remission
Serri et al. 1985[25]	21	8.9 (5–11)	3/21 (14%)	basal GH < 5 ng/ml GH (OGTT) < 2.5 ng/ml
Roelfsema et al. 1985[22]	43	3.3 (0.5–7)	0/43 (0%)	basal GH < 5 mU/l GH (OGTT) ⩽ 2.5 mU/l
Arafah et al. 1987[1]	30	7.6 (?–?)	5/30 (16%)	basal GH < 5 ng/ml
	21	8.1 (?–?)	0/21 (0%)	GH (OGTT) < 2 ng/ml
Artia et al. 1988[2]	41	? (0.25–6.2)	2/41 (5%)	basal GH < 5 ng/ml abnormal GH (TRH/LRH)
	20	? (0.25–6.2)	0/20 (0%)	basal GH < 5 ng/ml normal GH (TRH/LRH)
Grisoli et al. 1988[11]	60	? (2–6)	6/60 (10%)	basal GH < 5 ng/ml normal GH (TRH/LRH)
Landolt et al. 1988[14]	169	4.1 (0.1–14)	4/169 (2%)	basal GH ⩽ 5 ng/ml or SmC ⩽ 300 ng/ml
Losa et al. 1989[15]	12	2.9 (0.5–3.8)	0/12 (0%)	GH (OGTT) < 1 ng/ml
This series	61	6.1 (1.5–14)	4/61 (7%)	basal GH < 5 ng/ml
	43	6.1 (1.5–14)	0/43 (0%)	GH (OGTT) < 2 ng/ml

on for *Cushing's disease* the recurrence rate (Table 3) ranges from 6%[17] to 21% (our data). It should, however, be noted that the length of follow-up periods varies considerably and that different criteria were used to document persistent normalisation or recurrent disease. Furthermore different surgical procedures were carried out, ranging from strict selective adenomectomy to total hypophysectomy. Surgical pathology clearly demonstrates that an extraglandular extension of the adenoma found at primary surgery constitutes a major risk factor for a later recurrence[5,17]. Reoperations demonstrated that the recurrent tumours were frequently situated in the same or adjacent to the original location[5,18]. One of the endocrinological risk factors was an early eucortisolism after primary surgery, i.e. the patients do not require hydrocortisone replacement therapy and correspondingly show an ACTH and cortisol increase soon after surgery when stimulation tests with CRH are carried out[5,12]. The authors believe that the repeated determination of the suppressibility of cortisol following a low dose of dexamethasone is a very sensitive tool for the early detection of recurrences of Cushing's disease. Measurement of free urinary cortisol offers an alternative effective method. There was no neuroradiological evidence of residual tumour tissue after surgery in any of the cases described in this report. We thus feel able to exclude a case that parallels the one described by Wrightson et al.[26] in whom persisting tumour tissue was found at autopsy although endocrinological postoperative testing had revealed a normal growth hormone secretion pattern.

Table 3. *Recurrences After Transsphenoidal Surgery for Cushing's Disease – a Survey of the Recent Literature*

Authors	Number of patients followed-up	Follow-up period mean (range) in years	Recurrence rate absolute (%)	Operative procedure
Hardy 1982[13]	63	1.75 (?–?)	2/63 (3%)	selective adenomectomy, partial or total hypophysectomy
Nakane et al. 1987[18]	86	3.2 (?–?)	8/86 (9%)	selective adenomectomy
Derome et al. 1988[7]	124	3.8 (0.5–17)	19/124 (15%)	selective adenomectomy
Guilhaume et al. 1988[12]	42	2.0 (0.5–7)	6/42 (14%)	selective adenomectomy
Mampalam et al. 1988[17]	141	3.9 (?–?)	8/141 (6%)	selective adenomectomy
Pieters et al. 1989[19]	16	4.0 (1.5–7.5)	4/16 (25%)	selective adenomectomy
This series	66	8.2 (5–14)	14/66 (21%)	selective adenomectomy

References

1. Arafah BM, Rosenzweig JL, Fenstermaker R, et al (1987) Value of growth hormone dynamics and somatomedin C (insulin-like growth factor I) levels in predicting the long-term benefit after transsphenoidal surgery for acromegaly. J Lab Clin Med 109: 346–354
2. Artia N, Mori S, Saitoh Y, et al (1988) Transsphenoidal surgery for acromegaly – Follow-up results. In: Landolt AM, et al (eds) Progress in pituitary adenoma research. Pergamon Press, London, pp 265–266
3. Bertrand G, Tolis G, Montes J (1983) Immediate and long-term results of transsphenoidal microsurgical resection of prolactinomas in 92 patients. In: Tolis G, et al (eds) Prolactin and Prolactinomas. Raven Press, New York, pp 441–452
4. Buchfelder M, Lierheimer A, Schrell U, et al (1985) Recurrence of hyperprolactinaemia detected in long-term follow-up of surgically normalized microprolactinomas. In: Auer LM, et al (eds) Prolactinomas. De Gruyter, Berlin New York, pp 183–187
5. Buchfelder M, Fahlbusch R (1990) Recurrences in Cushing's disease – prediction and prevention? In: Lüdecke DK, et al (eds) ACTH, Cushing's syndrome, and other hypercortisolaemic states. Raven Press, New York, pp 281–288
6. Ciccarelli E, Ghigo E, Miola C, et al (1990) Long-term follow-up of 'cured' prolactinoma patients after successful adenomectomy. Clin Endocrinol 32: 583–592
7. Derome PJ, Delalande O, Visot A, et al (1988) Short and long term results after transsphenoidal surgery for Cushing's disease; incidence of recurrences. In: Landolt AM, et al (eds) Progress in pituitary adenoma research. Pergamon Press, London, pp 375–379
8. Faglia G, Moriondo P, Travaglini P, et al (1983) Influence of previous bromocriptine therapy on surgery for microprolactinomas. Lancet I: 133
9. Fahlbusch R, Buchfelder M, Müller OA (1986) Transsphenoidal surgery for Cushing's disease. J Roy Soc Med 79: 262–269
10. Fahlbusch R, Buchfelder M, Schrell U, et al (1988) Recurrences in hormonally active pituitary adenomas. In: Shizume K, et al (eds) Recent issues on pituitary adenomas. Sandoz Japan, Tokyo, pp 20–28
11. Grisoli F, Leclercq T, Jaquet P, et al (1985) Transsphenoidal surgery for acromegaly – Long-term results in 100 patients. Surg Neurol 23: 513–519
12. Guilhaume B, Bertagna X, Thomsen M, et al (1988) Transsphenoidal surgery for the treatment of Cushing's disease: results in 64 patients and long term follow-up studies. J Clin Endocrinol Metab 66: 1056–1064
13. Hardy J (1982) Cushing's disease: 50 years later. Can J Neurol Sci 9: 375–380
14. Landolt AM, Illig R, Zapf J (1988) Surgical treatment of acromegaly. In: Lamberts SWJ (ed) Sandostatin in the treatment of acromegaly. Springer, Berlin Heidelberg New York, pp 23–35
15. Losa M, Oeckler R, Schopohl J, et al (1989) Evaluation of selective transsphenoidal adenomectomy by endocrinological testing and somatomedin-C measurements in acromegaly. J Neurosurg 70: 561–567
16. Maira G, Anile C, De Marinis L, et al (1989) Prolactin-secreting adenomas: surgical results and long-term follow-up. Neurosurgery 24: 736–743
17. Mampalam TJ, Tyrrell JB, Wilson CB, et al (1988) Transsphenoidal microsurgery for Cushing's disease. Ann Int Med 109: 487–493
18. Nakane T, Kuwayama A, Watanabe M, et al (1987) Long term results of transsphenoidal adenomectomy in patients with Cushing's disease. Neurosurgery 21: 218–222
19. Pieters GFFM, Hermus ARMM, Meijer E, et al (1989) Predictive factors for initial cure and relapse rate after pituitary surgery for Cushing's disease. J Clin Endocrinol Metab 69: 1122–1126
20. Quabbe HJ (1982) Treatment of acromegaly by transsphenoidal operation, 90-yttrium implantation and bromocriptine: Results in 230 patients. Clin Endocrinol 16: 107–119
21. Rodman EF, Molitch ME, Post KD, et al (1984) Long-term follow-up of transsphenoidal selective adenomectomy for prolactinoma. JAMA 252: 921–924
22. Roelfsema F, van Dulken H, Frölich M (1985) Long-term results of transsphenoidal pituitary microsurgery in 60 acromegalic patients. Clin Endocrinol 23: 555–565
23. Schlechte JA, Sherman BM, Chapler FK, et al (1986) Long term follow-up of women with surgically treated prolactin-secreting pituitary tumors. J Clin Endocrinol Metab 62: 1296–1301
24. Serri O, Rasio E, Beauregard H, et al (1983) Recurrence of hyperprolactinaemia after selective transsphenoidal adenomectomy in women with prolactinoma. N Engl J Med 309: 280–283
25. Serri O, Somma M, Comtois R, et al (1985) Acromegaly: Biochemical assessment of cure after long term follow-up of transsphenoidal selective adenomectomy. J Clin Endocrinol Metab 61: 1185–1189
26. Wrightson P, Holdaway IM, Synek BJL (1984) Criteria for cure in acromegaly: report of a case apparently cured in which persisting tumor was found at autopsy. Neurosurgery 14: 750–755

Correspondence: Dr. med. M. Buchfelder, Neurochirurgische Klinik mit Poliklinik der Universität Erlangen-Nürnberg, Schwabachanlage 6, D-W-8520 Erlangen, Federal Republic of Germany.

Acta Neurochirurgica, Suppl. 53, 77–88 (1991)
© by Springer-Verlag 1991

Surgical Strategies and Technical Methodologies in Optimal Management of Craniopharyngioma and Masses Affecting the Third Ventricular Chamber

M. L. J. Apuzzo, M. L. Levy, and **H. Tung**

Department of Neurological Surgery, University of Southern California School of Medicine, Los Angeles, California, U.S.A.

Summary

Management of craniopharyngiomas and masses affecting the third ventricular chamber represents one of the most challenging problems confronting contemporary neurological surgeons. Given the devastating sequelae of surgical complications involved in approaches to the deep cerebral midline, surgical management requires a combination of sophisticated imaging, diagnostic pathology and surgical technique including ventricular microsurgery and stereotaxy and its attendant refinements. Surgical and nonsurgical management is based upon the structural presentation of these masses as defined by detailed imaging studies. Operative objectives include histological definition, maximally feasible excision, cerebral spinal fluid diversion and relief of neurologic deficits created by masses affecting the third venticular chamber.

Keywords: Surgical strategy; operative technique; craniopharyngioma; colloid cyst; Foramen Monroi; third ventricle.

Introduction

The topic of deep cerebral midline masses and their management presents the surgeon with a multitude of difficulties and often taxes the intellectual and technical resources of contemporary neurological surgeons[2]. However, in consideration of the region and the possibilities for pathological involvements it is imperative that the managing surgeon has resources of absolutely contemporary imaging and pathological diagnostic methods at his disposal and that he personally possesses experience in contemporary techniques which include optimally not only ventricular microsurgery, but also stereotaxy and its attendant refinements. This discussion will present an overview of these methods develop a concept of their strategic application to craniopharyngiomas and other masses affecting the third ventricular chamber.

Pathology: The Abnormal Structural Substrate

In spite of a diverse spectrum of histological processes, the structural presentation of masses affecting the anterior and mid third ventricular region may be divided into three major groups with secondary divisions[12]. Development of this classification is pertinent to the selection of the appropriate surgical corridor for excision and direction of strategies for alternative management.

A. Extraaxial Intraventricular

These lesions are histologically benign masses with minimal areas of origin and adherence to elements of the ventricular walls. Microscopic surgical planes are, in general, well-defined. This category consists of lesions of developmental, neoplastic, vascular and infections etiologies and includes colloid cysts, craniopharyngiomas, epidermoids, dermoids, teratomas, papillomas, cystercercosis cysts, ependymal cysts, granuloma, and arteriovenous malformations.

B. Intraaxial with Ventricular Component

These lesions have origin within or neural or supportive elements adjacent to the ventricle with concomitant mass producing ventricular compression or an exophytic component growing primarily into the ventricular cavity. Within this group are lesions which have extended to the region by local metastasis or by remote metastasis. Examples of the group include the spectrum of glial tumors which may affect the thalamus, hypothalmus, or optic structures, medulloblastomas and germinomas.

C. Basal

These lesions have origin from structures within the skull or brain bases and extend superiorly to involve the third ventricular cavity. These are most commonly histologically benign, potentially excisable, lesions with various extents of origin and involvement of the basal structures. Such lesions are, in general, developmental, neoplastic, vascular, or infectious in origin and include pituitary adenomas, craniopharyngiomas, chordomas, epidermoids, meningiomas, germinomas, arachnoid cysts, cystcercosis cysts, and aneurysms.

It is important to consider that these processes may be secondarily subdivided into lesions which elevate the third ventricular floor and disrupt the third ventricular floor in their evolution. Those lesions which disrupt the third ventricular floor are clearly visualized through the foramen of Monro.

Operative Objectives

With recognition and imaging definition of such a structural process the surgeon must direct his efforts to achieve four major goals:

1. Histological definition of the process.
2. Maximally feasible excision of the lesion.
3. Relief of alterations in cerebrospinal fluid dynamics.
4. Relief of local signs and symptoms attendant to regional mass.

General Technical Principles of Transcranial Approaches to the Third Ventricle

The overlying objectives in surgery of this region relate to obtaining maximal exposure and intraoperative flexibility for lesion access and manipulation. These objectives are to be obtained with minimal manipulation, injury or sacrifice of normal neural and vascular structures. Consideration of a number of principles is essential for a satisfactory outcome:

1. *Corridor Selection.* Multiple alternatives are available for access of the third ventricular chamber. However, for an individual lesion usually one corridor offers optimal exposure and maximal intraoperative flexibility. Selection of the corridor is dependent upon *adequate structural definition on imaging studies* as well

as possibly angiographic assessment. Proper selection of the operative corridor will minimize the "bottom line" neural manipulation, injury or sacrifice.

2. *Craniotomy Flap Position.* The craniotomy flap position should approximate skull base or midline to *minimize brain retraction and maximize exposure corridors.* Ventricular or spinal drainage as well as osmotic agents should be employed to reduce the mass of retracted tissues and need for excessive retractor pressure. Only self-retaining retractor systems should be employed.

3. *Incision of Neural Structures.* In view of the fact that the third ventricular chamber can be reached only with neural transit, neural incision is frequently required. The incision which is required in the lamina terminalis corpus callosum, or forniceal raphe should be minimized within limits of safe or adequate exposure.

4. *Venous Preservation.* The number of veins which are sacrificed during transit and at the site of pathology should be minimized. This principle applies to both parasaggital veins and veins of the galenic and paraventricular systems. Techniques of alternate routes of access as well as displacement should be employed prior to sacrifice. Cortical injury and deep venous thrombosis are a potential cause of major neurological deficit.

5. *Arterial Preservation.* All arterial structures in the region of a mass displacement should be preserved. Vessels should be displaced from the tumour capsule. Numerous important arteries are encountered in removing tumors of the third ventricle. The posterior circle of Willis and basilar apex appear below the floor. Perforating branches of the anterior circle are intimately associated with the anterior wall. The posterior cerebral, pericallosal, superior cerebellar and choroidal arteries are adjacent to the posterior wall. Both anterior and posterior cerebral arteries supply the roof. The internal carotid, anterior choroidal, anterior communicating and posterior communicating arteries supply perforating branches to the walls. Disorders of memory, personality and consciousness are the cost of otherwise technically adequate procedures in the face of minimal vascular injury or sacrifice.

6. *Lesion Management.* Every effort should be made to minimize trauma and transmission of pressure to normal structures in the region of pathology. This may be achieved not only by obtaining adequate and comfortable exposure, but also by utilizing careful principles of lesion excision. *Mass presence should be*

minimized initially by internal decompression. Initially, aspiration should be undertaken. Next the capsule should be opened, a biopsy obtained, and intracapsular removal completed at high-power magnification by microsurgical tech-nique with or without microsurgical adjuvants. *Only after this is completed should an effort be made to separate the capsule from the neural and vascular structures.* With decompression, a combination of brain pulsation, microirrigation, and microdissection most often will produce satisfactory dissection planes.

Operative Options

A number of operative techniques are available and of safe and proven value. Each must be performed appropriately from the technical standpoint and applied properly to the structural and histological substrate is optimization of result is to be realized[4].

Major operative options include:

I craniotomy by either basal, superior, or combined approaches
II imaging guidance stereotaxy
III cerebral spinal fluid diversion.

I. Craniotomy

A. Basal

Masses with basal components and origin are appropriately exposed by a number of alternative routes. All are essentially extraaxial corridors.

1. Transsphenoidal

This approach offers excellent and rapid access to the sella. In the event that this structure is enlarged by mass even greater suprasellar access is available in vectors that are in the line of sellar distension. Visual system and third ventricular region masses are readily decompressed, particularly if lesions are cystic or soft.

Lesion excision and surgical expectations are limited in the event that angular frontal or temporal masses exist, or when masses are solid in texture. In addition, excision of dense capsular components which may be adherent to vascular and neural structures are rarely complete and undertaken with risk. Therefore, tumor excision is generally limited to removal of tissue within the tumor capsule, permitting the capsule to retract from neural and vascular elements.

A number of potential complications must be considered with a transsphenoidal exposure:

a. stretch injury of infraorbital nerve, secondary to sublabial manipulation and speculum insertion,
b. olfactory injury with misdirection of superior dissection,
c. optic nerve injury with optic foramen fracture secondary to forceful retractor opening,
d. multiple cranial nerve (optic, oculomotor, trochlear trigeminal, abducers) and carotid artery injury with cavernous sinus trauma,
e. carotid, trigeminal, optic nerve injury with forced retractor opening and forceful manipulation in the sphenoid sinus,
f. optic nerve chiasmal, circle of Willis and hypothalamic injury with excessive manipulation during tumor excision, and
g. cerebrospinal fluid fistula with arachnoid disruption.

2. Transcranial

a. Subfrontal. Basal midline tumors with suprasellar extension may be readily approached by the subfrontal route either unilaterally or bilaterally. This approach may be undertaken along midline or oblique frontal corridors. With the midline corridor, angulation for visualization of the optic nerves and carotid arteries is perhaps the best in terms of general anatomical comprehension. The surgeon can work between the optic nerves and easily identify the pituitary stalk and carotid arteries. The arachnoid of the anterior chiasmatic cistern is opened. Retraction and manipulation of the optic nerves and chiasm is minimized. Following internal decompression of the mass by initial techniques of needle aspiration and microsurgical reduction of the interior of the mass, microdissection of the capsule is undertaken.

b. Pterional. The pterional approach offers the shortest transit from scalp to sella as well as good anterolateral visualization of the ipsilateral carotid-neurovisual pathway. With opening of the medial Sylvian fissure, and the employment of the *optico-carotid* and *lateral carotid* corridors *visualization of the retrosella space* is realized. Such exposures are effective in suprasellar tumors where the chiasm is prefixed. The opticocarotid corridor is utilized in the event that asymetrical superolateral extension of the mass distends the interval between the optic nerve and carotid artery, particularly if the chiasm appears prefixed. Care must be taken to preserve perforating branches from the internal carotid artery to the visual system.

In employing this exposure it must be considered that the opposite carotid artery and optic nerve are not fully visualized initially. Tumor removal is often difficult because of the obstructing disposition of major neural and vascular structures with various nerves and arteries positioned at a peculiar angle that is difficult to conceptualize without considerable experience.

c. Subtemporal. The subtemporal corridor offers optimal exposure for lesions in the posterior, parasella, dorsum sella and posterior perforated space region. If sufficient mass is present, exposure of such a lesion may be gained via the pterional opticocarotid approach. However, direct access for posterior suprasella lesions is optimized subtemporally. The major consideration with this approach is the *posterior communicating artery* with its perforating branches to the region. In addition, medial angulation of the tentorium may limit exposure. This approach requires extensive temporal retraction and provides poor visualization of structures in the prepontine cistern. The surgeon may visualize the ipsilateral posterior cerebral and superior cerebellar arteries, but the contralateral structures are not fully visualized. In addition, the ipsilateral third and fourth nerves are in the line of the approach.

All of the basal approaches, although providing access to basal components of an offending mass, provide limited superior access or visualization.

B. Superior

These approaches offer exposure of the third ventricle via superior entry through the trunk of the corpus callosum or the frontal cortex. These corridors are employed for exposure and excision of intraventricular lesions or intraventricular components of basal lesions that are not accessible from a basilar approach.

1. Transcortical

Originally described by Walter Dandy, this approach classically is undertaken through the right middle frontal gyrus and is optimally employed in the presence of ventriculomegaly which enhances exposure without the need for excessive brain excision,

retraction, or manipulation. It offers excellent visualization of the ipsilateral foramen of Monro with a satisfactory visual alignment for lesions of the mid and mid anterior sections of the third ventricular chamber. It provides the optimum angulation for employment of the *subchoroidal exposure*, but a less satisfactory visual alignment for the interforniceal maneuver or visualization of the contralateral foramen. Aside from the sacrifice of neural tissue required, it is considered to have a higher incidence of seizure complications than the transcallosal exposure. Guidance during the pial-ependymal transit may be enhanced expedited by employing real time ultrasonography.

2. Transcallosal

The transcallosal corridor, gained by interhemispheric exposure of the body of the corpus callosum in the pericoronal region followed by a 2–3 cm incision, offers the major advantages of constant anatomy, shorter transit to the diencephalic roof and flexibility of exploration within the *entire third ventricular* cavity through the optimum access provided by interforniceal exposure simultaneously with visualization of both foramen of Monro. There is no disruption of hemispheric tissue and, importantly, *ventricular size is irrelevant*.

Section of the collosal trunk has been extensively evaluated and does not carry a physiological cost which is currently considered to be measurable or recognizable (7). However, the interhemispheric exposure carries the risk of contralateral hemiparesis. The incidence of such a complication may be reduced by utilization of preoperative angiography as an adjunct to operative planning and refinement of operative technique. Mutism, a rare complication, may be related to bilateral cingulate retraction.

As noted, both superior approaches offer exposure of the foramen of Monroe and diencephalic roof with optimal maneuvers for third ventricular entry including (1) transforamenal, (2) transforamenal with ipsilateral forniceal column section, (3) subchoroidal visualization and (4) interforniceal visualization.

The goal of surgery is total excision with minimal trauma to adjacent neural tissues. The amount of exposure required to accomplish this end will vary with the nature of the pathological process and the skill and experience of the operator. Requirements for exposure are variable, but knowledge and familiarity with each method of exposure of the third ventricular chamber is imperative in order to expand the spectrum of options and thus safety of the operative endeavor.

Each of these methods and options carries certain advantages and disadvantages.

a. Transforamenal Visualization. Transforamenal exposure may be optimized by the presence of a large lesion which distends the foramen, although this is not a dependable feature of third ventricular lesions. In such a case, in the event that the angulation of exposure is satisfactory, excision may be accomplished with minimal midline manipulation. This is dependant in all cases on the texture of the individual lesion and its resistance to methods of excision initiated by the operator. Often, especially in the presence of a firm lesion, inadequate access of the posterior and anterior superior component necessitates further exposure maneuvers.

b. Transforamenal Exposure With Unilateral Section of the Ipsilateral Column of the Fornix. This method of enlargement of the area of exposure has been advocated in the past. However, it is not recommended as other maneuvers afford greater exposure without the sacrifice of neural elements.

c. Subchoroidal Visualization. This technique, which takes advantages of the natural plane at the region of the lamina affixa, allows mobilization of both forniceal bodies from ipsilateral to medial. This approach provides access to the central portion of the ventricle by the latter displacement via the velum interposition. It is suited for lesions in the superior half of the third ventricle adjacent to the roof and posterior to the foramen. This exposure is expanded to directly include the foramen of Monro by sacrifice of the thalamostriate vein at the foramen – a maneuver which has not been recognized to initiate complicating events. This tolerance confirms the capacity of collateral connections to shunt blood from the deep medullary to the superficial subependymal venous systems. These collaterals are apparent in certain pathological processes. In patients with a direct lateral tributary to the internal cerebral vein both the septal and thalamostriate vein may be safely sacrificed. The region drained by the direct lateral veins is similar to the thalamostriate vein; both receive transverse caudate tributaries, although the direct lateral vein enters the internal cerebral vein one to two cm posterior to the thalamostriate. With the presence of mass and inadequate foramen exposure, this maneuver will often provide satisfactory exposure without active retraction of the fornix. Lines of visualization for this maneuver are optimized by the *transcortical approach.* In our

experience the transcallosal approach may be employed as an initial stage prior to this maneuver, but it is somewhat less satisfactory. A drawback of this technique is that if a lesion is small or moderately sized, *retraction of the thalamus may be required* to gain adequate working visualization with the transcortical corridor.

d. Interforniceal Visualization. This maneuver takes advantage of a natural plane of division between the columns and body of the fornices which opens into the diencephalic roof. This division is occasionally apparent with biventricular exposure in the presence of a mass and is clearly evident in the presence of a cavum septum pellucidum or septal leafs. It is readily defined by the passage of a microinstrument at the line of the septal insertion in the presence of a mass. When combined with the transcallosal approach this maneuver affords complete exposure of the third ventricular chamber and midline basal structures. In the presence of a significant mass active retraction is not required; the internal cerebral veins are displaced by the mass or may be retracted for inferior or posterior visualization as required. This maneuver is undertaken only if transforamenal exposure is inadequate or if manipulation seems excessive. This exposure with bilateral foramenal exposure as afforded by the transcallosal technique provides the most extensive exposure of the third ventricular chamber.

Although a number of problems related to the hypothalamic region and its elegant functional components are possible, *the major complication experienced with micromanipulation of the midline diencephalic structures is transient memory loss. This problem is observed with each of the above techniques and is generally transient. It is considered to be related to direct and transmitted trauma to the deep midline and paramedian structures.*

C. Combined

It is important to appreciate that a single corridor is occasionally inadequate in terms of exposure for satisfactory safe excision of basal masses with simultaneous third ventricular involvement. In such cases consideration must be given to an approach which combines features of both basal and superior exposures.

II. Imaging Guidance Stereotaxy

The combination of principles of stereotaxy, radiographic imaging techniques and microinstrumentation has added a new and vital dimension to the management of intracranial mass lesions. The deep midline structures of the third venticular region are particularly accessible by this approach with a precision and inherent safety that has not been available in the past[3,10].

A number of stereotactic devices that provide capability for translation of imaging data in a rapid and useful fashion to the operating room are currently commercially available. Our experience with the Brown-Roberts-Wells System (BRW) and Cosman-Roberts-Wells System (CRW) at the University of Southern California Medical Center Hospitals in over 3,500 procedures attests to the value, safety and flexibility of such systems with appropriate support that is a resource in major medical centers.

Access to the target point is achieved readily, rapidly and safely with local anesthesia and an anesthesiologist standing by in all but selected pediatric patients where general anesthesia is required. Access of the target point is usually attained within sixty minutes from the time of initiation of the procedure with all trajectory settings and target locales verified extracranially on a phantom simulator.

Multiple microinstrumentation capabilities at the target point allows for:

1. histological and microbiological assay
2. cyst and abscess aspiration
3. installation of permanent or temporary drainage conduits
4. point source or colloid based brachytherapy (or other methods of intralesional therapy)
5. cerebroscopy and ventriculoscopy with biopsy, aspiration or excision

Ventriculoscopy is performed with local anesthesia and standby. An imaging based *target* is selected at the right foramen of Monroe for cystic lesions presenting in the anterior component of the chamber. An *entry point* is centered one centimeter anterior to the coronal suture and lateral to the pupillary line. An 18 mm burr hole is prepared and after cruciate opening of the dura a 1 cm cortical window is designed at the point of entry of the ventriculoscope sheath. We have employed a 6.2 mm endoscope sheath with a blunt obturator which is introduced to the target. With removal of the obturator an angled ventriculoscope is introduced which allows for capabilities of visualization, irrigation (Ringers lactate solution), aspiration and introduction of instrumentation for biopsy, cyst perforation and aspiration, or quartz

fiber for conduction of Argon Laser energy. The sheath is introduced through a rigid bushing directed by the arc guidance component of the BRW or CRW Systems with precise placement to the foramen. Minor adjustments and changes in angulation may be made by adjustment of four angulation settings on the arc which allow infinite degrees of motion.

At the University of Southern California Medical Center Hospitals histological verification of a process was attained in over 95% of cases, and realization of objectives of a procedure was achieved in over 98%. These objectives included biopsy, biopsy with culture, biopsy with aspiration, biopsy with installation of Rickham drainage systems, point source or colloid brachytherapy, endoscopic visualization with biopsy and endoscopic excision. Operative morbidity was less than 0.1%, while only one death occurred in this series. Craniotomy was indicated or ultimately required in less than 10% of those undergoing the initial stereotactic procedure.

These methods are particularly valuable in the assessment, management, and logical development of treatment plans in the individuals with lesions affecting the third ventricular chamber. They should be considered part of the management armamentarium for the following reasons:

1. The histological nature of intraaxial lesions may be rapidly and safely assessed, often circumventing the need for craniotomy.
2. Cystic lesions of basal or intraaxial origin may be drained with precise control with permanent conduits placed for later treatment with colloid brachytherapy or other intralesional methods.
3. Intraventricular cystic lesions may be aspirated under endoscopic visualization (colloid cyst) or totally excised (cysticercosis cyst).
4. Basal lesions with superior extension, to or above the foramen of Monroe, may be evaluated by ventriculoscopy to assess disruption of the hypothalamic floor prior to developing a primary surgical strategy.
5. Third ventriculostomy may be performed in cases of aqueductal or fourth ventricular outlet, atresia or stenosis.

III. Cerebral Spinal Fluid Diversion

Biventricular shunting offers a method of management for lateral ventriculomegaly and its attendant symptomatology secondary to bilateral foramen of Monroe obstruction. At times third ventricular masses permit communication between the lateral ventricles via the formina-anterior third ventricular complex. This may be indicated on imaging studies or be established by ventriculostomy followed by metrizamide ventriculography. Internalized *ventriculoperitoneal* or *jugular shunting* is occasionally required after direct management of third ventricular masses. At craniotomy, *third ventriculostomy* is accomplished with translamina terminalis exposures with lesion excision or perforation of the region of the tuber cinereum. Silastic conduits may be established from the prepontine cistern through the ventricle and midline corridor 'to a subgaleally placed Rickham reservoir. Internal measures of fluid diversion can be judged competent only by close observation of the patient with ICP monitoring over a 48–72 hour period, followed by frequent clinical and radiographic assessment.

Fenestration of the septum pellucidum is advisable with all direct third ventricular exploration to preclude the need for bilateral shunting procedures.

Memory

In the microsurgical era, surgery of the third ventricle with associated manipulation of midline basal cerebral structures is often attended by postoperative manifestations of an amnestic syndrome[6,11]. Fortunately this complication is usually transient (days to several weeks duration). This striking complication is observed in what is, in most cases an otherwise functionally intact patient, generating considerable concern and providing a major obstruction to optimal patient performance. The *fornix*, the major interconnecting limbic pathway and major component of the diencephalic roof is by "tradition" considered to be the primary focus of neural injury in such cases. However, the substance of this belief may be challenged. There is no agreement in the literature whether or not fornix integrity is required for normal memory. Although this structure represents a major limbic pathway, significant comparable fiber bundles would remain intact following isolated forniceal injury. Importantly, nearly all hippocampal connections with the associated cortices would be structurally patent. More logically, current data would appear to indicate that *diffuse multifocal midline injury to a number of areas concerned with the memory process are collectively required*. These probably include (1) basal forebrain nuclei, (2) thalamic nuclei and the (3) inferior thalamic peduncle.

Craniopharyngioma

Surgical Pathology

Although comprising between 1 and 4% of all primary intracranial neoplasms, this histological entity represents one of the more common surgical problems in the third ventricular region. Great variability in size is evident, with components of the lesions often involving the sella, suprasella and third ventricular compartments with combinations of cystic and solid components. As craniopharyngiomas are classically considered to arise from rests of buccal epitheleum which accompany migration of Rathke's pouch from the premature stomadeum upward to join the infundibulum and form the pituitary gland and its stalk, the spectrum of compartmental and structural variability is broad. Lesions may be totally intrasellar, intrasellar and extrasellar, suprasellar only, or intraventricular only. The most common structural manifestation relates to suprasellar mass with displacement and/or disruption of the floor of the third ventricular chamber. These lesions may be totally extraarachnoid, but may also be intrapial with finger like projections invading neural tissue. It is important to consider that the presence of this intrapial component may be attended by *intense glial reaction* in adjacent brain. This reaction acts as an impediment to establishing dissection planes in some cases and, particularly in cystic lesions with fine membranes, may further complicate efforts at excision. This response is variable in intensity and extent and, in certain cases, may provide a "buffer area" which allows dissection exclusive of functioning neural tissue.

A major technical issue relates to involvement of the components of the circle of Willis with elements of the neoplasm. Such intimate adherence often provides the major limitation in excision[1,5,8,9].

Operative Techniques (Suprasellar)

For the purposes of this discussion the operative considerations for a suprasellar craniopharyngioma without temporal or major frontal component will be described. This may be considered, with some modification, a "traditional" basal frontal exposure.

In the event that hydrocephalus is present a left frontal ventriculostomy is established. Bilateral ventriculostomies may be required in the event that complete obstruction of the right foramen is present. Components of a right basal frontotemporal exposure or a complete frontopterionotemporal craniotomy may be performed. We have preferred a right frontal craniotomy which incorporates the entire frontal floor from the midline to the sphenoid wing. This craniotomy is accomplished by incising of the temporalis muscle parallel to the frontal floor to the region of the pterion, then extending the incision at right angles to the base along the line of the coronal suture. A free bone flap is turned with the crescent of temporal muscle at the posteroinferior base. This exposure offers options of pterional and lateral wing excision and opening of the Sylvian fissure for added basilar and lateral exposure. The approach to the lesion is extraáxial via a number of optional angular corridors. The medial subfrontal approach offers optimum visualization of both optic nerves, but poor angulation for appreciation of the lateral component of the optic nerve, carotid artery and optic tract anatomy. The laterofrontal corridor afforded by the posterior (lateral) exposure affords such exposure and adds another intraoperative option.

Anatomic maintenance of the *pituitary stalk* is a major objective in any microsurgical dissection in the sellar region and is a requirement for normal pituitary function. By employing high power magnification the stalk is readily recognized by a distinctive striate pattern (Portal System) that is directed vertically from the inferior hypothalamic surface to the diaphragma region. This structure is most often identified in the posterior or posterolateral tumor margins. At completion of the excision, angular dental mirrors or endoscopes aid in regional visualization.

Although considerable variability of opinion exists regarding the resectability of such lesions, available data would imply that initial direct exploration is the most appropriate management, especially in lesions with solid components. Such action is required to properly assess the *operability of these lesions*. Major objectives in the procedure include decompression of the visual system and reduction of local mass effect at the foramen of Monroe. With attainment of these goals the procedure should probably be terminated in the event that microdissection planes are obscure.

Radiation therapy should be initiated in the postoperative period if operative knowledge or postoperative imaging indicate the presence of tumor or residual calcium[13,15]. Early recurrence (months) is most commonly cystic and should be managed by imaging stereotactic methods with conduit/reservoir placement for drainage and consideration of colloid based radionuclide installation[3,14].

Reoperation is not to be precluded by the events of previous operations and radiation treatment. However, surgical expectations are less optimistic and risks increased in relation to the initial procedure when dissection planes are optimal. In the event that reoperation is required, it is worthwhile to consider an alternate corridor.

Colloid (Neuroepithelial) Cyst

Development and Surgical Pathology

Colloid cysts of the third ventricle are relatively rare lesions accounting for 0.5 to 1.0% of primary intracranial neurally derived tumours. Many terms have been applied to these lesions including neuroepithelial cysts, neuroepithelial tumours, paraphyseal cysts, ependymal cysts, epithelial cysts, choroid plexus cysts and cysts of the foramen of Monroe.

Although the first documented case of a colloid cyst of the third ventricle was reported by Wallmann in 1858, it was not until 1933, that Dandy described the radiological definition and surgical management of these lesions.

There has been considerable debate and controversy over the origin of the cyst. In 1910, Sjovall suggested that the cyst was a remnant of the *paraphysis*. The paraphysis is a constant feature of human embryos in the 17–100 mm stage and lies at the rostral end of the diencephalic roof. This widely accepted concept carried with it the belief that such cysts occurred only at the anterior part of the third ventricle. In 1955, Kappers suggested that while occasional examples are paraphyseal in origin, most arise from *diencephalic ependymal pouches*. The *choroid plexus* has been proposed as an alternate site of origin of such cysts. The term *neuroepithelial cyst* was proposed by Shuangshoti and Netsky in 1966. They proposed that these lesions may occur anywhere along the course of the central nervous system from the choroid plexus or ependyma, both being derived from a common neuroepithelium.

Most commonly, colloid cysts arise in the anterior superior part of the third ventricle immediately posterior to the foramen of Monroe. They generally project inferiorly into the third ventricle and vary in extent superiorly and rostrally. Attachments of various dimensions are present with the tela choroidea of the third ventricular roof. Occasionally, the forniceal column superior to the anterior commissure will be separated by the mass presence. This separation may involve the leaves of the septum pellucidum. Generally, the cyst is well circumscribed, smooth and spherical with dimensions varying from 0.3 to 9 cm. The wall of the cyst is composed of a layer of epithelial cells, either low columnar or cuboidal and surrounded by a connective tissue capsule. The cyst is filled with homogeneous viscous material containing cellular debris. This material is variable in viscosity as not only various numbers of desquammated epithelial cells, but also leucocytes, red cells, gitter cells and cholesteral pigment have been described in the colloid material.

It is important to recognize that these lesions may occur posterior to the foramen of Monro and that they may be attended by various degrees of aqueductal stenosis.

Symptomatology

Numerous perspectives relating to symptomatology are available in the literature. Symptom complexes include the following:

a. *Acute* and *intermittent increases in intracranial pressure.* This the "classical" history of paraxcismal headache with changes in head position. These episodes may be attended by vertigo, vomiting, alterations in conscience level, alterations in mentation, seizure activity, vital sign aberrences or CSF rhinorrhea. The predisposition to *acute demise* has been repeatedly stressed.

b. *Chronically increased intracranial pressure.* In this complex chronic dementia alone, or in combination with gait disturbances and urinary incontinence are encounted.

c. *Local pressure effects* related to mass including sensorimotor, extrapyramidal, autonomic disturbances, and memory disorders.

It should be stressed that *identification of the presence of these lesions by the "classical presentation" is unusual.* Long standing, intermittent, nonspecific headache without attendant postural exacerbations is the most frequently encountered complaint.

Radiology

As has been noted previously, imaging studies provide the primary indicator toward suspicion of this lesion with masses generally presenting in the anterior third ventricle with attendant lateral ventriculomegaly with CT scanning. The spheroid masses are usually slightly hyperdense, but may be isodense. The lesion generally shows some elements of uniform enhancement with contrast media, but no enhancement or ring enhancements have been described. Attendant structural alterations include enlargement of the septum pellucidum and collapse of the posterior third ventricle. Fullness of the posterior third ventricle may be present in the event that aquaductal stenosis is present.

Occasionally, such a lesion may be disclosed as a truely "incidental" finding with no evidence of lateral ventriculomegaly. Focal enhancement may indicate the presence of a xanthogranulomatous component.

Management

In spite of its benign histological character *these lesions provide a menace to life.* Although the absolute risk of demise has not been accurately determined, there is no doubt that because of their location and repeated documentations of rapid and fatal neurological deterioration, definitive management to either reduce the cyst mass and/or maintain normal CSF dynamics is most appropriate.

An element of controversy exists regarding the best method for treatment. Arguments exist for the following management options:

1. Biventricular shunting
2. Stereotactic aspiration
3. Direct excision.

It should be stressed that because of the potential incidence of aqueductal stenosis (20%) some method of CSF diversion may be required if options 2 or 3 are exercised initially.

Endoscopic Stereotactic aspiration employing imaging guided techniques may be accomplished at small risk and offers an apparently plausible management option if experienced individuals are available. In our experience (more than 25 cases) lesions of less than 1 cm in diameter may be difficult to puncture and aspirate; however, with special instrumentation cysts may be perforated and compressed with microforceps to express contents. Published experience would indicate that reduction of cyst volume is possible in more than 80% of lesions. Use of this technique should be attended by a meticulous and vigilant monitoring of ventricular size and/or intraventricular pressure with a consideration of ventriculography postaspiration to assess patency of the aqueduct of Sylvius. It must be stressed that this technique requires expertise in the utilization of such instrumentation and should not be undertaken by individuals who are not experienced in methods of stereotaxy, endoscopy, and ventricular microsurgery. In the event that *craniotomy* is undertaken, with identification of the mass, at the foramen aspiration should be undertaken with a #20 needle or #3F suction after incision of the capsule. Miniature currettes may be introduced within the cyst cavity to assist with reduction of the content volume. At all times, care is taken to avoid traction or manipulation of the cyst attachment at the tela choroidea adjacent to the foramen with potential venous or arterial injury. Following evacuation of cyst contents the wall may be coagulated and gently delivered in fragments through the foramen. In the event that the foramen is small or adequate access for manipulation is not available added exposure may be gained via subchoroidal or interforniceal corridors (Table 1).

Following cyst excision ventricular exploration may be afforded by fiberoptic endoscopy or direct visualization in the event that addition corridors have been established. The development of a third ventriculostomy in the region of the tuber cinerium may be considered at that time with or without a silastic conduit led through the main operative corridor to a Rickham reservoir.

Subchoroidal or interforniceal corridors may be developed in the event that the cyst is not apparent at the foramen in order to identify the pathology and provide a route for manipulation and excision. In our experience "complete" third ventricular exploration is

Table 1
___

A. Extraaxial Intraventricular Mass

 ALT. 1. (i) Transcallosal (solid)
    (ventricular size irrelevant)
    a. biforaminal
    b. interforniceal
    c. subchoroidal
   (ii) Stereotactic (cystic)

 ALT. 2. Transfrontal
    (with ventriculomegaly)
    a. foraminal
    b. subchoroidal
    c. interforniceal

 ALT. 3. CSF diversion (permanet)

B. Intraaxial ventricular Mass

 ALT. 1. Stereotactic
    a. CSF diversion (malignant, major intraaxial
     or component)
    b. ALT. 2, 3 (benign minor intraaxial component)

 ALT. 2. Transcallosal
    (ventricular size irrelevant)
    a. biforaminal
    b. interforniceal

 ALT. 3. Transfrontal
    (with ventriculomegaly)
    a. foraminal
    b. subchoroidal

 ALT. 4. CSF diversion (permanent)

C. Basal Mass

 I(a) *Intrasellar-suprasellar (solid)*
  (A) *Enlarged sella with midline extension*
    ALT. 1. Transsphenoidal
    ALT. 2. Subfrontal
  (B) *Enlarged sella with frontal or temporal extension*
    Subfrontal, subtemporal, or fronto temporal
    craniotomy
  (C) *Normal sella with midline extension*
    ALT. 1. Consider suprasellar alternatives
    ALT. 2. Transsphenoidal
  (D) *Normal sella with frontal or temporal extension*
    Frontal, temporal or fronto temporal craniotomy

 I(b) *Intrasellar-suprasellar (cystic)*
  ALT. 1. Stereotactic
  ALT. 2. Transsphenoidal

 II(a) *Suprasella (Solid)*
  (A) *Mass midline suprasellar*
    subfrontal
    1. *Chiasm prefixed*
     (a) transsphenoidal
     (b) translamina terminalis
    2. *Chiasm normal*
     (a) subchiasmatic
     (b) translamina terminalis
  (B) *Mass midline retrosellar*
    ALT. 1. Peterional
       opticocarotid
       lateral carotid
    ALT. 2. Subtemporal
  (C) *Mass frontal*
    subfrontal
  (D) *Mass temporal*
    1. Subtemporal
    2. Pterional-subtemporal

 II(b) *Suprasella (cystic)*
  ALT. 1. Stereotactic
  ALT. 2. Consider other suprasellar (solid) alternatives

 III. *Superior extension (third ventricular)*
  (A) *Mass foraminal or supraforaminal (broad midline*
    base 2.5 cm)
    combined basal and transcallosal*
    a. biforaminal
    b. interforniceal
    c. subchoroidal
  (B) *Foraminal or supraforaminal (narrow midline*
    base 2.5 cm)
    ALT. 1. Transcallosal**
      a. biforaminal
      b. interforniceal
    ALT. 2. Combined basal and transcallosal
      a. biforaminal
      b. interforniceal
___

* Consider stereotactic endoscopy.
** Prior stereotactic endoscopy.

optimally accomplished via the transcallosal interforniceal approach.

Following cyst excision, monitoring of intracranial pressure is required for 48 to 72 hours.

Biventricular shunting as a definitive treatment may be considered. However, it should be recognized that greater than 80% of the patients will be unnecessarily shunt-dependent when the capabilities of other operative methodologies are considered.

Our current method of management of these lesions is to attempt endoscopic aspiration in all cases. If unsuccessful, primary excision is offered to individuals less than fifty years old and biventricular CSF diversion to those declining direct surgical excision or greater than fifty years old. Craniotomy is undertaken with a transcallosal corridor with foraminal or forminal exposure augmented by the interforniceal approach.

Management Summary

As has been noted, the selection of an appropriate surgical procedure generally rests on the structural substrate as defined by detailed modern imaging. Many factors may modify this generally including the individual patient, surgeon, and institutional factors.

The following summary represents our guidelines for management as practiced at our institution[4].

A. *Extraaxial Intraventricular*

Predominantly solid lesions confined within the third ventricle are approached via a transcallosal corridor which offers maximal options for midline exploration irrespective of ventricular size. In the event that foraminal exposure is inadequate, interforniceal or subchoroidal exposure is easily initiated. Cystic lesions presenting at the foramen of Monro are initially evaluated by stereotactic endoscopy where biopsy, aspiration or excision is undertaken. Cerebrospinal fluid diversion (ventriculoperitoneal) although occasionally indicated because of patient factors is not frequently employed as a primary management mode. All ventricular catheter placements are accomplished by stereotactic methods with imaging control.

B. *Intraaxial Intraventricular*

In general, these lesions are often either radiosensitive or manageable means after stereotactic biopsy. However, treatment is governed by data derived from stereotactic biopsy and includes cerebral spinal fluid diversion with radiochemotherapy for malignant lesions and transcallosal third ventricular exploration when a defined and separate intraventricular component is present with histologically benign lesions. Such surgery may occasionally make shunting unnecessary. Cerebrospinal fluid diversion without tissue assessment is considered generally imprudent and rarely practiced.

C. *Basal Masses*

1. Intrasellar Suprasellar

In the event that enlargement of the sella turcica and midline suprasellar extension is present, a *transsphenoidal route* is optimal. This is particularly true with cystic lesions. If sellar contour and volume are normal a subfrontal approach is generally the most effective.

2. Suprasellar

Suprasellar masses with *midline* subfrontal superior extension are managed by a *subfrontal exposure* that allows options initiated on the basis of chiasmal position. *Midline retrosellar* masses are exposed optimally through a *pterional corridor* with *temporal* extension necessary according to the amount of mass in the region of the dorsum sella and retrodorsal space. *Cystic* lesion (7) in these regions may be managed by experienced *stereotacticions*, however, in general initial effort at direct microexcision of wall and solid component it is indicated in these usually bengin lesions.

3. Superior Extension

In the event that extension is evident on imaging studies which is superior to the foramen of Monro and midline base is more than 25 mm in an exposure that allows combined basal and superior approaches is appropriate. Subfrontal exposure and exploration is undertaken initially with the superior approach either during the same procedure or after postoperative imaging is obtained and such a corridor is considered necessary.

From the technical standpoint lesions with a base of less than 25 mm may be completely excised via a superior corridor. We have used this approach rarely as an initial procedure, but have found it useful in cases where reoperation is necessary.

References

1. Al-Mefty O, Hassounah M, Weaver P, Sakati N, Jinkins JR, Fox JL (1985) Microsurgery for giant craniopharyngiomas in children. Neurosurgery 17: 585–595
2. Apuzzo MLJ (ed) (1987) Surgery of the third ventricle. Williams and Wilkins, Baltimore
3. Apuzzo MLJ, Chandrasoma P, Zelman V, vonHanwehr R (1987) Application of computerized tomographic guidance stereotaxis. In: Apuzzo MLJ (ed) Surgery of the third ventricle. Williams and Wilkins, Baltimore, pp 751–792
4. Apuzzo MLJ, Zee CS, Breeze, RE (1987) Anterior and med ventricular lesions: surgical overview. In: Apuzzo, MLJ (ed) Surgery of the third ventricle. Williams and Wilkins, Baltimore, pp 495–542
5. Baskin DS, Wilson CB (1986) Surgical management of craniopharyngiomas. J Neurosurg 65: 22–27
6. Block GA, Posner JB (1987) Anatomy and physiology of consciousness: Syndromes of altered consciousness related to third ventricular lesions. In: Apuzzo MLJ (ed) Surgery of the third ventricle. Williams and Wilkins, Baltimore, pp 213–223
7. Bogen JE (1987) Physiologic consequences of complete or partial commissural section. In: Apuzzo MLJ (ed) Surgery of the third ventricle. Williams and Wilkins, Baltimore, pp 175–194
8. Carmel PW (1980) Surgical syndromes of the hypothalamus. Clin Neurosurg 27: 133–159
9. Carmel PW (1985) Craniopharyngiomas. In: Wilkins RH, Sett SR (eds) Neurosurgery. McGraw-Hill, pp 905–916
10. Chandrasoma P, Apuzzo MLJ (1989) Stereotactic brain biopsy. Igaku-Shoin, New York
11. Damasio A, Van Hoesen G (1987) Anatomy and physiology of memory. In: Apuzzo MLJ (ed) Surgery of the third ventricle. Williams and Wilkins, Baltimore, pp 195–208
12. Davis R (1986) Pathological lesions of the third ventricular region. In: Apuzzo MLJ (ed) Surgery of the third ventricle. Williams and Wilkins, Baltimore
13. Hoff JT, Patterson RH Jr (1972) Craniopharyngiomas in childeren and adults. J Neurosurg 36: 299–302
14. Kobayashi T, Kageyama N, Ohara K (1981) Internal irradiation for cystic craniopharyngioma. J Neurosurg 55: 896–903
15. Richmond IL, Wara WM, Wilson CB (1980) Role of radiation therapy in the management of craniopharyngiomas in children. Neurosurgery 6: 513–517
16. Ryder JW, Kleinschmidt-DeMaster BK Keller TS (1986) Sudden deterioration and death in patient with benign tumors of the third ventricle area. J Neurosurg 64: 216–223

Correspondence: Prof. M.L.J. Apuzzo, Department of Neurological Surgery, University of Southern California School of Medicine, 1200 N. State Street, Suite 5046, Los Angeles, CA 90033, U.S.A

Acta Neurochirurgica, Suppl. 53, 89–91 (1991)

Transzygomatic Approach to Tumours of the Parasellar Region. Technical Note

D. Becker, M. Ammirati, K. Black, R. Canalis, and **J. Andrews**

Division of Neurosurgery and Head and Neck Surgery, University of California at Los Angeles, Calif., U.S.A.

Summary

A simple transzygomatic approach to the middle fossa centered on the inferior retraction of the temporal muscle hinged on the transected zygomatic arch is described. This approach allows a very low basal exposure of the middle and temporal fossa minimizing the amount of temporal lobe retraction needed to approach intra and extradural lesion in this location. The upper portion of the infratemporal fossa is also reached after removal of the middle fossa skull base. This approach is simple, easily performed, does not require extensive skull base removal, and still offers excellent visualization of the middle fossa and of the upper infratemporal fossa.

Keywords: Parasellar tumours; transzygomatic approach.

Introduction

There have been a variety of surgical approaches to the middle and temporal fossa described in the last 15 years. In many of these approaches the exposure of the middle and temporal fossa represented part of a wider infratemporal fossa exposure that was generally required for a combined neurosurgical otolaryngolocic approach to large skull base tumours[3]. These approaches require extensive skull base removal and occasionally opening of the paranasal sinuses[2,4,6–8]. However there are situations in which a low basal approach to the middle and temporal fossa is all that is required to minimize the amount of temporal lobe retraction to reach extra and/or intradurally the medial middle cranial fossa and the lesser wing of the sphenoid. In these instances a less involved approach may be useful. A few approaches have been reported which fulfill some of these criteria: in these approaches the basal exposure is obtained by sectioning the coronoidal attachment of the temporal muscle and, by superior or posterior reflection, of the temporal muscle[1,5]. We describe a transzygomatic approach

that enabled us to successfully remove parasellar lesions with minimal amount of temporal lobe retraction, with limited skull base removal, and with preservation of the temporalis muscle tendinous attachment to the coronoid process.

Surgical Technique

The patient is positioned supine with the head turned to the contralateral side and secured in a 3 point head fixation device. A preauricular question mark skin incision extending to the tragus of the ear is executed. The temporalis muscle is completely exposed by reflecting the scalp flap subgaleally except the anterior one-fourth of the temporalis muscle where the scalp flap is dissected between the 2 layers of the superficial temporalis fascia as described by Yaşargil[9] in order to preserve the facial nerve branches to the frontalis, orbicularis oculi and corrugator muscles. The dissection is then continued in a subcutaneous plane caudally to a point approximately 2 cm below the zygomatic arch, being careful not to injure the parotid, the facial nerve or the trunk of the superficial temporal artery. In such a way the zygomatic arch is completely exposed from immediately in front of the glenoid fossa to the zygomatic bone. The attachment of the masseter muscle to the inferior portion of the zygomatic arch is exposed and left undisturbed. The root of the arch and its anterior edge are cut using an oscillating saw. The temporalis is then horizontally incised 1–2 cm below the superior temporal line, subperiostally separated from the temporalis fossa, and inferiorly retracted hinged on the sectioned zygomatic arch through its fascial attachments. Having so

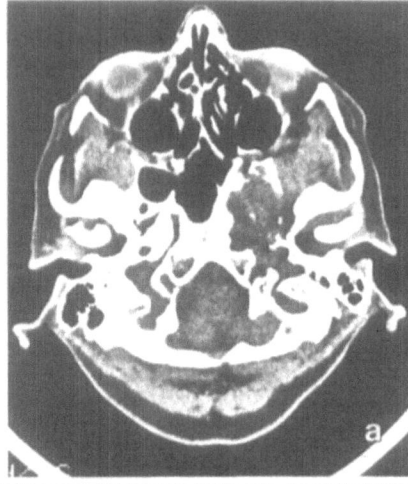
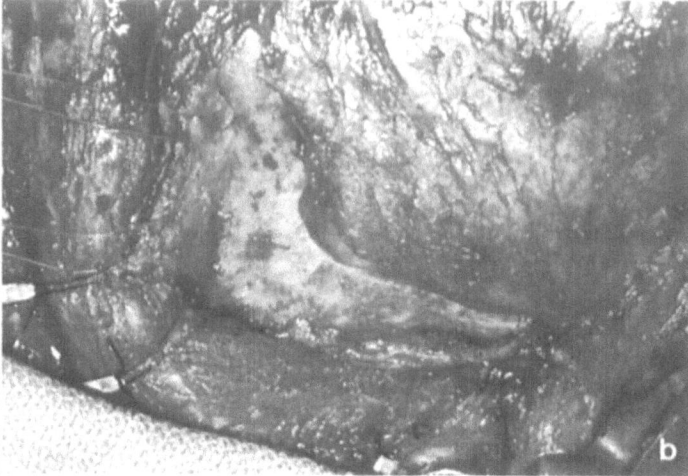
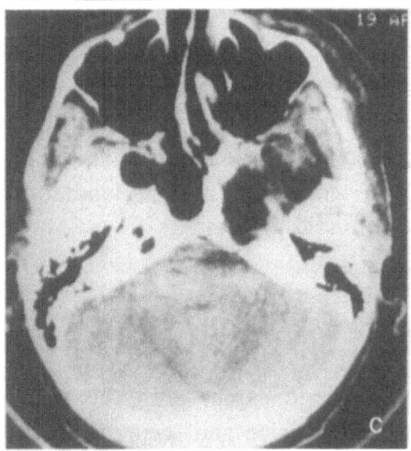

Fig. 1. CT scan shows a large lesion involving the parasellar and the infratemporal fossa on the left (a). The zygomatic arch and the lateral orbital rim are fully exposed (b). Postoperative CT scan shows no evidence of tumour; the resection cavity is filled with fat (c)

exposed the temporalis fossa the appropiate craniotomy or craniectomy is executed. When the skull base of the middle fossa is removed good exposure of the upper infratemporal fossa is achieved. At the end of the procedure the zygomatic arch is reapproximated using wires. The rest of the wound is closed as usual.

Illustrative Case

This 60 year old lady presented with facial numbness on the left. Neurological exam was positive for decreased sensation to cold temperature and light touch over all 3 distributions of the left trigeminal nerve. CT scan showed a tumor in the left middle and infratemporal fossa (Fig. 1 a). At surgery a chondrosarcoma of the left middle and infratemporal fossa was totally removed via a transzygomatic approach (Fig. 1 b). The second and third division of the trigeminal nerve were involved by tumour and needed to be sacrificed; the resection cavity was filled with abdominal fat. Postoperative course was uneventful. Patient received postoperative radiation therapy and remains clinically and neuroradiologically (Fig. 1 c) recurrence-free 18 months postoperatively.

Discussion

Extensive skull approaches are not always necessary when dealing with intra and extradural lesions mainly located in the parasellar area and/or in the middle fossa. Still, low basal surgical routes to the parasellar area are useful to minimize the amount of temporal lobe retraction and to improve tumour exposure. Simple low basal approaches to the parasellar area require detachment of the temporalis muscle from the temporal fossa. Posterolateral displacement of the temporal muscle as done in an interfascial pterional craniotomy is inadequate in fully exposing the temporal fossa, especially its posterior and inferior extent. Superior reflection of the temporal muscle requires transection of its tendinous attachment to the coronoid process with possible limitation of jaw opening. In addition, the vascular supply of the superiorly retracted muscle is totally dependent on anastomotic periosteal channels due to the inevitable anatomical compromise of the middle temporal and anterior and posterior deep temporal arteries inherent to this surgical approach. Our approach employing inferior retraction of the temporal muscle hinged through its superficial fascia on the cut zygomatic arch preserves the middle temporal artery vascular pedicle; in addition leaving part of the superior temporal muscle still attached to the temporal squama preserves some periosteal collaterals. Moreover the integrity of the temporal muscle tendon to the coronoid process is not compromised minimizing the amount of postoperative malfunction of the temporal muscle[1,5]. Contrary to what has been previously reported, we have found that the bulk of the inferiorly retracted temporal muscle does not hinder the low basal surgical exposure if the zygomatic arch is adequately mobilized[1].

References

1. Al-Mefty O, Anand VK (1990) Zygomatic approach to skull-base lesions. J Neurosurg 73: 668–673
2. Attia EL, Bentley KC, Head T (1984) A new external approach to the pterygomaxillary fossa and parapharyngeal space. Head Neck Surg 6: 884–891
3. Fish U, Pillsbury HC (1979) Infratemporal fossa approach to lesions in the temporal bone and base of the skull. Arch Otolaryngol 105: 99–107
4. Fujitsu K, Kuwabara T (1985) Zygomatic approach for lesions in the interpeduncular cistern. J Neurosurg 62: 340–343
5. Gates GA (1988) The lateral facial approach to the nasopharynx and infratemporal fossa. Otolaryngol Head Neck Surg 99: 321–325
6. Hakuba A, Liu S, Nishimura S (1986) The orbitozygomatic infratemporal approach: a new surgical technique. Surg Neurol 26: 271–276
7. Pellerin P, Lesoin F, Dhellemmes P, Domazzan M, Jomin M (1984) Usefulness of the orbitofrontomalar approach associated with bone reconstruction for frontotemporosphenoid meningiomas. Neurosurgery 15: 715–718
8. Sekhar LN, Schramm VL, Jones NF (1987) Subtemporal-preauricular infratemporal fossa approach to large lateral and posterior cranial base neoplasms. J Neurosurg 67: 488–499
9. Yasargil MG, Reichmann MV, Kubik S (1987) Preservation of the frontotemporal branch of the facial nerve using the interfascial temporalis flap for pterional craniotomy. J Neurosurg 67: 463–466

Correspondence: D. Becker, M.D., Division of Neurosurgery, Room 74-140CHS, University of California at Los Angeles, Los Angeles, CA 90024, U.S.A.

Acta Neurochirurgica, Suppl. 53, 92–97 (1991)
© by Springer-Verlag 1991

Clinoidal Meningiomas

O. Al-Mefty[1] and S. Ayoubi[2]

[1]Division of Neurological Surgery, Loyola University Medical Center, Chicago, Illinois, USA and [2]Hurstwood Park Neurological Center, Haywards Heath, Uk

Summary

Clinoidal meningiomas have distinguishing clinical, radiological, and surgical considerations. They present a surgical challenge and have a notorious rate of recurrence. The best chance of their cure comes through total removal, but the fear of injury to cerebral vessels has led most surgeons to accept subtotal removal. We classify these tumours into three groups according to the presence or absence of an interfacing arachnoid membrane between the tumour and cerebral vessels. The presence or absence of this membrane depends on the origin of the tumour and its relation to the naked carotid segment lying outside the carotid cistern. In Group I, total removal is impossible and results are disappointing. In Groups II and III, total removal is possible and results are good despite arterial encasement by the tumour.

Keywords: Meningioma; anterior clinoid; sphenoid ridge; cavernous sinus.

Introduction

Clinoidal meningiomas, also known as sphenocavernous meningiomas, originate from the dura of the cavernous sinus, the anterior clinoid process and the internal part of the sphenoid wing.

They are frequently grouped with sphenoid ridge or suprasellar meningiomas[6,13,14,22,29,30] but should be defined as a separate entity having distinguishing clinical, radiological, and surgical considerations. They correspond with what Cushing referred to as meningiomas of the "deep or clinoidal third"[9], with the Group A sphenoid ridge meningiomas in Bonnal and colleagues' classification[7], and with the first category of Ojemann's sphenoid ridge meningiomas[21].

Clinoidal meningiomas have always presented a surgical challenge and had an ominous outcome and a notorious rate of recurrence[6,8,13,14,22,29,30]. Only a few patients have had excellent results, as defined by total removal combined with complete clinical remission and no clinical or radiological signs of recurrence[7,9,25]. A striking difference in mortality, morbidity, failure of total removal, and recurrence is evident when comparing clinoidal meningiomas to middle and lateral sphenoidal tumours or tuberculum sellae tumours[6,7,9,15,16,22,30]. Recent advances in cranial base and cavernous sinus surgery have markedly improved the incidence of total removal and good outcome[2,3,11,24,27]. We herein update our experience with this tumour, emphasizing the impact of their classification on surgical difficulties, success of total removal and morbidity.

Anatomical Considerations and Classification

Based on intraoperative anatomical observation related to the presence of an arachnoid membrane between the tumour and cerebral vessels, we have distinguished 3 groups of clinoidal meningiomas.

As the carotid artery emerges from the cavernous sinus inferomedial to the anterior clinoid process, it enters the subdural space to be vested in the carotid cistern. The arachnoid membrane of the carotid cistern does not follow the internal carotid artery (ICA) into the cavernous sinus space nor is it attached to the anterior clinoid process. There are 1 or 2 mm of naked artery between the investment of the carotid cistern and the dura of the cavernous sinus[32].

Group I includes meningiomas with origins proximal to the end of the carotid cistern, as is the case in meningiomas originating at the inferior aspect of the anterior clinoid process. These tumours enwrap the carotid artery, adhering to the adventitia and lacking an interfacing arachnoid membrane (Fig. 1).

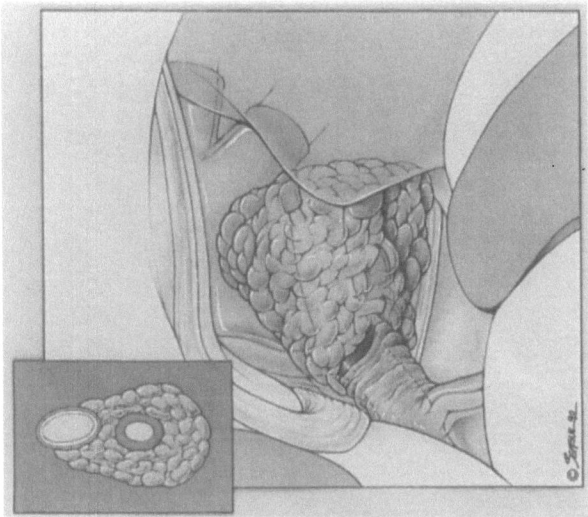

Fig. 1 A. Artist's illustration of a Group I tumour. The tumour encases the carotid artery and its branches with direct attachment to the adventitia. The optic nerve maintains an arachnoidal plane from the chiasmatic cistern. (Reproduced with permission from Al-Mefty O: Clinoidal meningiomas. J Neurosurg 73: 840–849, 1990)

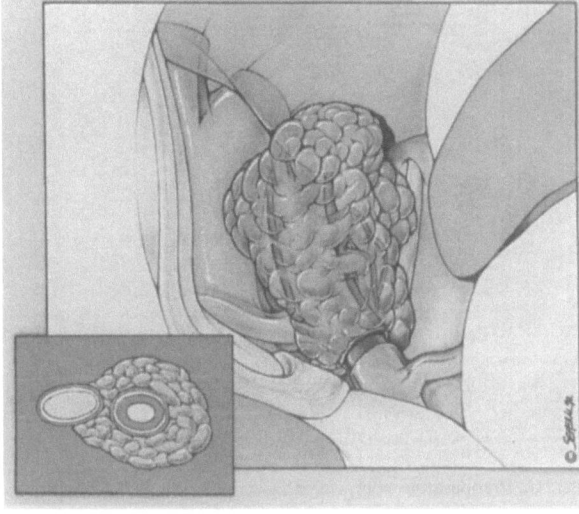

Fig. 2 A. Artist's illustration of a Group II tumour. The tumour encases the carotid artery and its branches. An arachnoidal membrane of the carotid cistern separates the tumour from the adventitia, making dissection possible. The optic nerve maintains an arachnoidal membrane from the chiasmatic cistern. (Reproduced with permission from Al-Mefty O: Clinoidal meningiomas. J Neurosurg 73: 840–849, 1990)

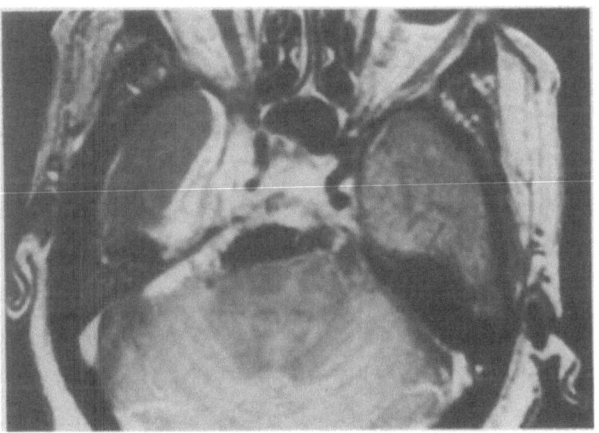

Fig. 1 B. MR image of a Group I tumour

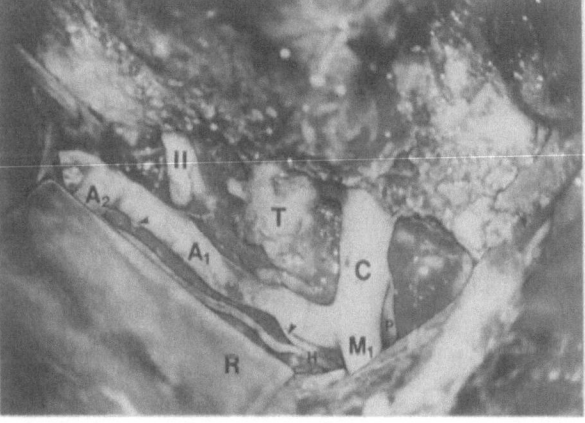

Fig. 2 B. Retouched operative photograph of a Group II tumour. The optic nerve (II), the anterior cerebral artery (A_1), the middle cerebral artery (M_1), and part of the internal carotid artery (C) are dissected free from the encasing tumour (T). The dissection was relatively easy, owing to the presence of an arachnoid membrane of the carotid cistern

Their direct attachment to the vessel wall continues as the tumour grows to the carotid bifurcation and along the middle cerebral artery.

Group II includes meningiomas originating above the segment of the carotid artery invested in the carotid cistern, as is the case in meningiomas originating from the superior and/or lateral aspects of the anterior clinoid process. As the tumour grows, an arachnoid membrane separates it from the arterial adventitia, making microsurgical dissection feasible despite total arterial encasement by the tumour (Fig. 2).

In both groups, the optic nerve and chiasm are wrapped in the arachnoid membrane of the chiasmatic

cistern, making microdissection of the nerves and chiasm from the tumour relatively easy. In patients having had previous surgery, the arachnoidal membrane may be violated, making dissection of a Group II tumour as difficult as dissection of a Group I tumour.

Group III includes meningiomas originating at the optic foramen, extending to the optic canal and the tip of the anterior clinoid process. The arachnoid membrane is present between the tumour and vessels,

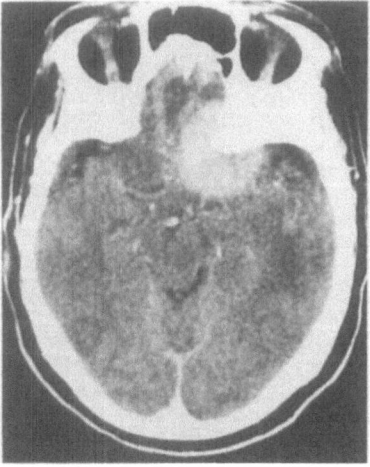

Fig. 2 C. Preoperative contrast enhanced CT scan of a Group II clinoidal meningioma

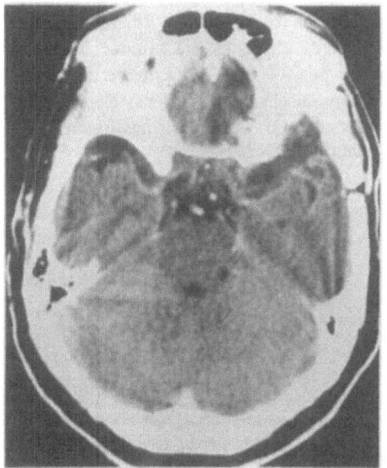

Fig. 2 D. Postoperative CT scan after total removal

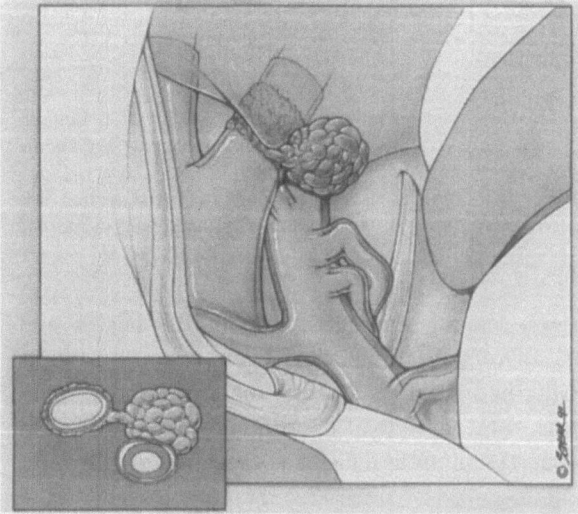

Fig. 3 A. Artist's illustration of a Group III tumour. The origin of the tumour is the optic foramen. The tumour is small, separated from the carotid by the carotid cistern, but it extends into the optic canal. (Reproduced with permission from Al-Mefty O: Clinoidal meningiomas. J Neurosurg 73: 840–849, 1990)

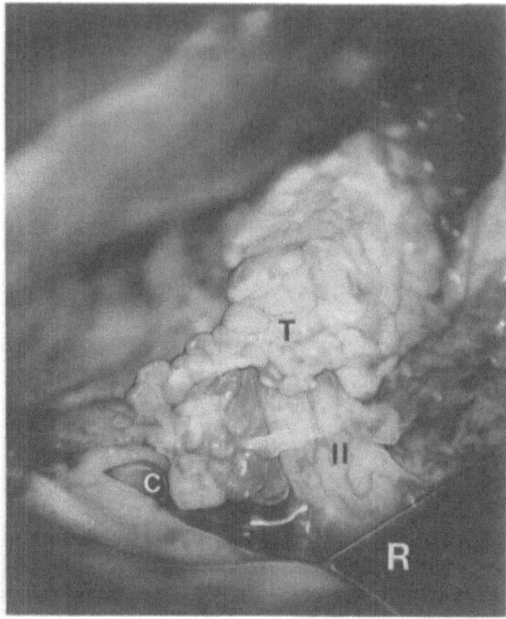

Fig. 3 B. Retouched operative photograph of a Group III tumour. The carotid cistern is intact. The tumour is small and extends into the optic canal. *T* Tumour; *II* optic nerve; *C* carotid artery; *R* retractor on the frontal lobe

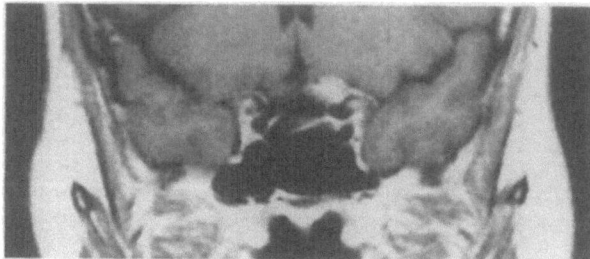

Fig. 3 C. Contrast enhanced MR image of a Group III tumour

but may be absent between the optic nerve and the tumour (Fig. 3).

Case Material

Twenty-eight cases qualifying as clinoidal meningiomas were operated on over an 8 year period; some have been included in an earlier report[3]. There were seven other patients who did not have surgery. Excluded were meningiomas with origins (as described intraoperatively) on the tuberculum sellae, diaphragm sellae, planum sphenoidale, and middle and lateral sphenoid ridge, as well as hyperostosing *en plaque* meningiomas. Ages of patients ranged from 26 to 76 years (mean: 50 years); seven were males and 21 were females. The symptoms of two females presented during pregnancy. Five patients had previous surgery on their tumours.

Visual disturbances were present in 86% of cases, similar to the typical findings described for tumours at this site (initial unilateral visual loss). Seven patients experienced loss on one side only; 12 experienced optic atrophy, and six had papilledema. Foster-Kennedy syndrome was documented in only one case. Six patients had impairment of the oculomotor or trigeminal nerve and seizures occurred in three patients. Two patients were admitted in a comatose state with giant tumours and underwent emergency surgery. Visual loss preceded diagnosis in a range of 2 to 44 months (average: 25 months).

Computized tomography (CT) scans revealed the presence of the tumour and its extensions in all cases. Magnetic resonance (MR) images with gadolinium enhancement were used in the last seven cases. All patients underwent cerebral angiography to delineate the anatomy of cerebral circulation, arterial displacement, encasement of major vessels, and blood supply. According to the aforementioned classification, there were three Group I tumours, 21 Group II tumours, and four Group III tumours.

The carotid, middle cerebral, and anterior cerebral arteries, as well as the optic apparatus, were all intimately involved with the tumour, being displaced, adherent, or totally engulfed. The carotid artery was totally encased in 12 patients; the branches of the middle cerebral artery were encased in seven; the anterior cerebral artery was encased in three, and the optic nerve was encased in ten. Cavernous sinus invasion occurred in 12 patients.

Surgical Technique

We use the cranio-orbital approach, described elsewhere[2] to remove clinoidal meningiomas.

The sphenoid ridge is completely drilled, unroofing the superior orbital fissure and removing the anterior clinoid process extradurally. This maneuver intercepts the arterial feeders coming from the middle meningeal artery while the involved bone is removed. It also prepares for exposure of the superior aspect of the cavernous sinus. The dura is opened with a semicircular incision centered on the pterion, and a branching incision is carried out posteriorly and inferiorly toward the floor of the temporal fossa.

Brain relaxation is achieved by slowly draining 35 to 50 ml of cerebrospinal fluid (CSF). The drain is then closed to keep the arachnoid cisterns open and facilitate dissection. The arachnoid of the sylvian fissure is opened; this opening is extended on the frontal side to preserve the middle cerebral veins. Retracting the frontal lobe 1.5 cm is adequate for tumour removal. The olfactory nerve is dissected for some distance from the base of the frontal lobe and preserved.

Both moderate and large tumours are encountered upon opening the sylvian fissure. Microdissection is carried out in a plane between the tumour and the frontal and temporal lobes. After debulking the tumour with an ultrasonic aspirator, the distal branches of the middle cerebral artery are followed and dissected, removing the tumour capsule from the arterial wall. This dissection is carried out along the bifurcation of the ICA and along the anterior cerebral artery. Dissection is then continued to free the ventriculostriate arteries, the perforators of the

anterior cerebral artery, the ICA branch to the optic apparatus, and along the posterior communicating and anterior choroidal arteries before sacrificing any arterial branches. The surgeon must be certain that an arterial twig, and not a vital perforator, is supplying the tumour. The third nerve is then freed from the tumour. In most cases, the Liliequist membrane is intact, making dissection of the interpeduncular fossa and the posteriorly displaced basilar artery relatively easy. If a tear occurs in a cerebral vessel, temporary vascular clips are applied proximal and distal to the bleeding point, which is then sutured using 10–0 nylon.

The optic nerve may be displaced inferiorly and medially, elevated, or engulfed by the tumour. In all cases, the presence of an arachnoid membrane facilitates dissection of the optic apparatus. If the tumour extends into the optic canal, the canal should be unroofed and the tumour removed. The arterial supply to the optic apparatus should be preserved, particularly the inferior group, which is the sole supply to the central decussating fibers of the chiasm. The optic nerve should not be sacrificed even in patients having total blindness as visual recovery has been reported[4,19,23].

If the cavernous sinus is involved, the intrapetrous ICA is exposed for proximal control, and the cavernous sinus is entered through the lateral or superior wall[5].

After gross tumour removal, the dura around the anterior clinoid process is evaporated using the CO_2 laser. Any further hyperostosis is drilled, and a piece of fascia is applied over the drilled bone to avoid CSF leakage. The dura is closed watertight, the bone flap secured, and the skin closed in two layers.

Results

In Group II, total removal (tumour, dura and bone), as judged by intraoperative inspection and confirmed by postoperative CT scans, was achieved in all 21 cases but two, in which a small nub of tumour was left in the cavernous sinus and the medial wall of the sella respectively. There was one death nine days postoperatively, due to pulmonary embolism, in a patient who was in excellent condition and was ready to be discharged. One patient lost vision in one eye in which she had been able to count fingers preoperatively from a one-foot distance.

Preoperative visual impairment improved in four patients. One patient had permanent third cranial nerve palsy. Three patients had transient diabetes insipidus and one patient had permanent diabetes insipidus. One patient was readmitted for repair of a CSF leak and one required a CSF shunt for hydrocephalus. One other patient had a pulmonary embolism. The one semicomatose and one fully comatose patient at admission both made impressive recoveries postoperatively.

Postoperative follow-up ranged from seven months to seven years, with an average of 57 months. There was only one asymptomatic recurrence which was observed to be without change via a CT scan three years later in one of the patients with subtotal removal. In Group I, only partial but extensive removal was possible in all three patients. One patient developed delayed postoperative vasospasm 7 days postoperatively, which was confirmed by angiography, with a deteriorating ischemic neurological condition and eventual death 4 months later. The second patient had postoperative hemiplegia and was treated for pulmonary embolism. A gradual increase of tumour size over a three-year period was documented by CT scan. Radiation therapy was administered upon the patient's refusal of a second operation. The third patient showed some recovery of extraocular movement and received radiation therapy, showing no changes in his MR image 2 years later.

The four patients in Group III had no complications and two patients showed improvement in their visual findings in postoperative follow-up.

Discussion

The surgical mortality of anterior clinoid meningiomas has remained unacceptably high. A mortality of 32% was reported by Uihlein and Weyand in 1953[31], and a mortality of 42% was reported by Bonnal in 1980[7]. The major operative cause of death is injury to a major cerebral vessel[7,9,13,22,31], prompting most surgeons to recommend subtotal removal[6,7,9,10,12,13,17,26,30].

On the other hand, the extent of surgical removal is the determining factor in tumour progression or recurrence[1,20,28]. Incomplete removal of tumours carries a higher recurrence rate and the results from a second operation are discouraging[22].

Microsurgical techniques have improved operative mortality, morbidity, and chance of total removal[3,11,18,19,26,29]. The presence of an arachnoid membrane has a great impact on the surgical outcome, as is seen in our Group I. In patients of Groups II and III, in which the arachnoid membrane was present, total removal was possible and the morbidity was minimal.

Acknowledgement

The authors thanks Julie Hipp for her editorial assistance.

References

1. Adegbite AB, Khan MI, Paine KWE, Tan LK (1983) The recurrence of intracranial meningiomas after surgical treatment. J Neurosurg 58: 51–56
2. Al-Mefty O (1989) Surgery of the cranial base. Kluwer Academic Publishers, Boston
3. Al-Mefty O (1990) Clinoidal meningiomas. J Neurosurg 73: 840–849
4. Al-Mefty O, Holoubi A, Rifai A, Fox JL (1985) Microsurgical removal of suprasellar meningiomas. Neurosurgery 16: 364–372
5. Al-Mefty O, Smith RR (1988) Surgery of tumours invading the cavernous sinus. Surg Neurol 30: 370–381
6. Andrews BT, Wilson CB (1988) Suprasellar meningiomas: The effect of tumour location on postoperative visual outcome. J Neurosurg 69: 523–528
7. Bonnal JP, Thibaut A, Brotchi J, Born J (1980) Invading meningiomas of the sphenoid ridge. J Neurosurg 53: 587–599
8. Brihaye J, Brihaye-van Geertruyden M (1988) Management and surgical outcome of suprasellar meningiomas. Acta Neurochir (Wien) [Suppl] 42: 124–129
9. Cushing H, Eisenhardt L (1938) Meningiomas: Their classification, regional behaviour, life history and surgical end results. Charles C Thomas, Springfield, Illinois, pp 224–249, 298–319
10. David M, Mahoudeau D (1935) Les méningiomes de la petite alle du sphénoide (Considerations anatomo-cliniques et thérapeutiqués). Gazette Medical de France, pp 111–130
11. Dolenc VV (1979) Microsurgical removal of large sphenoidal bone meningiomas. Acta Neurochir (Wien) [Suppl] 28: 391–396
12. Fischer G, Fischer C, Mansuy L (1973) Pronostic chirurgical des méningiomas de l'arête sphénoïdale. Neurochirurgie 19: 323–346
13. Fohanno D, Bitar A (1986) Sphenoidal ridge meningioma. In: Symon L et al (eds) Advances and technical standards in neurosurgery, Vol 14. Springer, Wien New York, pp 137–174
14. Grant FC (1947) Intracranial meningiomas, surgical results. Surg Gynecol Obstet 85: 419–431
15. Guyot JF, Vouyouklakis D, Pertuiset B (1967) Méningiomes de l'arête sphénoïdale: A propos de 50 cas. Neurochirurgie (Paris) 13: 571–584
16. Jan M, Bazeze V, Saudeau D, Autret A, Bertrand P, Gouaze A (1986) Devenir des méningiomas intracrâniens chez l'adulte: Etude rétrospective d'une série medico-chirurgicale de 161 méningiomes. Neurochirurgie 32: 129–134
17. Kempe LG (1968) Sphenoid ridge meningioma. In: Operative neurosurgery, Vol 1. Springer, New York, pp 109–118
18. Konovalov AN, Fedorov SN, Faller TO, Sokolov AF, Tcherepanov AN (1979) Experience in the treatment of the parasellar meningiomas. Acta Neurochir (Wien) [Suppl] 28: 371–372
19. Koos WTh, Kletter G, Schuster H, Perneczky A (1975) Microsurgery of suprasellar meningiomas. Adv Neurosurg 2: 62–67

20. Mirimanoff RO, Dosoretz DE, Linggood RM, Ojemann RG, Martuza RL (1985) Meningioma: Analysis of recurrence and progression following neurosurgical resection. J Neurosurg 62: 18–24

21. Ojemann RG (1980) Meningiomas of the basal parapituitary region: Technical considerations. Clin Neurosurg 27: 233–262

22. Olivecrona H (1967) The surgical treatment of intracranial tumours. In: Olivecrona H, Tönnis W (eds) Handbuch der Neurochirurgie. Springer, Berlin Heidelberg New York, pp 1–301

23. Parent AD, Al-Mefty O (1988) Poster: Visual recovery after blindness from compressive optic neuropathy. American Association of Neurological Surgeons Annual Meeting, Toronto, Canada, 24–28 April

24. Pellerin P, Lesoin F, Dhellemmes P, Donazzan M, Jomin M (1984) Usefulness of the orbitofrontomalar approach associated with bone reconstruction for frontotemporosphenoid meningiomas. Neurosurgery 15: 715–718

25. Pompili A, Derome PJ, Visot A, Guiot G (1982) Hyperostosing meningiomas of the sphenoid ridge – clinical features, surgical therapy, and long-term observations: Review of 49 cases. Surg Neurol 17: 411–416

26. Probst C (1987) Possibilities and limitations of microsurgery in patients with meningiomas of the sellar region. Acta Neurochir (Wien) 84: 99–102

27. Sekhar LN, Sen CN, Jho HD, Janecka IP (1989) Surgical treatment of intracavernous neoplasms: A four-year experience. Neurosurgery 24: 18–30

28. Simpson D (1957) The recurrence of intracranial meningiomas after surgical treatment. J Neurol Neurosurg Psychiatry 20: 22–39

29. Symon L, Rosentein J (1984) Surgical management of suprasellar meningioma. Part I: The influence of tumor size, duration of symptoms, and microsurgery on surgical outcome in 101 consecutive cases. J Neurosurg 61: 633–641

30. Ugrumov VM, Ignatyeva GE, Olushin VE, Tigliev GS, Polenov AL (1979) Parasellar meningiomas: diagnosis and possibility of surgical treatment according to the place of original growth. Acta Neurochir (Wien) [Suppl] 28: 373–374

31. Uihlein A, Weyand RD (1953) Meningiomas of anterior clinoid process as a cause of unilateral loss of vision: surgical considerations. Arch Ophthalmol 49: 261–270

32. Yaşargil MG (1984) Operative anatomy. In: Microneurosurgery, Vol 1. Georg Thieme, New York, pp 26–32

Correspondence: Prof. O. Al-Mefty, M.D., Division of Neurological Surgery, Loyola University Medical Center, 2160 S. First Avenue Maywood, Illinois 60153, U.S.A.

Acta Neurochirurgica, Suppl. 53, 98–100 (1991)

Invading Meningiomas of Sphenoid Wing. What Must we Know Before Surgery?

J. Brotchi, M. Levivier, C. Raftopoulos, and **J. Noterman**

Department of Neurosurgery, Erasme Hospital, Free University of Brussels, Brussels, Belgium

Summary

Sphenoid wing meningiomas are very invasive tumours. The only permanent treatment is total eradication. But quality of life should also be taken into account. Several surgical approaches have been proposed with more and more aggressivity. We have raised a list of 9 questions which is not exhaustive. We recommend solving them before surgery and to be sure to have an answer before a surgical decision is made. This would be of great benefit for more efficacious results with less sequelae.

Keywords: Sphenoid wing meningioma.

Introduction

The removal of invading meningiomas of the sphenoid wing remains a challenge even in the hands of very skillful neurosurgeons[1,2,8]. The aim of this paper is not to present our results, which have been published elsewhere[3,4,5], but to emphasize some details which could have a major influence on the surgical results. Based on our personal experience of 93 cases, we shall ask some specific questions about which one must think and find answers before surgery.

What Must we Know Before Surgery?

1. *Is it a Meningioma?*

One must remember that the best neuroradiological investigation never gives a certainty about the histology. Some surprizes can happen. A cavernous angioma can mimic an intracavernous meningioma[7,8]. One must focus attention on the bony aspect. One must remember that meningiomas induce an hyperostotic bony reaction. So, if for example, the anterior clinoid process is missing, a metastasis rather than a meningioma must be suspected, as we have observed twice (Fig. 1).

2. *Blood Supply of the Tumour?*

The tumour may be vascularized by the external carotid artery only, by the internal carotid alone, or may be fed by both. It is very important to have a supraselective angiogram prior to surgery in order to discuss the possibility of pre-operative embolization. On the other hand, knowing all the feeding arteries, the surgeon may occlude them, without injuring by mistake any branch of the internal carotid artery.

3. *Meningioma-arterial Relationships?*

We know that an artery may be enveloped by the meningioma. The angiogram is unable to differentiate

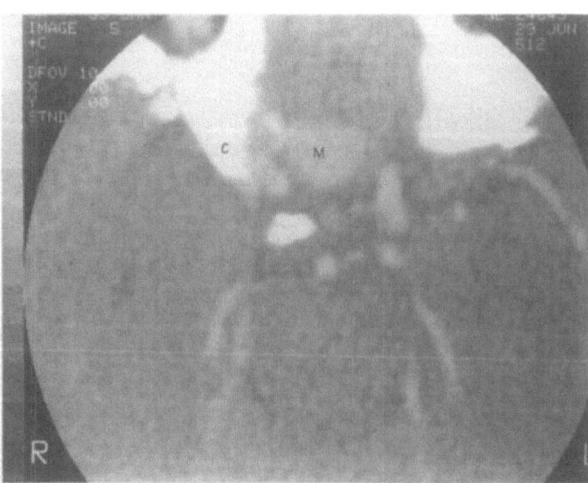

Fig. 1. Enhanced CT scan of a breast cancer metastasis (*M*) eroding the right anterior clinoid process (*C*) and simulating a meningioma

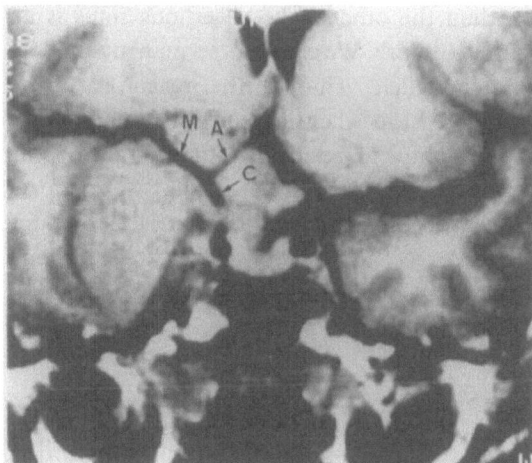

Fig. 2. Gadolinium enhanced MRI. Coronal view showing the internal carotid (C), anterior (A) and middle (M) cerebral arteries embedded within the meningioma

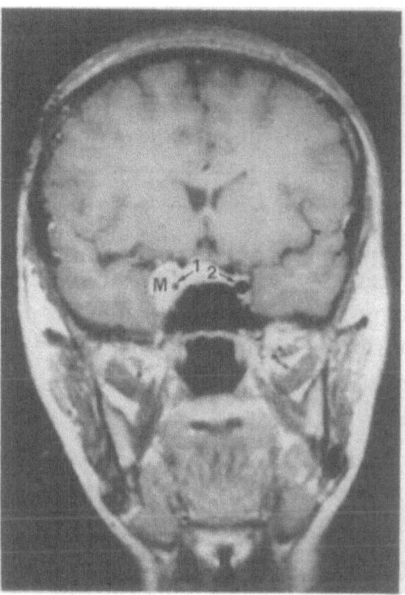

Fig. 3. Gadolinium enhanced MRI. Coronal view demonstrating normal left carotid artery (2) and narrow right carotid artery (1) due to a cavernous meningioma with a midline extension (M)

between a stretched or an encased artery. When a major vessel or its branches are shifted or stretched, great care must be taken in the surgical approach in order to avoid injury to the vessels. We have shown[3] that, when such an angiographic picture is associated with an ipsilateral loss of vision or optic atrophy, this is in favour of a deep-seated meningioma which surrounds the internal carotid artery. Prior to surgery, it is very important to know if the vessel is embedded or stretched only. Angiography is unable to give the answer. Stretched and encased vessels have the same angiographic profile[5]. Magnetic resonance imaging (MRI) is of great help, since it nicely shows the vessels inside and around the meningioma, thus providing great safety during the dissection. Moreover, the intracavernous carotid artery – meningioma relationships are well defined with gadolinium – enhanced MRI (Fig. 2).

4. Are the Optic Nerve and Tract Involved?

When there is some visual impairement, one may deduce that the meningioma has close relationships with the optic nerve or tract. Normal vision however does not mean that the tumour lies far away from the optic nerves. Again, gadolinium-enhanced MRI is able to give an answer, showing a tumoural extension in front of the optic chiasma, or on both sides of the optic nerves, in patients with normal vision.

It is of great benefit to know before surgery the potential intimity between the meningioma and the optic nerves in order to avoid visual postoperative sequelae.

5. Why Exophtalmia?

Exophtalmia may be due to bony hyperostosis, which actually means a bone invasion as we have shown previously[3]. It may be due either to an invasion of the orbit by the tumour, or to a cavernous sinus involvement. It is very important to know if the cavernous sinus is implicated. Its tumoural invasion may be encountered without any cranial nerve deficit. One must understand before surgery the cause of the exophtalmos. The combination of CT scan with bony windows and MRI in coronal views gives much information and very often the answer (Fig. 3).

6. Why Diplopia?

The two major causes are orbital and cavernous sinus invasion. But sometimes, diplopia may be due to a tumoural bud, as we have observed several times, herniated into the posterior fossa between the upper brain stem and the tentorial free edge. In such a situation, the fourth and the third cranial nerves may stick to the tumour. Careful dissection will avoid any nerve rupture, which may happen when the tumour is mobilized and one does not pay attention. Cautious investigations by the new generation CT scans nicely illustrate this trap[5].

7. *Extent of the Dural Invasion?*

The dural invasion may be very extensive in "en plaque" meningiomas, as in our groups B and C[3]. Gadolinium enhanced MRI nicely shows an hyperintense zone of the dura, which most of the time corresponds to the tumoural invasion. However, enhancement does not necessarily mean invasion. It could be only hypervascularization. Sekhar (10) has made extensive biopsies and in several cases has not found any tumour. That means that today we are unable to answer this question. We need better radiological definitions.

8. *Extent of the Skull Base and Cranio-facial Cavities Invasion?*

With the development of new surgical approaches[1,2,6,9,11], we see that surgical limits are extending. Coronal sections (CT Scan, MRI) are the best way to see the extent of a cranio-facial cavities invasion. Since hyperostotic bone means bone invaded by the meningioma, it should always be removed by a wide margin to avoid recurrence. It is therefore important to assess the extent of the bone lesion. Moreover, it is important, before surgery, to know if the sphenoid sinus is involved, in order to manage surgery without any CSF leakage.

9. *How Much Do we Succeed in the Total Removal of the Tumour While Respecting the Quality of Life?*

Firstly, by answering the eight previous questions berfore surgery. It is better to raise these questions before operation than after disappointing surgery. We recommend to try to eradicate these tumours at the first surgical procedure. Total removal must be our aim. But, quality of life depends on the surgeon's experience. Those who have a great mastership of skull base tumour surgery will be able to go further with

less risk than the others. The cavernous sinus is an important landmark. We consider permanent diplopia as a major deficit. That is the reason why we recommend to stop when it is obviously impossible to make a complete removal without injuring the cranial nerves. In such a situation, we perform radiosurgery on the small residual part of the tumour in order to respect the quality of life of the patient, even if today, it is too early to draw any conclusion on the efficacy of such a policy.

References

1. Al-Mefty O (1986) The supraorbital-pterional approach to skull base lesions. Neurosurgery 21: 474–477
2. Al-Mefty O (1989) Surgical technique for the juxtasellar area. In: Al-Mefty O (ed) Surgery of the cranial base. Kluwer Academic Publishers, Boston, pp 73–89
3. Bonnal J, Thibaut A, Brotchi J, Born J (1980) Invading meningiomas of the sphenoid ridge. J Neurosurg 53: 587–599
4. Bonnal J, Brotchi J, Born J (1987) Meningiomas of the sphenoid wings. In: Sekhar LN, Schramm VL Jr (eds) Tumours of the cranial base: diagnosis and treatment. Mount Kisco, Futura Publishing, New York, pp 373–392
5. Brotchi J, Bonnal J (1991) Lateral and middle sphenoid wings Meningiomas. In: Al-Mefty O (ed) Meningiomas. Raven Press, New York, pp 413–425
6. Derome PJ, Visot A (1987) Bony lesions of the anterior and middle cranial fossa. In: Sekhar LN, Schramm VL (eds) Tumours of the cranial base: diagnosis and treatment. Mount Kisco, Futura Publishing, New York, pp 295–309
7. Meyer FB, Lombardi D, Scheithauer B, Nichols DA (1990) Extra-axial cavernous hemangiomas involving the dural sinuses. J Neurosurg 73: 187–192
8. Rigamonti D, Pappas CTE, Spetzler RF, Johnson PC (1990) Extracerebral cavernous angiomas of the middle fossa. Neurosurgery 27: 306–310
9. Samii M (1989) Surgery of space-occupying lesions of the middle skull base. In: Samii M, Draf W (eds) Surgery of the skull base. Springer, Berlin Heidelberg New York, pp 273–358
10. Sekhar LN (1990) Personal communication
11. Sekhar LN, Schramm VL, Jones NF (1987) Subtemporal-preauricular infratemporal fossa approach to large lateral and posterior cranial base neoplasms. J Neurosurg 67: 488–499

Correspondence: Prof. J. Brotchi, Department of Neurosurgery, Erasme Hospital, Free University of Brussels, route de Lennik 808, B-1070 Brussels, Belgium.

Acta Neurochirurgica, Suppl. 53, 101–112 (1991)
© by Springer-Verlag 1991

Management of Tumours Involving the Cavernous Sinus

L. N. Sekhar, Sh. Pomeranz, and **Ch. N. Sen**

Department of Neurological Surgery, University of Pittsburgh School of Medicine, Pittsburgh, Pennsylvania, U.S.A.

Summary

The operative experience with 137 tumours of the cavernous sinus at the University of Pittsburgh during the past 7 years is reported. The importance of the normal and tumour-infiltrated cavernous sinus anatomy and imaging is delineated. 63% of the tumours are benign, primarily meningiomas, for which an anatomical grading system is presented. The various operative approaches to the cavernous sinus are described. 88% of the meningiomas were totally resected. There was a 1.5% operative mortality and 1.5% severe morbidity rate. Initial ipsilateral opthalmoplegia progressively improved in the majority of patients. For all patients with at least 6 months of follow up of benign tumours, the intracavernous tumour recurrence rate was 3% and total recurrence rate was 6%.

Keywords: Cavernous sinus; tumour; operative approaches; internal carotid artery.

Introduction

The cavernous sinus (CS) contains an intricate combination of important blood vessels and cranial nerves. This anatomy, together with the location of the CS relative to the brain, adjacent blood vessels and nerves, and the cranial base have historically made this region a surgical no-man's land. Improved understanding of this anatomy[13,22,24,28,29], better imaging modalities[14], knowledge of CS pathology[12,14,30,37,38,39], and evolving neurosurgical experience[23,25,27,30] have led to numerous publication in the last decade describing successful surgery of CS lesions. Today several groups world-wide regularly operate on CS lesions[1,4,5,6,10,11,16,31,34]. This paper will outline our experience with 137 tumours of the CS during the years 1983–1990. During the same period, exposure of the CS was performed during the management of approximately 25 aneurysms of the internal carotid artery or the basilar artery. These are not discussed in this article.

Anatomy

The CS anatomy has been described[12,13,14,15,22,29,30,32,37,38,39]. The dural/periosteal walls of the CS border the sphenoid sinus and sella turcica medially, the petrous bone apex posteriorly, the middle cranial fossa floor inferiorly, Meckel's cave and the medial aspect of the temporal lobe laterally, and the carotico-optic arachnoidal cisterns superiorly (Fig. 1). Anteriorly the CS is continuous with the superior orbital fissure and orbital apex. Between the lateral sinus wall layers are cranial nerves (CN) III,

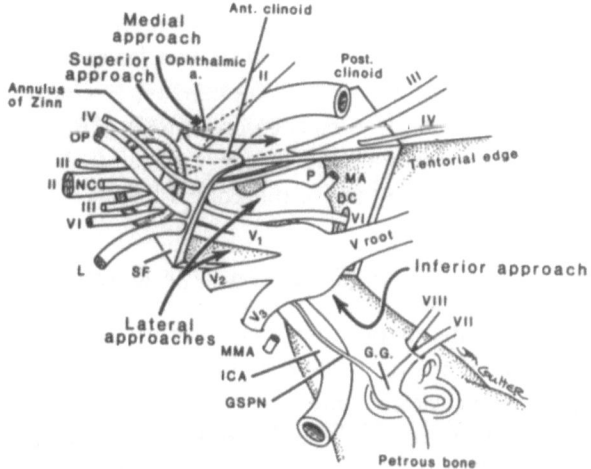

Fig. 1. Scheme of cavernous sinus as viewed from anterio-superiolaterally. The relationship of the cavernous sinus to the Gasserian ganglion orbital apex and petrous apex can be seen. The inferior, lateral, and superior surgical approaches to the cavernous sinus are demonstrated with arrows. *II–VIII* cranial nerves, *ICA* internal carotid artery, *MMA* middle meningeal artery, *MA* meningohypophyseal artery, *P* pituitary gland, *DC* Dorello's canal, *GSPN* greater superficial petrosal nerve, *GG* geniculate ganglion, *SF* superior orbital fissure, *NC* naso ciliary nerve, *L* lacrinal nerve. (With permission)

IV, V_1, and usually V_2. Within the CS are CN VI entering through Dorello's canal and the sympathetic branch which accompanies the internal carotid artery in the petrous bone.

The internal carotid artery (ICA) lies within the CS in a "S" shaped configuration. The ICA is anchored by three periosteal or dural rings at the entrance and exit from the CS. The intracavernous ICA gives off the meningohypophyseal trunk, and the inferolateral trunk, and occasionally, a capsular artery, the ophthalmic artery, and other unnamed vessels. Most of the CS volume is a venous plexus with rich collaterals that cross the midline around the pituitary gland. This plexus communicates anteriorly with the ophthalmic veins and posteriorly with the petrosal sinuses and the basilar plexus of veins. The venous plexus may contain smaller and larger caliber vessels, the latter leading to the erroneous impression of a "sinus".

Imaging

Magnetic resonance imaging (MRI) is the prime modality for demonstrating CS lesions[14]. It is the only modality that can demonstrate with high resolution the relationship between tumour and the internal carotid artery (ICA) and is the most sensitive for demonstrating minute lesions. Thin section computerized tomography with "bone windows" demonstrate the osseous anatomy and calcifications. CT scans with soft tissue algorithms are useful for postoperative follow up. Cerebral angiography is best for assessing the vascular configuration of CS lesions and is required for CS lesion interventional neuroradiology. MRI, CT, and angiography are complementary and all three are needed for optimal visualization of CS lesions[14].

Pre-operative Functional Assessment of the ICA

75% of the population can tolerate prolonged occlusion of one ICA. The rest may suffer a minor or major stroke within minutes to years of the occlusion and even death[2,4,9,20,40]. In addition, secondary increased flow in the contralateral ICA predisposes to aneurysm formation, growth, and rupture in that vessel[6,8].

Since any CS surgery has a significant probability of temporary or permanent ICA occlusion, it is important to assess the patient's tolerance of such an occlusion preoperatively. The traditional Matas test[17,18,19] of manually compressing the cervical vessels by external pressure is inadequate. The degree

of occlusion and which vessels (common carotid, ICA, external carotid, or a combination thereof) are occluded are unknown. In addition, beyond the 10% of patients who have clinical cerebral ischemia within 15 minutes of unilateral ICA occlusion, 15% will have significantly decreased cerebral blood flows (CBF) of below 30 cc/100 g/min during the test, with an increased probability of delayed cerebral ischemic phenomena[3,18,21].

The patients planned for CS surgery at our center undergo a 15 minute balloon test occlusion (BTO) of the ipsilateral ICA. The balloon is immediately deflated if any clinical expression of cerebral ischemia is observed, and the patient is considered to have failed the test (high risk group). If there were no clinical manifestations, a CT stable xenon CBF is performed before and after balloon occlusion. Patients having a CBF of less than 30 cc/100 g/min on balloon occlusion are considered to belong to a moderate risk group and those having higher flows constitue a low risk group[7,30]. This information allows preoperative evaluation of the risk of CS surgery, intraoperative preparation for brain protection, and planning of alternative revascularization in the event of ICA occlusion.

Cavernous Sinus Tumours

The histology of the 137 operated CS tumours is outlined in Table 1. Approximately 40 patients with intracavernous lesions were evaluated during the same period and were not operated since they failed to meet

Table 1. *Surgical Management of Cavernous Sinus Neoplasms 1983–1990*
Histology: Total 137

Benign tumors		Malignant tumors	
Meningioma	60	Meningioma	3
Neurilemmona	12	Pituitary adenoma	8
Juvenile angiofibroma	6	Chordoma	12
Craniopharyngioma	1	Chondrosarcoma	12
Epidermoid cyst	2	Adenoid cystic Ca	5
Chondroblastoma	1	Osteosarcoma	2
Teratoma	1	Squamous cell Ca	4
Hemangioma	3	Basal cell Ca	1
	—	Malignant melanoma	1
	86	Plasmacytoma	1
		Malignant fibrous histocytoma	1
		Hypernephroma	1
			—
			51

Table 2. *Classification of Intracavernous Neoplasms* (From Reference 30)

Grade	Cavernous sinus involvement	Intracavernous ICA
I	One area only (A, P, L, or M)	Not involved
II	More than one area	Displaced, not totally encased
III	Entire CS	Totally encased, at least a short length
IV	Entire CS	Encased, with narrowing, pseudoaneurysm or occlusion
V	Bilateral CS	Encased

Abbreviations: ICA, = Internal Carotid Artery, A = Anterior, P = Posterior, L = Lateral, M = Medial, CS = Cavernous Sinus.

our criteria for an operation. Sixty-three percent of the operated tumours are benign, primarily meningiomas (44% of total), neurilemmomas and juvenile angiofibromas. Chondrosarcomas and chordomas are the predominant low grade malignancies, composing 17% of the total. Basal and squamous cell carcinoma and metastatic neoplasm are the commonest high grade malignancies, and in general, were rare lesions in this series. In some patients, the histology was unsuspected preoperatively.

Tumour spread within the CS is classified anatomically[30] into four regions (anterior, posterior, lateral and medial) and according to the relationship of the tumours to the ICA (from not involved to totally encased) to give a grading of I–V (Table 2)[30]. The higher graded meningiomas are technically more difficult to remove, and had a higher recurrence rate prior to the use of ICA vein grafting. Tumour spread outside the CS in the imaging modalities should be observed when planning surgery. Specifically in the smaller meningiomas it can often be determined whether the tumour originated from within or outside the cavernous sinus, the latter group being significantly easier to resect.

The indication for resection of benign CS tumours is progressive growth observed on imaging studies and/or progression of cranial nerve deficits. The management decisions regarding the ICA are based on the preoperative BTO, and have been previously published[30]. The BTO high risk group with tumour configuration suggesting complete encasement of the intracavernous ICA are poor surgical candidates. In such cases, when surgery is strongly indicated, it may be undertaken with ICA revascularization[35], under brain protection with moderate hypothermia

(30–33°C) and barbiturate or Etomidate induced coma.

Low grade malignancies such as chondrosarcomas and chordomas are usually soft, do not generally invade vascular and neural structures, and are relatively easier to resect from the CS. Intracavernous operation to remove these tumours is performed if total removal is a goal of the operation. During the removal of these tumours, it is justifiable to enter both cavernous sinuses if necessary, if total tumour resection can be accomplished.

The removal of high grade malignancies involving CS is attempted in an en bloc fashion, without entering the cavernous sinus. It can be done if the CS is involved unilaterally, and the resection includes all tumour tissue. The ICA may be reconstructed if necessary[35]. Such surgery is undertaken as part of a treatment regimen that includes adjuvant therapy. Bilateral CS invasion by such malignancies precludes operative resection.

Anesthesia, Monitoring, and Positioning

General endotracheal anesthesia is performed with an inhalation agent to allow intraoperative neurophysiological monitoring. A constant infusion of sodium pentothal at 2 mg/Kg/min decreases the need for inhalational anesthetics and appears to relax the brain.

Somatosensory evoked potentials, auditory brain stem evoked potentials, electroencephalography, and electromyographic monitoring of functioning cranial nerves III and VI are routinely performed. When intraoperative occlusion of the ICA performed on high or medium risk BTO group patients, electroencephalographic burst suppression is attained with thiopental or etomidate coma, and arterial hypertension is induced (30–40 torr).

The patients are positioned supine, with the head turned 45° contralaterally and moderately raised so that it is above the heart. The neck is slightly extended.

Operative Technique

The key elements of the operation include: a basal approach to minimize brain retraction, adequate tumour exposure, proximal and distal ICA control, complete tumour resection including from within the cavernous sinus, vascular and cranial nerve reconstruction as needed, and cranial base reconstruction to prevent cerebrospinal fluid leakage.

Proximal control of the ICA may be attained either cervically or in the horizontal petrous bone segment[33], the latter being more difficult but necessary for a graft ICA reconstruction or when the petrous bone is invaded by tumour.

The skin incision is either bicoronal or frontotemporal, extending below the zygomatic arch close to the external ear canal (Fig. 2). A frontotemporal craniotomy is followed by an orbito-zygomatic osteotomy. The orbital roof is resected extradurally anterior to the anterior clinoid process and the optic canal. The zygomatic osteotomy is anterior to the condylar fossa if ICA reconstruction is not needed, but includes the condylar fossa, if saphenous vein graft reconstruction of the cavernous ICA is planned. Extradural middle fossa dissection is performed to identify and divide the greater superficial petrosal nerve (GSPN) and the middle meningeal artery (MMA) and to identify and unroof the mandibular (V_3) and maxillary (V_2) nerves at the foramen ovale and rotundum respectively. the horizontal petrous ICA is exposed posteromedial to V_3, medial to the MMA, and inferior to the GSPN under the microscope utilizing a micro-drill and fine rongeurs[29,31,34]. Exposure of the remainder of the petrous ICA requires the opening of the temporo-mandibular joint with excision of the mandibular condyle and eustachian tube, and is performed for tumours with extensive petroclival bone involvement.

The CS may be entered extradurally or intradurally (Figs. 1 and 3). The extradural approaches are appropriate for extradural tumours (i.e., petrous apex, sphenoid, or clival) with a relatively small intracavernous portion so that these resections are primarily directed at the extracavernous portion. The *inferior extradural approach* follows the petrous ICA into the cavernous sinus. The *anterolateral extradural approach* follows the divisions of the trigeminal nerve into the CS. The *medial extradural approach* is either through the sphenoid sinus in a basal frontal (Fig. 2 d) or through the sella turcica around the pituitary gland if tumour resection is followed from one CS to the contralateral CS.

An intradural approach (Fig. 3) is utilized for tumours that are predominantly within the CS, tumours that have a large intradural component, and all meningiomas. If the intradural tumour is small, upon opening the dura the optic nerve and supraclinoid ICA are initially exposed and then the Sylvian fissure is split. For large tumours, the Sylvian fissure is split initially to avoid injury to tumour encased or displaced ICA or middle cerebral artery (MCA), and the MCA branches are followed medially. If excessive temporal lobe retraction will be required for tumour exposure, the anterior 2 centimeters of the inferior temporal gyrus is resected to minimize retraction and postoperative temporal lobe swelling. The subdural portion of the tumour is resected before approaching the CS.

In the *superior approach* (Fig. 4 a), the optic canal is unroofed, the anterior clinoid process resected, and the dural sleeve along the optic nerve opened. The dural rings anchoring the ICA at its exit from the CS are incised. The CS is entered medial to CN III to give good exposure of the superior and medial CS including those aspects of the horizontal intracavernous ICA and the anterior genu. Venous bleeding is controlled by packing with oxidized cellulose, and if necessary, elevation of the head.

In the *lateral approach* the CS is entered between CN III and IV, CN IV and V_1 (Parkinson's triangle) or between V_1 and V_2. For tumours that are readily dissectable from the involved nerves and vessels (chordoma, chondrosarcoma, and neurilemmona) a horizontal incision in the outer layer of the cavernous sinus wall is made, the outer layer partially peeled away, and a vertical incision is made crossing the initial incision. CN IV may be exposed directly between the CS wall layers but CN III is better initially exposed at its entry or exit from the sinus wall. A *trans-trigeminal approach* is sometimes necessary, between the rootlets of CN V, or after splitting the trigeminal ganglion between V_2 and V_3 or between V_1 and V_2. This exposes the blind spot in the CS medial to the trigeminal nerve.

The ICA and CN VI are also more easily exposed and dissected if they can be traced into the CS rather than initially found within the sinus. Electromyographic monitoring of the extraocular muscles can assist in locating CN VI within the CS. In resecting meningiomas, which tend to adhere to the nerves and vessels and are more fibrous in consistency, the lateral CS wall is completely excised before continuing tumour resection within the CS.

In Grade III or IV meningiomas, when the ICA is encased, it must often be excised to insure total tumour resection. Simple lacerations of the ICA may be directly sutured, usually under temporary trapping, but significant ICA injuries must be patch repaired, grafted, or the artery sacrificed (Fig. 4).

We utilize the saphenous vein of the thigh as a graft between the horizontal petrous ICA (end-to-end) and

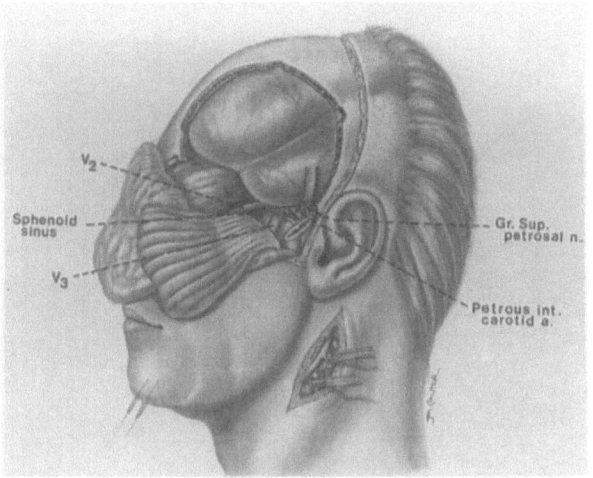

Fig. 2 a. Following elevation of the carniotomy flap, an orbito-zygomatic osteotomy is performed and resection of the infratemporal bone to mobilize CN V$_2$ and V$_3$. (With permission)

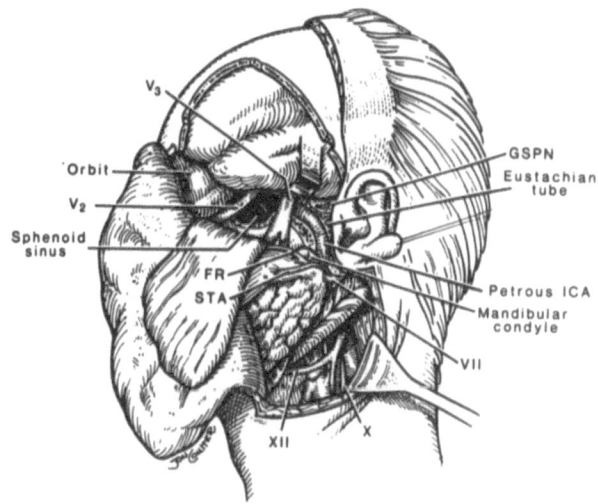

Fig. 2 b. The scalp and cervical incisions may be united, exposing the extracranial CN VII and mandibular condyle, which can be disarticulated and resected to provide additional exposure. The greater superficial petrosal nerve (*GSPN*) is found extradurally on the floor of the middle fossa and transected to avoid traction on the geniculate ganglion. The GSPN serves as a guide for locating the horizontal petrous internal carotid artery (*ICA*) which is under the nerve. To expose the curve of the vertical petrous ICA to become the horizontal petrous ICA the eustachian tube must be transected. The frontal branch of CN VII (*FR*) and the superficial temporal artery (*STA*) can be seen. (With permission)

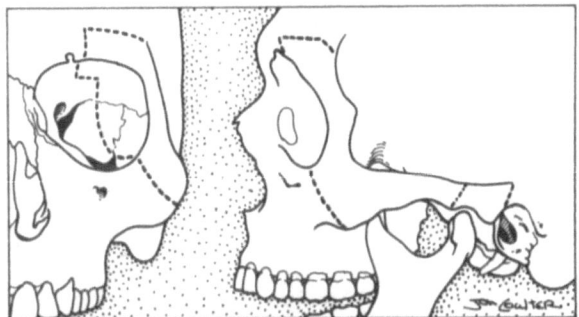

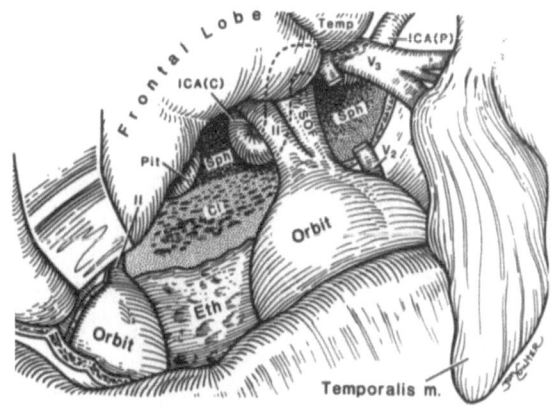

Fig. 2 d. Frontobasal view following bifrontal craniotomy and biorbital-zygomatic osteotomy demonstrating an extradural medial approach to the cavernous sinus. *C* cavernous, *P* petrous, *Pit* pituitary gland, *Sph* sphenoid sinus, *Eth* ethnoid sinuses, *Temp* temporal lobe. (With permission)

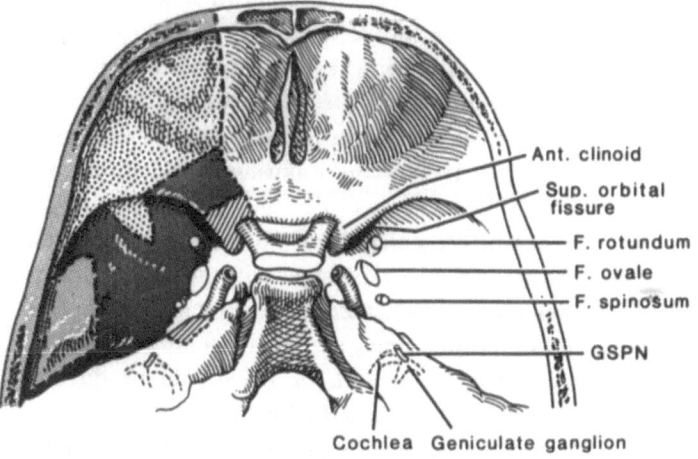

Craniotomy
Cut
Drilled
Rongeured

Fig. 2 c. Extent of orbitozygomatic osteotomy (insets: anterior and lateral views) and the bone resection of anterior and middle fossa floors

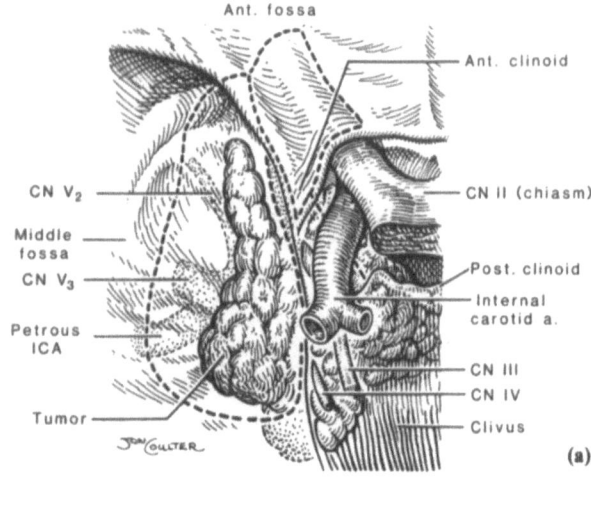

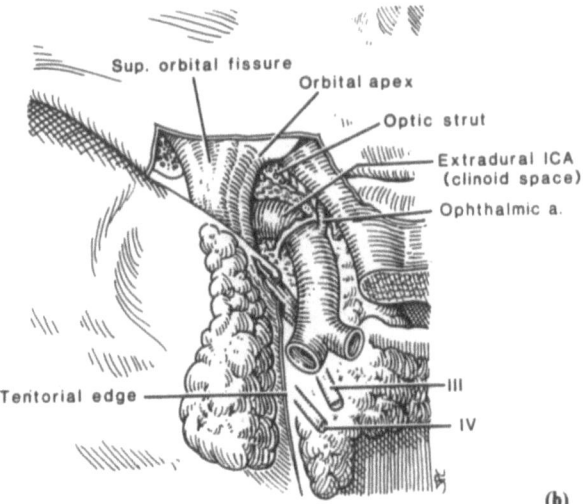

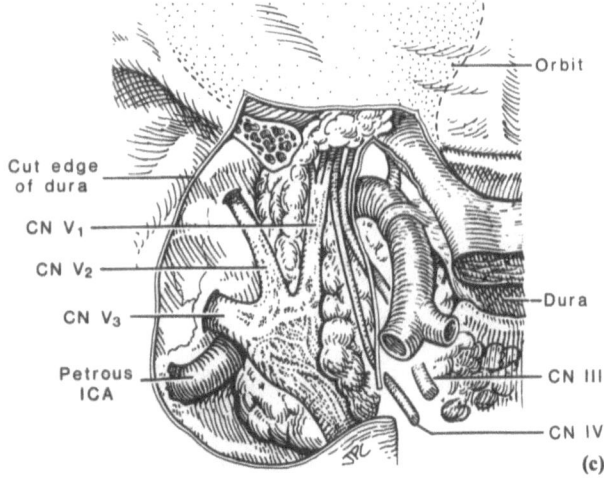

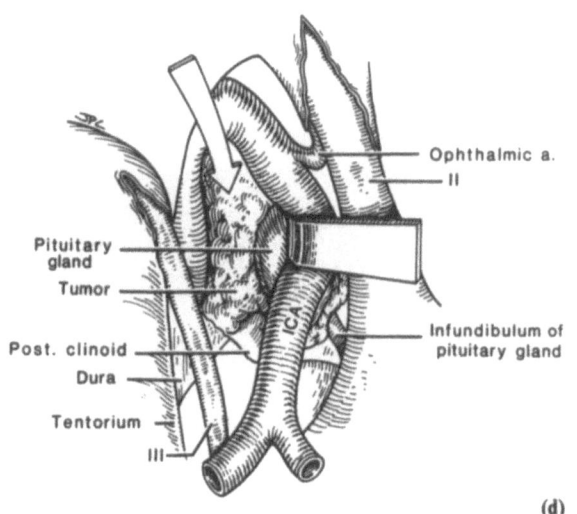

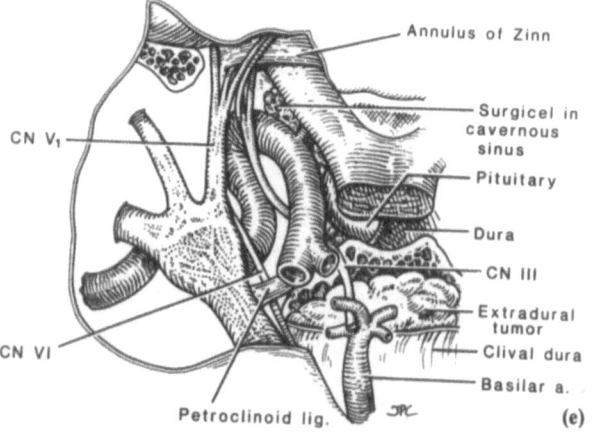

Fig. 3. The steps in approaching a benign cavernous sinus tumour after splitting the Sylvian fissure. a) Resection of the dura and underlying anterior clinoid (*dotted lines*) and lateral cavernous sinus wall (*dotted lines*). b) Resection of the optic strut and exposure of the orbital apex. c) Piecemeal resection of the tumour to expose CN V and its branches, CN III, and CN IV. d) A schematic view of the superior approach (*arrow*) to a cavernous sinus tumour. e) Completion of tumour resection to expose the intracavernous ICA and CN VI. (With permission)

the supraclinoid ICA (usually end-to-side), to provide retrograde perfusion of the ophthalmic artery. The vessel is sutured with 8–0 nylon or 7–0 prolene interrupted sutures. This technique was first developed in anatomical studies by Sekhar *et al.*, and subsequently used patients by Fukushima and by Sekhar *et al.*[29,35,36].

Following completion of the tumour resection within the CS any extensions into adjacent regions (i.e., sella turcica, sphenoid sinus, orbital apex, controlateral cavernous sinus, upper clivus) are resected.

Lacerated CN V_1, VI, or III should be directly anastomosed or cable grafted with a sural nerve or a greater auricular nerve segment. CN IV loss usually produces minimal deficits and is not generally reconstructed unless it can be easily performed.

Difficult cavernous sinus tumour resections, especially with ICA grafts, are often staged to avoid performing the critical parts of surgery when the

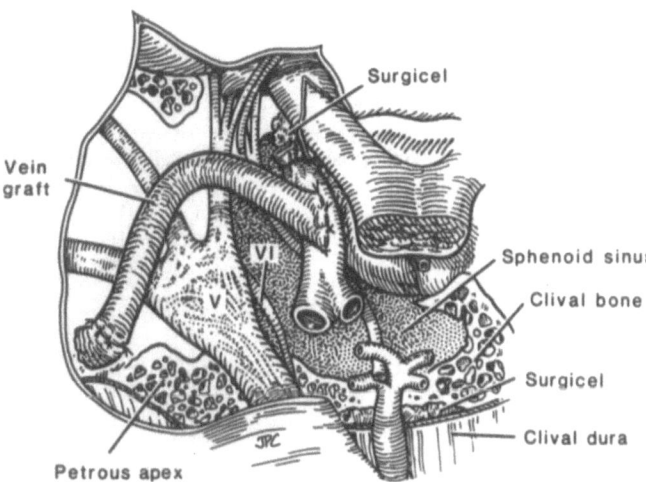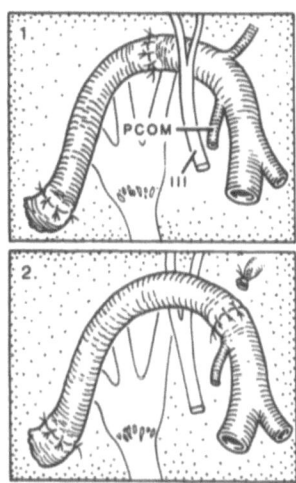

Fig. 4 a. If the tumour infiltrates or encases the ICA, the artery may be resected and a saphenous vein graft interposed between the petrous ICA (end-to-end) and supraclinoid ICA (end-to-side) to maintain ophthalmic artery flow. (With permission). Insets: Variations of the distal vein graft – ICA anastomosis. *1* End-to-end proximal to the ophthalmic artery (often impractical due to ICA invasion by the tumour in the CS). *2* End-to-end with exclusion of the ophthalmic artery

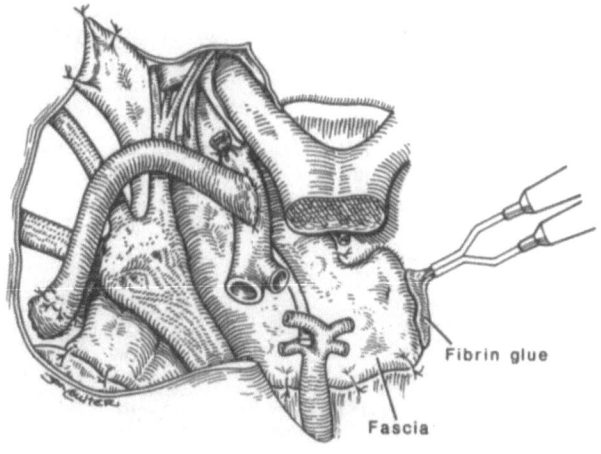

Fig. 4 b. Reconstruction: to prevent cerebrospinal fluid leakage via the sphenoid sinus, a fascia lata graft is tacked down and its edges sealed with fibrin glue

surgeon is exhausted. The completion of the operation is usually performed approximately two weeks following the first stage.

The primary objective of cranial base reconstruction following the resection of CS tumours is to avoid CSF leakage with the danger of ensuing infection (Fig. 4 b). The sites of possible leakage are the eustachian tube, the facial air sinuses, the middle ear and the naso-pharynx. If the eustachian tube has been opened it is packed with fat and suture tied. The air sinuses are stripped of mucosa and packed with fat. Dural defects are closed with fascia lata or pericranium. Dural gaps that cannot be sutured closed are packed with fat. The temporalis muscle can be rotated

subtemporally to fill a large defect infratemporally and/or in the sphenoid sinus. A large bifrontal peri-cranial or galeopericranial vascularized flap should be rotated subfrontally to line the sphenoid sinus if a large opening into it is present at the end of the operation. The defect is thus closed by three layers: pericranium, autologous fat, and free fascial graft.

Postoperative Care

The initial postoperative care is in an intensive care unit, the majority of the patients being extubated soon after the operation. When barbiturate coma is utilized for brain protection, the patient may take up to 72 hours to be fully awake and extubated.

A CT scan is attained on the first postoperative day and before discharge. An ICA arteriogram is usually performed before discharge. Periodic MRI or CT scans are the primary means of follow up imaging after discharge. Vein grafts are followed with MRI angiography.

Outcome – Cavernous Sinus Tumours

The spectrum of the types and frequency of the 137 CS tumours in our series are listed in Table 1. Many of the meningiomas involved areas other than the cavernous sinus (Table 3). Of the 137 CS tumours, 52 of the 60 benign meningiomas were totally resected from all areas as seen via the operative microscope and postoperative imaging (MRI or CT) (Table 3)[32]. Residual tumour found on postoperative imaging was

Table 3. *Benign Cavernous Sinus Neoplasms 1983–1990.*
Extent of Resection *vs* Recurrence or Regrowth

Neoplasm	Number	Cavernous sinus only				All areas			
		Total (recurrence)		Partial (regrowth)		Total (recurrence)		Partial (regrowth)	
Meningioma	60	56	(1)	4	(1)	52	(2)	8	(1)
Neurilemmona	12	12	(0)	–	–	11	(0)	1	(1)
Juvenile angiofibroma	6	6	(0)	–	–	5	(0)	1	(0)
Chondroblastoma	1	1	(0)	–	–	1	(0)	–	–
Hemangioma	3	3	(0)	–	–	3	(0)	–	–
Craniopharyngioma	1	1	(0)	–	–	1	(0)	–	–
Teratoma	1	1	(0)	–	–	1	(0)	–	–
Epidermoid cyst	2	2	(0)	–	–	2	(0)	–	–
Total	86	82	(1)	4	(1)	76	(2)	10	(2)

Table 4. *Maligant Cavernous Sinus Neoplasms 1983–1990.*
Extent of Resection *vs* Recurrence or Regrowth

Neoplasm	Number	Cavernous sinus only				All areas			
		Total (recurrence)		Partial (regrowth)		Total (recurrence)		Partial (regrowth)	
Meningioma	3	2	(0)	1	(0)	2	(0)	1	(0)
Pituitary adenoma	7	5	(0)	2	(0)	4	(0)	3	–
Chordoma	12	8	(1)	4	(3)	7	(2)	5	(3)
Chondrosarcoma	10	10	(0)	2	(0)	8	(0)	4	(0)
Adenoid cystic carcinoma	5	3	(0)	2	–	3	(1)	2	(1)
Basal cell carcinoma	1	1	(0)	–	–	–	–	1	(0)
Squamous cell carcinoma	5	2	(0)	3	(0)	2	(2)	3	(1)
Osteogenic sarcoma	2	2	(0)	–	–	2	(2)	–	–
Malignant fibrous histiocytoma	1	–	(0)	1	(0)	–	–	1	(0)
Plasmacytoma	1	–	–	1	(0)	–	–	1	(0)
Malignant melanoma	1	–	(0)	1	(1)	–	–	1	(1)
Hypernephroma (metastatic)	1	1	(0)	–	–	1	(0)	–	(0)
Total	49	34	(2)	17	(6)	29	(8)	22	(6)

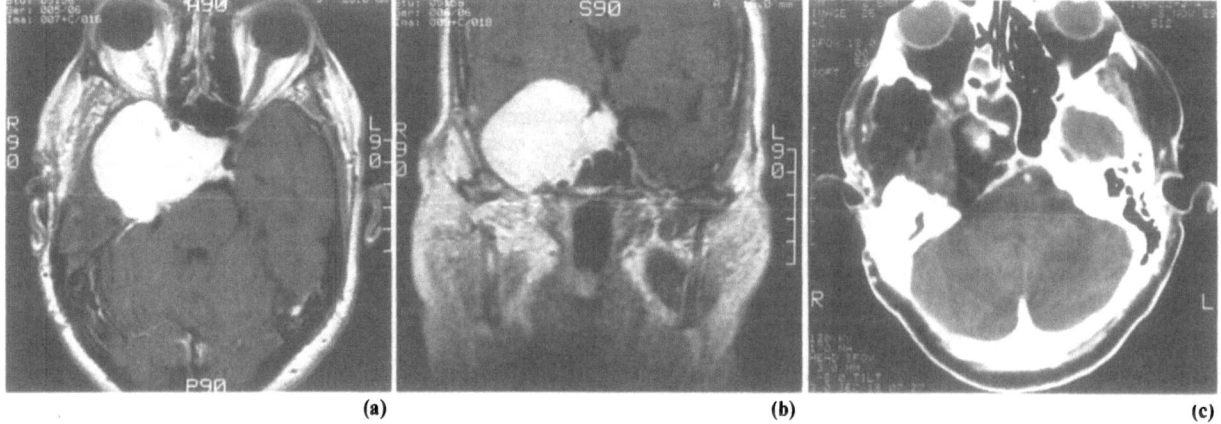

(a)　　　　　　　　　　　(b)　　　　　　　　　　　(c)

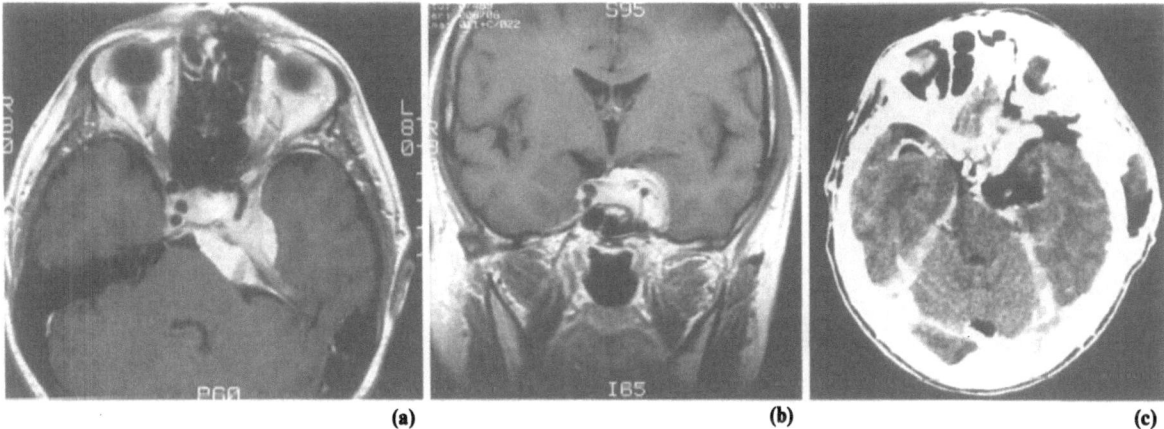

(a) (b) (c)

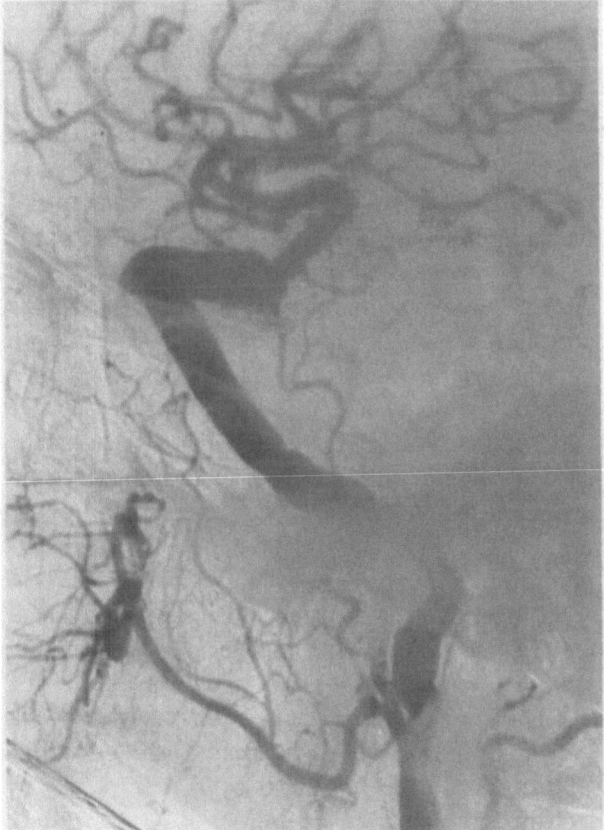

(d)

Fig. 6. G.W., 49-year-old woman with Grade IV cavernous sinus meningioma (ICA totally encased and narrowed). a) Preoperative axial and b) coronal T_1 weighted MRI with intravenous gadolinium. The cavernous ICA flow voids are prominent. c) Axial contrast enhanced CT demonstrating total tumour resection and the enhancing graft. The sphenoid sinus is packed with fat. d) Lateral angiogram of the graft

usually outside the cavernous sinus. Surgical experience and resection of the intracavernous ICA have decreased the frequency of residual CS tumours. Small residual tumour outside the CS was often treated by gamma knife radiotherapy. Tumour recurrence was treated by surgery with or without radiotherapy. In surgery on patients that had undergone previous surgery or radiotherapy, the ability to preserve cavernous region cranial nerve function was prominently diminished. Of the 49 malignant tumours, in 34, total initial CS resection was achieved, and in 29, total tumour resections was attained in all areas (Table 4). Chordomas and chondrosarcomas that underwent complete resection received no adjuvant therapy. All other malignant tumours received external beam radiotherapy. The squamous cell carcinomas progressed in spite of this combined treatment, whereas for the other malignant tumours this course of treatment appears promising.

Representative cases demonstrating the management of CS neoplasms are presented in Figs. 5–7.

The complications related to all 137 patients that underwent cavernous sinus tumour surgery are listed in Table 5. Two patients died, one of a hemispheric stroke. Two patients had minor cerebral infarctions with total resolution of their ensuing symptoms. Six patients had transient cerebral ischemia. The utilization of "cerebral protective" means during prolonged ICA clamping has virtually eliminated this complication. Three patients had temporal lobe edema, probably secondary to excessive retraction.

Fig. 5. G.G., 62 years old woman with Grade II cavernous sinus (ICA displaced but not totally encased) and middle cranial fossa meningioma. This patient had undergone previous tumour debulking and suboccipital craniectomy with section of CN VIII for vertigo. a) Preoperative axial and b) coronal T_1 weighted MRI following intravenous gadolinium administration, both cavernous ICAs are well visualized as black flow voids. c) Postoperative axial CT with intravenous contrast. The frontotemporal craniotomy can be seen, an orbitozygomatic osteotomy was also done as an approach. No evidence of tumour residual. The sphenoid sinus is packed with fat

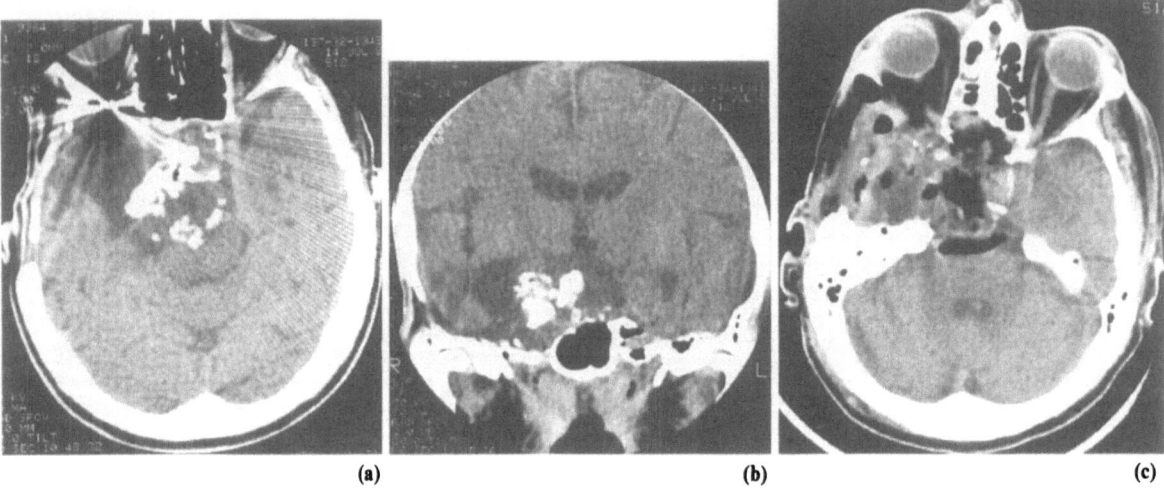

(a)   **(b)**   **(c)**

Fig. 7. J.O., 47 year old man with cavernous sinus and clivus chordoma following previous partial resection. a) Preoperative axial and b) coronal CT demonstrating tumour calcification. c) Postoperative axial CT demonstrating tumour resection

Table 5. *Operated Cavernous Sinus Tumours 1983–1990 Surgical Complications (137 Cases)*

Death (ICA dissection; sepsis and pulmonary embolism)	2
Cerebral infarction	
superior cerebellar artery occlusion, small infarct	1
Postoperative vasospasm, small caudate infarct	1
Cerebral ischemia	
temporary hemiparesis/aphasia, <1 week, no infarct	6
Hematomas	
frontal	1 (evacuated)
subdural	1 (evacuated)
Brain edema	
Temporal lobe	2
Temporal lobe herniation 2° excessive CSF drainage	1 (reoperation)
CSF leak	
Wound	2
Sphenoid sinus	10 (8 reoperations)
Eustachian tube	2 (1 reoperation)
External ear canal	1 (reoperation)
Infections	
meningitis – following CSF leak	3
meningitis – without CSF leak	2
wound infection with carotid pseudoaneurysm	1
pneumonia	1
Seizures, postoperative	2
Diabetes insipidus, transient	6
Deep vein thrombophlebitis	2
Pulmonary embolism	4
Outcome of Surgical Complications	
Death	2
Disabled, requiring, assistance in daily life	2

All the major complications of CS surgery occurred in patients who had been previously operated on or had been previously irradiated. This indicates that the risks of cavernous sinus operation are much less in "virgin" tumours. Unfortunately, at least a third of the patients we treat have had prior incomplete resection or irradiation.

Fifteen patients had cerebrospinal fluid leakage and 3 of these developed meningitis. In 10 patients the leak was via the sphenoid sinus, 7 requiring a second operation to seal the leak. Two patients had leakage through the eustachian tube, one requiring reoperation. Two leaks via the operative wound resolved spontaneously and one through the external ear canal required reoperation. CSF leakage was more common when the tumour resection involved opening of the sphenoid sinus, in repeat operations, and following radiation, and was often associated with disturbed CSF absorption as expressed by hydrocephalus or increased intracranial pressure.

Virtually all patients undergoing resection of CS tumours have transient ophthalmoplegia or paresis. Many of these deficits start resolving within two months postoperatively, a good prognostic sign as to long term extraocular muscle function. Table 6 lists the permanent cranial nerve deficits following CS tumour resection, those expected due to the tumour invasion or surgical approach are so noted. Table 7 lists the outcome of extraocular muscle function relative to the preoperative function in patients with at least six months of follow up, four of the 34 with fair or poor preoperative function having significantly improved, and two with good or excellent preoperative function having significantly worsened. Few of the

Table 6. *Operated Cavernous Sinus Tumours 1983–1990* Permanent Cranial Nerve Palsies/Worsening (First 101 cases – minimum follow-up 6 months)

I	Olfactory	3 (expected)
III	Oculomotor	6
IV	Trochlear	11 (3 expected)
V_1	Ophthalmic	10 (expected)
V_2	Maxillary	7 (expected)
V_3	Mandibular	5 (4 expected)
VI	Abducens	10 (3 expected)

Table 7. *Extraocular Muscle Function.* All Cavernous Sinus Tumour 1983–1989 (First 91 cases)

	Excellent	Good	Fair	Poor
Preoperative	35	22	13	21
Postoperative				
Excellent	25	6	–	–
Good	7	11	2	2
Fair	–	2	7	1
Poor	–	–	2	15
*Indeterminate	3	3	2	3

* Indeterminate = Too early to evaluate, or orbital exenteration for malignant tumour.

patients with fair or poor preoperative function regain binocular vision, but it is apparent that the better the preoperative extraocular function, the better the resultant postoperative outcome.

Cranial nerve reconstruction was performed in several patients, listed in Table 8. The results of such reconstruction are encouraging, and our reconstruction techniques are improving.

Conclusion

Adequate treatment modalities are available today for most CS lesions. The mainstay of treatment of benign CS tumours is surgical, based on adequate anatomical knowledge and state-of-the-art micro-neurosurgical technique. However, careful patient selection is important to avoid unnecessary patient morbidity. For malignant CS tumours, total resection must be achieved and followed up by adjuvant therapy.

References

1. Al-Mefty O, Smith RR (1988) Surgery of tumors invading the cavernous sinus. Surg Neurol 30: 370–381
2. Barnett HJM (1978) Delayed cerebral ischemic episodes distal to occlusion of major cerebral arteries. Neurology 28: 769–774
3. Brackett CE (1953) The complications of carotid artery ligation in the neck. J Neurosurg 10: 91–106
4. Diaz FG, Ohaegbulam S, Dujovny M, Ausman JI (1988) Surgical management of aneurysms in the cavernous sinus. Acta Neurochir (Wien) 91: 25–28
5. Dolenc V (1983) Direct microsurgical repair of intracavernous vascular lesions. J Neurosurg 58: 824–831
6. Dyste GN, Beck DW (1989) De novo aneurysm formation following carotid ligation: Case report and review of the literature. Neurosurgery 14: 88–92
7. Erba SM, Horton JA, Latchaw RE, Yonas H, Sekhar LN, Schramm V, Pentheny S (1988) Balloon test occlusion of the internal carotid artery with stable xenon/CT cerebral blood flow imaging. AJNR 9: 533–538
8. Faria MA, Fleischer AS, Spector RH (1980) Bilateral giant intracavernous carotid aneurysms treated by bilateral carotid ligation. Surg Neurol 14: 207–210
9. German WJ, Black SPW (1965) Cervical ligation for internal carotid aneurysms: An extended follow-up. J Neurosurg 23: 572–577
10. Hakuba A, Nishimura S, Tskanoto M (1982) Surgical approaches to the cavernous sinus: Report of 19 cases. Neurol Med Chir (Tokyo) 22: 295–308
11. Hakuba A, Tanaka K, Suzuki T, Nishimura S (1989) A combined orbitozygomatic infratemporal epidural and subdural

Table 8. *Cranial Nerve Reconstruction During Cavernous Sinus Surgery*

Nerve	Reconstruction type	Preop function			Recovery			
		Good	Fair	Poor	Good	Fair	Poor	Too early
III	Resuture	–	1	–	–	1	–	–
	Graft	–	1	–	–	–	–	1
IV	Resuture	1	–	–	–	–	–	1
	Graft	1	–	–	–	–	–	1
V_1	Graft	3	–	–	–	2	–	1
V								
Root	Graft	–	1	–	–	1	–	–
VI	Resuture	1	–	–	1	–	–	–
	Graft	4	–	–	2	–	–	2

approach for lesions involving the entire cavernous sinus. J Neurosurg 71: 699–704

12. Harris FS, Rhoton AL (1976) Anatomy of the cavernous sinus, a microsurgical study. J Neurosurg 45: 169–180

13. Hayreh SS, Ramji D (1962) The ophthalmic artery, origin and intracranial and intracanalicular course. Br J Ophthalmol 46: 65–98

14. Hirsch WL Jr, Hryshko FG, Sekhar LN, Brunberg J (1988) Comparison of MR imaging, CT and angiography in the evaluation of the enlarged cavernous sinus. AJR 151: 1015–1023

15. Inoue T, Rhoton AL, Theele D, Barry ME (1990) Surgical approaches to the cavernous sinus: A microsurgical study. Neurosurgery 26: 903–932

16. Lesion F, Jonin M (1987) Direct microsurgical approach to intracavernous tumors. Surg Neurol 28: 17–22

17. Matas R (191,1) Testing the efficiency of the collateral circulation as a preliminary to the occlusion of the great surgical arteries. Ann Surg 53: 1–43

18. Matas R (1914) Testing the efficiency of the collateral circulation as a preliminary to the occlusion of the great surgical arteries. JAMA 63: 1441–1447

19. Matas R, Allen CW (1911) Occlusion of large surgical arteries with removable metallic bands to test the efficiency of the collateral circulation. JAMA 56: 233–239

20. Oldershaw JB, Voris HC (1966) Internal carotid artery ligation, follow-up study. Neurology 16: 937–938

21. Olivecrona H (1944) Ligature of the carotid artery in intracranial aneurysms. Acta Chir Scand 91: 353–368

22. Parkinson D (1964) Collateral circulation of the cavernous carotid artery: anatomy. Can J Surg 7: 251–268

23. Parkinson D (1965) Surgical approach to the cavernous portion of the carotid artery: Anatomic studies and case report. J Neurosurg 23: 474–483

24. Parkinson D (1979) Anatomy of the cavernous sinus. In: Pia HW, Langmaid C, Zierski J (eds) Cerebral aneurysms: advances in diagnosis and therapy. Springer New York, pp 62–66

25. Parkinson D (1979) Surgical approach to cavernous sinus aneurysms. In: Pia HW, Langmaid C, Zierski J (eds) Cerebral aneurysms: advances in diagnosis and therapy. Springer, New York, pp 224–228

26. Parkinson D, West M (1990) Lesions of the cavernous plexus region. In: Youmans JR (ed) Neurological surgery. W. B. Saunders, Philadelphia, pp 3351–3370

27. Perneczky A, Knosp E, Vorkapic P, Czech TH (1985) Direct surgical approach to infraclinoid aneurysms. Acta Neurochir (Wien) 76: 36–44

28. Rhoton AL Jr, Hardy DG, Chambers SM (1979) Microsurgical anatomy and dissection of the sphenoid bone, cavernous sinus and sellar region. Surg Neurol 12: 63–104

29. Sekhar LN, Burgess J, Atkin O (1987) Anatomical study of the cavernous sinus emphasizing operative approaches and related vascular and neural reconstruction. Neurosurgery 21: 806–816. (Also presented at the International Symposium on Cavernous Sinus, Ljubljana, Yugoslavia, 1986)

30. Sekhar LN, Linskey ME, Sen CN, Altschuler EM (1990) Surgical management of lesions within the cavernous sinus. In: Black Peter McL (ed) Clinical neurosurgery 37. Williams and Wilkins, Baltimore, MD, pp 440–489

31. Sekhar LN, Moller AR (1986) Operative management of tumors involving the cavernous sinus. J Neurosurg 64: 879–889

32. Sekhar LN, Pomeranz S, Sen CN (in press) Cavernous sinus lesions. In: Brock M (ed) Modern neurosurgery

33. Sekhar LN, Schramm VL Jr, Jones NF (1986) Operative exposure and management of the petrous and upper cervical carotid artery. Neurosurgery 19: 967–982

34. Sekhar LN, Sen CN, Jho HD, Janecka IP (1988) Surgical treatment of intracavernous neoplasms: A four-year experience. Neurosurgery 24: 18–30

35. Sekhar LN, Sen CN, Jho HD (1990) Saphenous vein graft bypass of the cavernous internal carotid artery. J Neurosurg 72: 35–41

36. Spetzler RF, Fukushima T, Martin N, Zabramski JM (1990) Petrous carotid-to-intradural carotid saphenous vein graft for intracavernous giant aneurysm, tumor and occlusive cerebro-vascular disease. J Neurosurg 73: 496–502

37. Taptas JN: The so-called cavernous sinus (1982) A review of the controversy and its implications for neurosurgeons. Neurosurgery 11: 712–717

38. Umansky F, Nathan H (1982) The lateral wall of the cavernous sinus, with special reference to the nerves related to it. J Neurosurg 56: 228–234

39. Willinksy R, Lasjaunias P, Berenstein A (1987) Intracavernous branches of the internal carotid artery (ICA): Comprehensive review of their variations. Surg Radiol Anat 9: 201–215

40. Winn HR, Richardson AE, Jane JA (1977) Late morbidity and mortality of common carotid ligation for posterior communicating aneurysms. A comparison of conservative treatment. J Neurosurg 47: 727–736

Correspondence: L. N. Sekhar, M.D., F.A.C.S., Department of Neurosurgery, Room 9402 PUH, 230 Lothrop Street, Pittsburgh, PA 15213, U.S.A.

Acta Neurochirurgica, Suppl. 53, 113–116 (1991)

Gd-DTPA-Enhancement Magnetic Resonance Imaging of the Cavernous Sinus

G. Rosseau, A. Mark, and **D. O. Davis**

Department of Neurological Surgery, George Washington University, Washington, D.C., U.S.A

Summary

Based upon our experiences with 7 cases and a literature review a survey is provided on the possibilities and limitations of pre-operative diagnosis of space-occupying lesions of the cavernous sinus using MRI with Gd-DTPA enhancement.

Advantages are, that in many cases arteriography is no longer necessary, and that the diagnostic sensitivity is higher as compared with CT. The pattern of enhancement does not allow for histological distinction among the various lesions.

Keywords: Cavernous sinus; tumour; MRI; Gadolinium enhancement; differential diagnosis.

Introduction

Magnetic Resonance Imaging (MRI) has been enthusiastically adopted by neurosurgeons because of the clarity of anatomic detail it provides. Since the introduction of MRI into widespread clinical use in 1983, a large experience has developed in correlating these images with a variety of neurosurgical conditions, via tissue obtained at operation.

Experience remains limited, however, in the diagnosis of lesions of the cavernous sinus by MRI. Gadolinium-DTPA (Gd-DTPA) has been recently introduced as a contrast agent for MRI. The pharmacokinetics are in part similar to that of iodinated contrast used for computerized tomography (CT). The normal cavernous sinus and both inflammatory and neoplastic conditions enhance with gadolinium on T1-weighted images. Rapidly flowing blood within the cavernous carotid artery produces a flow void resulting in excellent contrast between the artery and the cavernous sinus. We report our experience with 7 patients in whom masses of the cavernous sinus were studied pre-operatively with Gd-DTPA.

Materials and Methods

Seven patients with clinical symptoms (Table 1) referable to the cavernous sinus were evaluated by MRI without and with use of intravenous Gd-DTPA. The images were performed on a GE 1.5T superconducting unit. The post-injection images were obtained after infusion of Gd-DTPA in doses of .1 mmol/kg. Slice thickness ranged from 3 mm–5 mm. All patients were studied with T1- and T2- weighted images (T1WI, T2WI). Pathological correlation was available in every case. One patient with Tolosa-Hunt Syndrome had biopsy via open craniotomy which revealed normal dura and symptoms resolved following treatment with corticosteroids.

Results

All lesions were much more conspicuous after the administration of Gd-DTPA. Case 2 was a 52 year-old man with left facial and orbital dysesthesia. The pre-Gd-DTPA T1-weighted axial image suggested a mass in the left cavernous sinus. On post-Gd-DTPA images, the lesion enhanced markedly, producing a signal similar to that of the adjacent, normally-enhancing nasal mucosa. The mass represented local spread of nasopharyngeal carcinoma.

In case 4, a 40 year-old woman presented with right facial weakness and visual loss. Non-contrast MRI images revealed a large mass in the right cavernous sinus. Gd-DTPA-enhanced images demonstrated uniform uptake of the contrast by the mass, as well as subtle enhancement along the tentorium cerebelli, suggesting leptomeningeal spread. This lesion, after biopsy, was identified as a plasmacytoid lymphoma.

Case 6 was a 41 year-old man with headache and left facial numbness in the distribution of the maxillary nerve. A mass identified on T2-weighted images was of low signal intensity, mimicking a meningioma. At surgery, the lesion proved to be sarcoid (Fig. 1).

In case 7, a 61 year-old woman presented with left

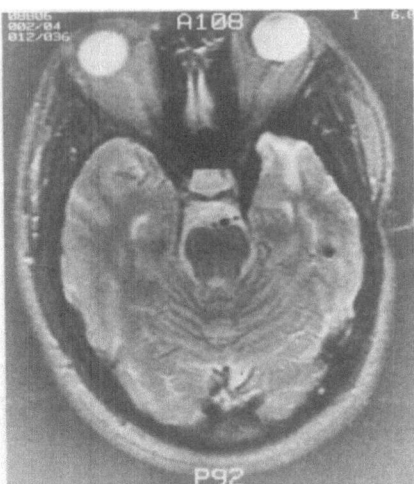

Fig. 1. Case 6, 41 y., male. A mass identified on T2 weighted images mimicked a meningioma, but at surgery turned out to be sarcoid

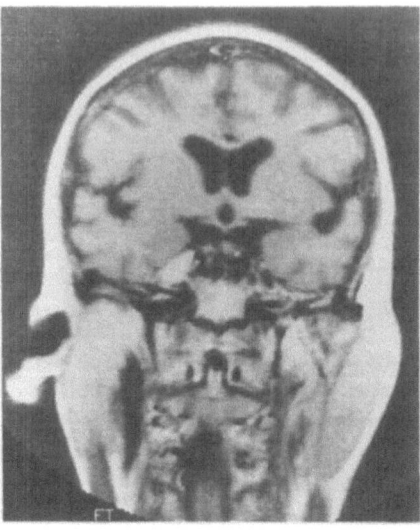

Fig. 2. Case 3, 55 y., female. Patient with a known malignant melanoma developed trigeminal neuralgia. The images without gadolinium were normal. The enhanced images, however, revealed a discretely and uniformly enhancing mass in the right cavernous sinus

eye blindness and proptosis. The increased signal intensity on the T2-weighted images could suggest an epidermoid tumour. After Gd-DTPA administration, however, the enhancing left cavernous sinus and sphenoid wing lesion was consistent with a meningioma, which is what the lesion proved to be at surgery.

In three patients, the lesion was only identifiable after contrast enhancement. In case 1, an otherwise healthy 55 year-old woman complained of diplopia, right forehead numbness and right facial weakness. Pre-contrast images were normal. Axial and coronal T1-weighted post-Gd-DTPA administration demonstrated enhancement and thickening of the dura of the cavernous sinus. Biopsy of the dural of the lateral cavernous sinus wall revealed inflammatory changes. The patient's symptoms resolved after a course of steroids, suggesting a diagnosis of Tolosa-Hunt Syndrome. The patient in case 3, a 55 year-old woman, had undergone local wide excision of a malignant melanoma. Subsequently, widespread multi-focal metastatic disease occurred. When she developed right-sided trigeminal neuralgia, an MRI was obtained. The pre-gadolinium images were normal. The enhanced images, however, revealed a discretely and uniformaly enhancing mass in the right cavernous sinus. Although this tumour is known to have a propensity to bleed, there was no evidence of changes consistent with focal hemorrhage, such as deoxyhemoglobin, methemoglobin or hemosiderin (Fig. 2).

In case 5, a 55 year-old woman with osteosarcoma of the right mandible presented with right facial numbness in the mandibular nerve distribution. The T1-weighted pre-gadolinium images were normal.

The coronal T1-weighted Gd-DTPA enhanced images demonstrated thickening of the right cavernous sinus and foramen ovale, consistent with perineural spread of the known mandibular carcinoma.

Discussion

Pathology in the cavernous sinus is suspected when dysfunction occurs in one or more of the cranial nerves which supply the extra-ocular muscles, especially when accompanied by ipsilateral changes in facial sensation, retro-orbital pain or visual loss. A variety of conditions may cause these signs and symptoms and prompt radiological evaluation and subsequent neurosurgical consultation.

The structure of the cavernous sinus was described by Winslow in 1732[29]. The work of Rhoton described the microscopic anatomy of the cavernous sinus and parasellar regions[23]. Advances in imaging over the past decade have contributed greatly to the understanding of the complex anatomy in this region[2,3-10,13-15,18,22,28,30,31].

Axial CT images may demonstrate the intra-orbital and intracranial abnormalities associated with a cavernous sinus lesion[11,12]. The coronal image, however, offers more detail and may reveal expansion of the sphenoid sinus as well as the relationship of the mass to the neural structures, the pituitary and the skull base[16]. CT remains the superior study for demonstration of skull erosion or hyperostosis[18]. The limitations of CT are well-known and include radiation exposure, iodinated contrast reactions, beam-hardening artifacts secondary to bone and dental amalgam and, most importantly, limited soft tissue resolution[21]. In particular, the diagnosis which appears to be most difficult on CT is that of the benign-appearing well-circumscribed mass with uniform enhancement[6].

The supremacy of CT and angiography has been challenged. The MR appearance of the normal and abnormal cavernous sinus has been described[2,7,10,14,15,17–20,24–27]. In a study comparing CT, angiography and MRI in cavernous sinus lesions, Hirsch et al. found MR superior to CT in defining the relation of the mass to the pituitary gland, optic chiasm, cranial nerves and infundibulum[18]. In addition, others have demonstrated its superior display of the impact of masses on the third ventricle, hypothalamus, cavernous sinus and carotid artery[30]. The internal carotid artery is easily recognized, due to flow void, and MRI has been shown to be better than angiography at demonstrating encasement of the cavernous carotid[18]. The T1-weighted coronal image is the single best study for the analysis of these relationships[18].

The limitations of MRI in the cavernous sinus include:

1) poor imaging of the medial wall,
2) the presence of lateral bowing which may be seen with or without invasion[9,10,21].
3) increased signal on T1-weighted images secondary to fat or slow blood which could be mistaken as neoplasm[2], and
4) potential to miss small isointense lesions, e.g. meningioma, especially if entirely intracavernous[18].

Gd-DTPA has recently been introduced as an MRI contrast agent. The pharmacokinetics are in part similar to that of iodinated contrast used for computerized tomography. No allergic reactions have been reported[2,9]. After gadolinium infusion, the T1 signal for normal pituitary stalk and cavernous sinus rapidly increases[2]. Meningiomas and neuromas tend to increase signal intensity by 300%–500%, while pituitary adenomas increase intensity by only 30%–50%, generally allowing distinction between the neoplasms[15].

In the current study, gadolinium enhancement was useful in the evaluation of masses due to nasopharyngeal carcinoma, lymphoma, central nervous

Table 1. 7 Patients with Cavernous Sinus Lesions Studied Preoperatively with Gd-DTPA

Case	Age/Genger	Signs and symptomas	Diagnosis
1	55/F	Diplopia, right forehead numbness, right facial weakness	Tolosa-Hunt Syndrome
2	57/M	Left facial and orbital dysesthesia	Nasopharyngeal carcinoma
3	55/F	Right trigeminal neuralgia, all divisions	Metastatic melanoma
4	40/F	Right facial weakness and visual loss	Plasmacytoid lymphoma
5	53/F	Right facial, numbness, V_3 distribution	Osteosarcoma of right mandible with perineural tumour spread to cavernous sinus
6	41/M	Headache: left facial numbness, V_2 distribution	CNS Sarcoid
7	61/F	Left eye blindness, proptosis	Meningioma

system sarcoidosis and meningioma. Gd-DTPA was essential in the detection of non-hemorrhagic metastatic melanoma, perineural spread of osteosarcoma, and dural inflammatory disease consistent with TolosaHunt Syndrome.

Conclusion

All lesions were much more conspicuous after the administration of Gd-DTPA and, in 3 patients (cases 1, 3 and 5), the lesion was only identifiable after contrast enhancement. In all cases, the mass could easily be separated from the cavernous and supraclinoid carotid artery on the basis of signal void. Patterns of enhancement did not allow for histological distinction among the various lesions.

The advantages of MR imaging in this region include:

1) obviating the need for arteriography, and
2) increased sensitivity in lesion detection as compared with CT. This sensitivity is further increased by the use of Gd-DTPA.

References

1. Bedford MA (1966) The "cavernous sinus". Br J Ophthalmol 50: 41–46
2. Berry I, Brant-Zawadski M, Osaki L, Brasch R, Murovic J,

Newton TH (1986) Gd-DTPA in clinical MR on the brain: 2. Extraaxial lesions and normal structures. AJNR 7: 789–793

3. Bradac GB, Riva A, Stura G (1987) Cavernous sinus meningiomas: An MRI Study. Neuroradiology 29: 578–581

4. Bydder GM, Kinopley DPE, Brown J, Niendorf HP, Young IR (1985) MR imaging of meningioma including studies with and without Gadolinium-DTPA. J Comput Assist Tomogr 9: 690

5. Chakeres DW, Curtin A, Ford G (1989) Magnetic resonance imaging of pituitary and parasellar abnormalities. Radiol Clin North Am 27:265–281

6. Chung CW, Chang KH, Han MH, Kim BH, Sang CS (1988) Computed tomography of cavernous sinus diseases. Neuroradiology 30: 319–328

7. Daniels DL, Czervionke LF, Bonneville JF, Catlin F, Mark LP, Peck P, Hendrix LE, Smith DF, Haughton VM, Williams AL (1988) MR imaging of the cavernous sinus: Value of spin echo and gradient recalled echo images. AJR 151: 1009–1014

8. Daniels DL, Peck P, Pojunas KW (1986) Magnetic resonance imaging of the trigeminal nerve. Radiology 159: 577–583

9. Davis P, Hoffman H, Spencer T, Tindall G, Braun I (1987) MR imaging of pituitary adenoma: CT, clinical and surgical correlation. AJR 148: 797–802

10. DeGroot J, Wilson CB (1988) MR imaging of cavernous sinus involvement by pituitary adenomas. AJR 151: 799–806

11. Delpassand ES, Kirkpatrick JB (1988) Cavernous sinus syndrome as the presentation of malignant lymphoma: Case report and review of the literature. Neurosurgery 23: 501–504

12. Freeman MP, Kessler RM, Allen JH, Price AC (1987) Craniopharyngioma: CT & MR imaging in nine cases. J Comput Assist Tomogr 11: 810–814

13. Goldberg R, Byrd S, Winter J, Takahasi M, Joyce P (1988) Varied appearance of trigeminal neuroma on CT. AJR 114: 57–60

14. Haughton VM (1985) Magnetic resonance imaging of the cavernous sinus. AJR 144: 1009–1014

15. Haughton VM, Mark L (1988) MRI of suprasellar and parasellar lesions. MRI Decisions: 17–27, March/April

16. Hayes WS, Sherman JL, Stern BJ (1987) Magnetic resonance and CT evaluation of intracranial sarcoidosis. AJR 149: 1043–1049

17. Hirabuki N, Muira T, Mitomo M, Harada K, Haskimoto T, Kawai R, Kozuka T (1988) MR imaging of dural arteriovenous malformations with ocular signs. Neuroradiology 30: 390–394

18. Hirsch WL, Hryshko FG, Sekhar LN, Brumberg J, Kanal E, Latchaw RE, Curtin H (1988) Comparison of MR imaging, CT and angiography in the evaluation of the enlarged cavernous sinus. AJR 151: 1015–23

19. Kao SCS, Yuh WTC, Saro Y, Barloon TJ (1987) Intracranial granulocytic sarcoma (chloroma): MR findings. J Comput Assist Tomogr 11: 938–41

20. Kwan ESK, Wolpert SM, Scott RM, Runge V (1988) MR evaluation of neurovascular lesions after endovascular occlusion with detachable balloons. AJNR 9: 523–531

21. Michael AS, Paige ML (1988) MR imaging of intrasellar meningioma simulating pituitary adenomas. J Comput Assist Tomogr 12: 944–6

22. Olson W, Brant-Zawadski M, Hades J, Norman D, Newton T (1987) Giant intracranial aneurysms: MR imaging. Radiology 163: 431–435

23. Rhoton A1, Harris FS, Renn WH (1977) Microsurgical anatomy of the sella regions and cavernous sinus. Clin Neurosurg 24: 54–85

24. Scotti G, Yu C, Dillon W, Norman D, Colombo N, Newton T, DeGroot J, Wilson CB (1988) MR imaging of cavernous sinus involvement by pituitary adenomas. AJR 151: 799–806

25. Sekhar L, Moller A (1977) Operative management of tumours involving the cavernous sinus. Clin Neurosurg 24: 54–85

26. Selman WR, Laws ER, Scheithauer BW, Carpenter SM (1986) The occurrence of dural invasion in pituitary adenomas. J Neurosurg 64: 402–407

27. Tomas JE, Yoss RE (1970) The parasellar syndrome: Problems in determing etiology. Mayo Clin Proc 45: 617–623

28. Tsuha M, Aoki H, Okamura T (1987) Roetgenological investigation of cavernous sinus structures with special reference to paracavernous cranial nerves. Neuroradiology 29: 462–67

29. Winslow JB: Exposition anatomique de la structure du corps humaine, Vol. 2. Prevost, London, pp 31 (Cited in Ref 25).

30. Yeakley JW, Kulkarni MV, McArdle CB, Hoar FL, Tang RA (1988) High-resolution MR imaging of juxtasellar meningioma with CT and angiographic correlation. AJNR 9: 279–285

31. Young SC, Grossman RI, Goldberg HI (1988) Magnetic resonance of vascular encasement in parasellar masses: Comparison with angiography and CT. AJNR 9: 35–38

Correspondence: Dr. G. Rosseau, Department of Neurological Surgery, George Washington University, 2150 Pennsylvania Ave., N.W. Washington, DC 20037, U.S.A.

Acta Neurochirurgica, Suppl. 53, 117–121 (1991)
© by Springer-Verlag 1991

Direct Surgery of the Cavernous Sinus: Patient Selection

O. Al-Mefty[1], **S. Ayoubi**[2], and **R. R. Smith**[3]

[1]Division of Neurological Surgery, Loyola University Medical Center, Chicago, Illinois, U.S.A., [2]Hurstwood Park Neurological Center, Haywards Heath, U.K., [3]Department of Neurosurgery, University of Mississippi Medical Center, Jadison, Mississippi, U.S.A.

Summary

The cavernous sinus is involved either in lesions arising primarily in the sinus or in lesions invading the sinus from surrounding structures. Experience with direct surgery of the cavernous sinus is encouraging, but no conclusive evidence exists concerning the roles of conservative, surgical, and radiological treatments in terms of effectiveness, morbidity, and long-term results. Consequently, management is individualized according to the patient and the lesions. We discuss these factors in patient selection for cavernous sinus surgery.

Keywords: Cavernous sinus; tumours; aneurysm; microsurgery.

Introduction

The appropriate management of lesions involving the cavernous sinus is still controversial. Current options in managing neoplastic lesions involving the cavernous sinus include observation only, surgical excision, and radiotherapy either alone or combined with surgery. The options are even more numerous for aneurysms[8]. Unfortunately, there are no conclusive data about the effectiveness, morbidity, and long-term results of these modalities. Although Krogius[12] directly approached an endothelioma in the cavernous sinus in 1895, the fear of profuse venous hemorrhage and injury to the cavernous portion of the internal carotid artery (ICA) as well as to the cranial nerves made this space a "no man's land" for many years. The modern direct approach to the cavernous sinus, based on thorough anatomical knowledge, should be credited to Parkinson[14]. His use of hypothermia, however, hindered the spread of his technique.

Several surgeons have reported favorable experience with direct exposure and removal of tumours of the cavernous sinus[9,11,17]. We share their enthusiasm and encouraging experience[4]. Patient selection remains the most crucial and highly debatable issue concerning direct surgery of the sinus. Perviously, patient selection depended on surgical ability. Hence, Zozulia and colleagues[19], in their report on 247 tumours involving the cavernous sinus (167 meningiomas and 80 pituitary adenomas), concluded that tumours involving only the lateral wall of the sinus could be surgically removed.

The major risk of cavernous sinus surgery stems from injury to the carotid artery with the subsequent need for permanent occlusion or prolonged temporary clipping. Because of this, Sekhar and colleagues[17] have justifiably advocated the safety of carotid occlusion with adequate collateral as the decisive factor in selecting patients for direct cavernous sinus surgery. This factor, however, might deprive patients with benign tumours of a potential surgical cure and may entice the surgeon to recommend surgery because of its relative safety to patients with malignant tumours who might have little or no long-term benefits from such major surgery.

On the other hand, Parkinson and West[15] have emphasized the nature of the lesion as the crucial factor in patient selection. He believed that only a preoperative diagnosis of an aneurysm, a meningioma, or a neurofibroma justifies a direct surgical approach to the cavernous sinus. We, however, take the potential benefit as the decisive factor when selecting patients for direct surgery. Parkinson's statement that a direct operative approach is indicated when it is anticipated that the lesion can be removed governs our practice and philosophy. The following is a review of our experience based on this principle.

Table 1. *Cavernous Sinus Lesions: 1983–1990 (154 cases)*

	Total	Cavernous sinus surgery	No cavernous sinus surgery
I. Benign tumours	89	45	44
meningioma	42	30	12
schwannoma	4	2	2
pituitary	35	8	27
craniopharyngioma	1	1	
myxochondrofibroma	2	2	
hemangioma	1	1	
juvenile angiofibroma	1	1	
plexiform neurofibroma	3		3
II. Malignant tumours	29	5	23
nasopharyngeal carcinoma	15		15
paranasal sinus carcinoma	4		3
adenocystic carcinoma	2	1	1
chordoma	1	1	
hemangiopericytoma	1	1	
metastasis	4		4
carcinoid	1	1	
aggressive desmoid fibromatosis	1	1	
III. Aneurysm	36	24	12
ophthalmic	19	19	
fusiform	13	3	10
traumatic aneurysm with fistula	4	2	2

Case Material

From 1983 to 1990, 154 patients with cavernous sinus lesions were evaluated for a direct surgical approach (Table 1). These lesions fall into 3 main categories: benign tumours, malignant tumours, and aneurysms. Each patient had a full preoperative work-up with computerized tomography (CT) and/or magnetic resonance (MR) images with multiple views, angiography, and evaluation of collateral circulation through one or several of the following techniques: cross-compression angiography, balloon occlusion tests, transcranial Doppler test with carotid compression, and recently, transcranial Doppler compression tests with brain SPECT scans. In the latter, we have oberserved that prompt reversal of flow in the anterior cerebral artery (ACA) and a drop in velocity in the middle cerebral artery (MCA) of less than 50% with symmetrical uptake on the SPECT scan signifies sufficient collateral flow. Conversely, the lack of reversal in the ACA and a drop in the MCA of more than 50% represents a high risk (Figs. 1–3).

There were 74 operated cases (Table 2). Two deaths occurred but were not related to cavernous sinus surgery *per se*. One patient died of sepsis from craniofacial resection of an adenocystic carcinoma; the other died following delayed vasospasm after removal of a clinoid meningioma. Complications are listed in Table 3. In our practice, benign tumours and aneurysms are obviously the prime candidates for direct surgery of the cavernous sinus.

Discussion

The selection of patients for direct surgery of the cavernous sinus is individualized according to factors related to the patient (condition, age, neurological

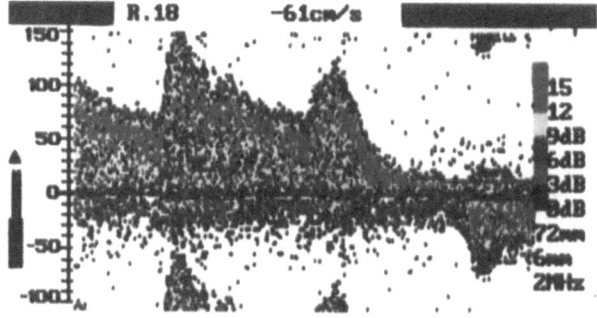

Fig. 1. Transcranial Doppler study taken during carotid compression test. Flow velocity in the ACA is promptly reversed, a favourable sign of adequate collateral circulation

deficit, and anatomy of the arterial circulation), to the tumour (pathology, behavior, previous treatment, and the extent of tumour involvement) and to the surgeon (conventions, experience and technique).

The authors, however, give more weight to a patient's benefit from cavernous sinus surgery than the mere grading of surgical risk. At present, we do not perform or advocate direct surgery of the cavernous sinus for highly malignant tumours such as nasopharyngeal carcinomas and squamous cell carcinomas of the paranasal sinus (Fig. 4). In the future, however, *en bloc* resection can be developed to excise

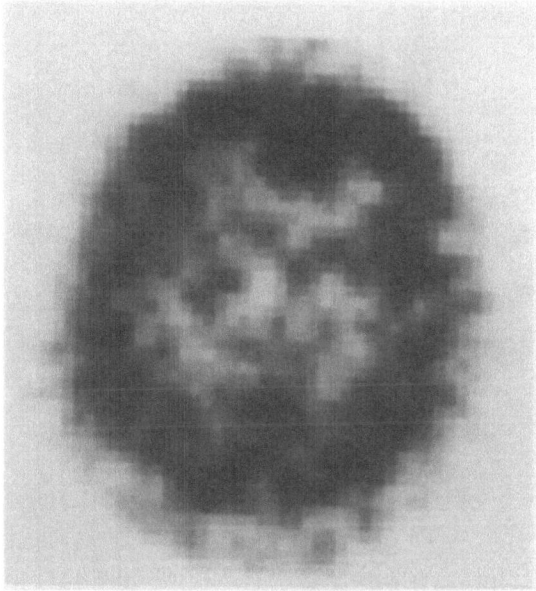

Fig. 2. SPECT scan with isotope injection during carotid compression and transcranial Doppler monitoring. Notice the symmetrical uptake

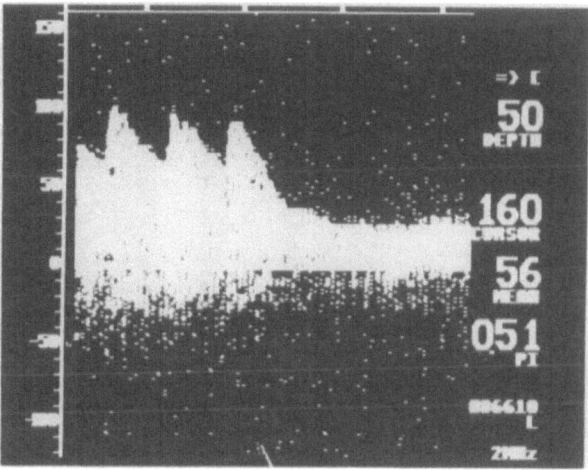

Fig. 3. Transcranial Doppler study showing the flow velocity of the MCA during carotid compression. The velocity dropped below 50% of the pre-compression value, a warning of poor collateral circulation

Table 2. *Surgery of the Cavernous Sinus (1983–1990) (74 cases)*

Meningioma	30
Schwannoma	2
Pituitary	8
Craniopharyngioma	1
Myxochondrofibroma	2
Hemangioma	1
Juvenile angiofibroma	1
Adenocystic carcinoma	1
Chordoma	1
Hemangiopericytoma	1 + reoperated
Carcinoid	1
Aggressive desmoid fibromatosis	1
Fusiform aneurysm	3
Ophthalmic aneurysm	19
Traumatic aneurysm with fistula	2

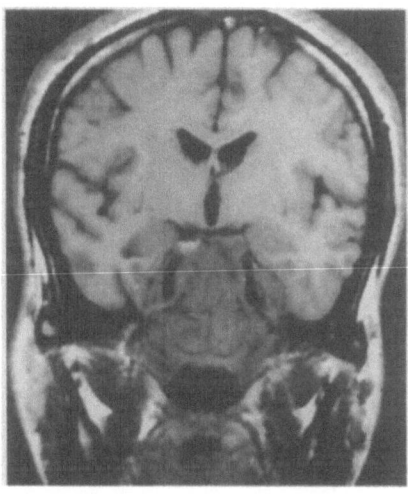

Fig. 4. MR image of a nasopharyngeal carcinoma invading the cavernous sinus. This is *not* recommended for direct surgery of the cavernous sinus

Table 3. *Complications Related to Cavernous Sinus Surgery (74 cases)*

	Transient	Permanent	Too early to tell
III nerve palsy	3	3	7
IV nerve palsy	1	1	7
V nerve palsy	9 (V2–V3)	1 (V2)	
VI nerve palsy	2	1	7
VII nerve palsy	1		
Hemiplegia	1		
CSF Leak	1		

the cavernous sinus area and reconstruct the carotid artery. Less aggressive radiation-resistant lesions, such as chordomas and chondrosarcomas, are recommended for surgical removal from the cavernous sinus[5,17]. Hemangiopericytomas are also recommended for surgical removal despite their malignancy (Fig. 5).

Among the benign tumours, schwannomas warrant aggressive surgical removal and yield the best results. Although some authors have expressed reservations about the successful removal of meningiomas[9,13], we pursue their aggressive removal, acknowledging that some meningiomas lack intervening dissecting planes

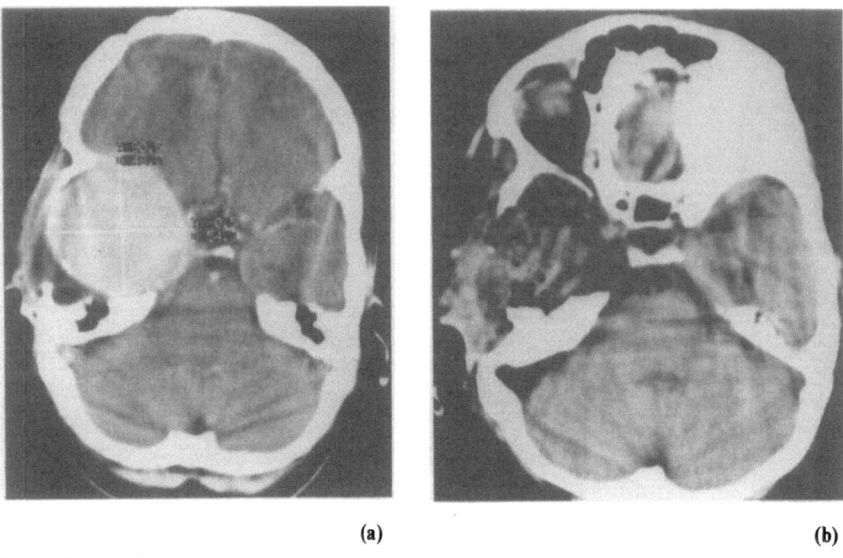

(a)   (b)

Fig. 5. Enhanced CT scan of a large recurrent hemangiopericytoma invading the cavernous sinus. a) Preoperative, b) postoperative

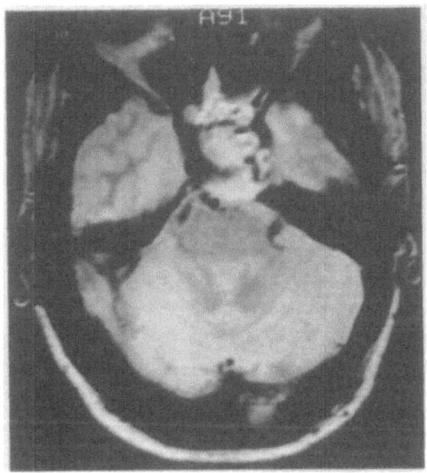

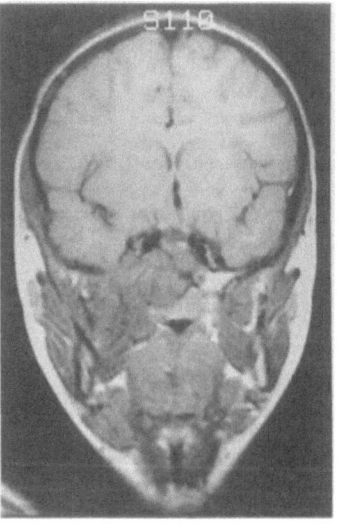

Fig. 6. MR image of a myxochondrofibroma invading the cavernous sinus. Diagnosis was made at the time of surgery and removal was total

Fig. 7. MR image of a juvenile angiofibroma invading the cavernous sinus but remaining extradural

and directly adhere to the carotid adventitia. In these cases, it is impossible to achieve total removal[1]. Prolactinomas are best treated initially with bromocriptine. Other pituitary tumours require thorough evaluation to compare the long-term outcome of direct surgery with the effects of radiation therapy. Craniopharyngiomas, myxochondrofibromas and hemangiomas are indications for a surgical approach; frequently, diagnosis is made at the time of surgery (Fig. 6). Angiofibromas and other rare lesions invade the cavernous sinus but remain extradural and may be approached extradurally[2] (Fig. 7).

Direct clipping of ophthalmic segment aneurysms has become a routine practice, owing to the understanding of their anatomy and advancements in cavernous sinus surgery[7,10]. With giant intracavernous aneurysms, however, the surgeon stands at a crossroads in selecting the optimal management from the competitive modalities of endovascular surgery[6,8], direct aneurysmal reconstruction or a cavernous sinus venous bypass graft[3,16,18]. Benign bilateral lesions and asymptomatic tumours are vexing, each requiring an independent management decision.

Acknowledgement

The authors thank Julie Hipp for her editorial assistance.

References

1. Al-Mefty O (1991) Clinoidal meningomas. In: Al-Mefty O (ed) Meningiomas. Raven Press, New York
2. Al-Mefty O, Anand VK (1990) Zygomatic approach to skull-base lesions. J Neurosurg 73: 668–673
3. Al-Mefty O, Khalil N, Elwany MN, Smith RR (1990) Shunt for bypass graft of the cavernous carotid artery: An anatomical and technical study. Neurosurgery 27: 721–728
4. Al-Mefty O, Smith RR (1988) Surgery of tumours invading the cavernous sinus. Surg Neurol 30: 370–381
5. Arnold H, Herrmann HD (1986) Skull base chordoma with cavernous sinus involvement: Partial or radical tumour removal? Acta Neurochir (Wien) 83: 31–37
6. Barrow DL, Spector RH, Braun IF, Landman JA, Tindall SC, Tindall GT (1985) Classification and treatment of spontaneous carotid-cavernous sinus fistulas. J Neurosurg 62: 248–256
7. Day AL (1990) Aneurysms of the ophthalmic segment. A clinical and anatomical analysis. J Neurosurg 72: 677–691
8. Diaz FG, Ohaegbulam S, Dujovny M, Ausman JI (1989) Surgical alternatives in the treatment of cavernous sinus aneurysms. J Neurosurg 71: 846–853
9. Dolenc VV (1989) Anatomy and surgery of the cavernous sinus. Springer, Wien New York
10. Dolenc VV (1985) A combined epi- and subdural direct approach to carotid-ophthalmic artery aneurysms. J Neurosurg 62: 667–672
11. Hakuba A, Tanaka K, Suzuki T, et al (1989) A combined orbitozygomatic infratemporal epidural and subdural approach for lesions involving the entire cavernous sinus. J Neurosurg 71: 699–704
12. Krogius A (1896) Om operativ behandlund of tumoren i fossa media cranii. Rev Chir 16: 434
13. Lesion F, Jomin M (1987) Direct microsurgical approach to intracavernous tumours. Surg Neurol 28: 17–22
14. Parkinson D (1965) A surgical approach to the cavernous portion of the carotid artery: Anatomical studies and case report. J Neurosurg 23: 474–483
15. Parkinson D, West M (1982) Lesions of the cavernous plexus region. In: Youmans JR (ed) Neurological surgery, Vol 5, 2nd ed. WB Saunders, Philadelphia, pp 3004–3023
16. Sekhar LN, Sen CN, Jho HD (1990) Saphenous vein graft bypass of the cavernous internal carotid artery. J Neurosurg 72: 35–41
17. Sekhar LN, Sen CN, Jho HD, et al (1989) Surgical treatment of intracavernous neoplasms: A four-year experience. Neurosurgery 24: 18–30
18. Spetzler RF, Fukushima T, Martin N, Zabramski JM (1990) Petrous carotid-to-intradural carotid saphenous vein graft for intracavernous giant aneurysm, tumour, and occlusive cerebrovascular disease. J Neurosurg 73: 496–501
19. Zozulia YA, Romodanov SA, Patsko YV (1979) Diagnosis and surgical treatment of benign craniobasal tumours involving the cavernous sinus. Acta Neurochir (Wien) [Suppl] 28: 387–390

Correspondence: Prof. O. Al-Mefty, M.D., Division of Neurological Surgery, Loyola University Medical Center, 2160 S. First Avenue, Maywood, Illinois 60153, U.S.A.

Acta Neurochirurgica, Suppl. 53, 122–126 (1991)

Management of Intracavernous Tumours: An 11-Year Experience

A. Sepehrnia, M. Samii, and M. Tatagiba

Hannover Medical School, Neurosurgical Clinic, Nordstadt Hospital, Hannover, Federal Republic of Germany

Summary

Seventy-one patients with tumours involving the cavernous sinus (CS) were operated upon between 1979 and 1989. Fifty-four patients underwent a direct approach to the CS. The average age of these latter patients was 47 (9–69) years. The lesions included 51 benign tumours (26 meningiomas, 16 [7 invasive] pituitary adenomas, 3 trigeminal neurinomas, one chordoma, one chondroma, one craniopharyngioma, one epidermoid tumour, and one cavernous haemangioma), and 3 malignant tumours (one chondrosarcoma, one adenoid cystic carcinoma and one metastatic adenocarcinoma).

Dissecting tumour away from the carotid artery was the management of choice for intracavernous tumours which involved the internal carotid artery, except when the carotid artery had already pre-operatively presented with advanced narrowing or occlusion by encasing tumour. Microsurgical technique facilitated dissection and preservation of the cranial nerves. Patients treated radically by direct CS surgery had improvement of their symptoms and signs more frequently than those patients treated by subtotal tumour removal. However, operative complications in direct CS surgery were higher than in subtotal tumour removal without CS entry.

Keywords: Cavernous sinus; cranial nerves; meningioma; neurilemmoma.

Introduction

Management of tumours involving the cavernous sinus (CS) has been considered a difficult challenge in neurosurgery because of the complex neurovascular anatomy in this region[1,4,6,11]. Interest in direct operative management of intracavernous lesions has increased in recent years[3,4,7,12]. Advances in surgical technique and increasing knowledge of topographic and pathological anatomy of the CS have allowed considerable progress in surgical removal of intracavernous tumours with reduced mobidity[3,11]. In order to contribute to the study of the clinical evolution and the surgical possibilities of neoplasms involving the CS, we report our experience of dealing with CS tumours since 1979.

Subjects and Methods

Between 1979 and 1989, 71 patients with tumours involving the CS were operated on in our department. In 54 cases tumour removal included the opening of the CS. The clinical, radiological and operative information was examined retrospectively. Clinical and radiological follow-up of these 54 patients was obtained retro- and prospectively.

Pre-operative angiographic studies were performed in all patients in order to evaluate the anatomy of the intracavernous internal carotid, the potential collateral circulation and the tumour vascularity. Despite its excellence in demonstrating the relations between tumour and soft neurovascular structures in the region of the cavernous sinus, MRI studies were well complemented by CT scans with soft tissue and bone algorithms.

Operative Technique

Different cranial intradural and extradural approaches can be chosen to reach the CS[12]. We have used the anteromedial, anterolateral, lateral and posterolateral intradural approaches, and the medial extradural approach[10]. A medial extradural approach (transethmoidosphenoidal) to the CS was made only once unintentionally during removal of a pituitary adenoma. This approach allows only limited exposure and therefore restrictive proximal and distal control of the carotid artery[1].

The anteromedial approach is the approach following a subfrontal craniotomy through the planum sphenoidale and the sphenoid sinus, this way reaching the opposite CS. For the lateral approach through the Parkinson's triangle[8], and the anterolateral approach by removing the anterior clinoid and the wall of the optic foramen, a frontotemporal craniotomy is performed. During the posterolateral approach the petrous apex is exposed via a combined retromastoid-subtemporal approach with preservation of the transverse sinus[9].

Results

Tables 1 and 2 summarize the presentation of the 71 neoplasms involving the CS. Sixty-eight benign and 3 malignant tumours were removed. A total of 34 tumours had their origin in the middle of the skull base and affected the CS laterally and medially (pituitary adenoma, tuberculum sellae and sphenoid

Table 1. *71 Tumours Affecting the Cavernous Sinus (1979–1989)*

Tumour pathology			
Benign	68	Malignant	3
Meningioma	35	Adenocarcinoma	1
V Neurinoma	4	Chondrosarcoma	1
Pituitary adenoma	21	Metastasis	1
Others: angiofibroma,	8	(hypernephroma)	
chemodectoma, chordoma,	(one		
chondroma, epidermoid,	each)		
craniopharyngeoma,			
cavernous haemangioma			

Table 2. *Major Clinical Findings in 71 Patients with Intracavernous Tumours*

Headache	35 (50%)
Visual deficit	28 (39%)
Amaurosis	11 (15%)
Ophthalmoplegia	17 (24%)
Exophthalmos	11 (15%)
Paresis of limbs	6 (8%)
Mental changes	4 (6%)

wing meningioma, and craneopharyngeoma). In 24 cases the tumours originated from the posterior skull base and involved the CS posterolaterally (petroclival meningioma, trigeminal neurinoma, chemodectoma, chordoma, chondroma and chondrosarcoma of the clivus, and epidermoid tumour). In 7 cases the tumours originated from the anterior skull base (meningioma,

adenocarcinoma, and juvenile angiofibroma). Six tumours were strictly intracavernous (meningioma, metastasis, and cavernous angioma). The most important clinical findings were headache and visual deficits. Eleven patients had already pre-operatively amaurosis and 17 patients had any grade of ophthalmoplegia.

In 54 of the 71 cases (76%) the CS was opened to allow further tumour removal (Table 3). The determining factors in surgical strategy for opening the CS were the side of tumour involvement, the tumour pathology and the clinical presentation of the patients. Table 4 shows the clinical presentation of the 54 patients who underwent direct CS surgery. The most frequent affected cranial nerves were the optic nerve (46%), the maxillary nerve (V-2) (37%), and the abducent nerve (35%). From these 54 neoplasms, 42 (78%) were completely removed. The 3 malignant tumours were subtotally removed.

After surgery, partial or temporary deficit affected most frequently following cranial nerves III, V-2, II and VI. Permanent or complete deficit affected most frequently IV, V-1 and V-2 cranial nerves.

The immediate postoperative status of the 17 patients whose operation did not include an opening of the CS was compared with the postoperative status of the 54 patients who under-went direct CS surgery (Table 5). The criteria of evaluation included motor function of the limbs and the fuctional status of these

Table 3. *Operative Management of 54 Intracavernous Tumours (1979–1989)*

| Tumour | Number | Resection | | Radiation | Recurrence | | Follow-up |
		Total	Subtotal		CS	Outside	(months)
Benign	51	42	9	2	1	2	
Meningioma	26	18	8	1	1	1	10 (6–13)
Neurilemmoma V	3	3					39 (8–72)
Pituitary Adenoma	16	15	1	1		1	28 (6–110)
diffusive	9						
invasive	7						
Haemangioma	1	1					14
Chemodectoma	1	1					12
Chordoma	1	1					24
Chondroma	1	1					30
Craniopharyngeoma	1	1					18
Epidermoid	1	1					4
Malignant	3		3	3			
Chondrosarcoma	1		1	1		1	14
Cylindroma	1		1	1			5
Metastasis (hypernephroma)	1		1	1			8
Total	54	42	12	5	2	5	

Table 4. *Clinical Presentation of 54 Patients with Intracavernous Tumours*

| Presentation | Preoperative status | Postoperative Status | |
		Temporary/partial deficit	Permanent/complete palsy
Headache	28		
Mental disturbances	3		
Motor impairment	6		
Cerebellar dysfunction	1		
Seizures	2		
Cranial nerve deficit			
I	4	0	9
II	25	10	3
III	15	13	4
IV	11	1	13
V_1	16	7	10
V_2	20	11	10
V_3	9	1	6
VI	19	10	5

Table 5. *Comparative Postoperative Neurostatus* of 71 Patients with Intracavernous Tumours*

	Without opening the CS (17 patients)	After opening the CS (54 patients)
Improved	4 (24%)	24 (44%)
Unchanged	8 (47%)	18 (33%)
Worse	5 (29%)	10 (19%)
Dead	0	2 (4%)

* Motor function of limbs, II, III, IV, VI and V cranial nerves.

cranial nerves II, III, VI, IV, and V. Patients with direct CS approach experienced after surgery more frequently an improvement of their preoperative neurostatus, compared with the group of patients without CS opening. However, while there were 2 deaths after direct CS approach, no patient treated without entry into the CS died after surgery.

Neurinomas

Four patients including one female and 3 male patients had trigeminal neurinomas. The average age of the 4 patients was 41 (28–62) years. Three neurinomas invaded the CS, and one neurinoma only compressed the lateral wall of the CS. The II, III, and VI cranial nerves were affected once, respectively. All tumours were completely removed through an intradural lateral approach. Follow-up studies ranging from 8 to 72 (mean 39) months demonstrated no tumour recurrence. Improvement of abducent paresis was reported once.

Meningiomas

Twenty-five female and 10 male patients had meningiomas involving the CS. The average age of the 35 patients was 51 (24–78) years. The sites of involvement included the sphenoid wing in 11 cases, the apex of pyramid in 12 cases (Fig. 1), the middle skull base and the lateral wall of the CS in 4 cases respectively, and the anterior skull base and the tentorial dura twice, respectively. Twenty-seven patients underwent direct CS surgery. The CS was not opened in 9 cases. Minimal cranial nerve deficits and a growing infiltrative tumour constituted the most important factors for deciding against a direct CS approach. In 18 cases the meningiomas were completely removed. One from 8 patients whose tumour was only subtotaly removed underwent radiotherapy. The mean follow-up period of 10 months showed 2 recurrences outside the CS and one recurrence within the CS. Five patients experienced improvement of their visual function after surgery due to decompression of the optic nerve. The cranial nerves III–VI, however, failed to demonstrate any improvement of function at the immediate postoperative period.

Pituitary Adenomas

Twenty-one patients, including 14 males and 7 females had pituitary adenoma. The average age was 44 (9–69) years. Nine tumours had diffuse growth demonstrating a radiographically enlarged sella and localized sellar erosion. Seven tumours were invasive adenomas (Fig. 2) showing radiographically extensive

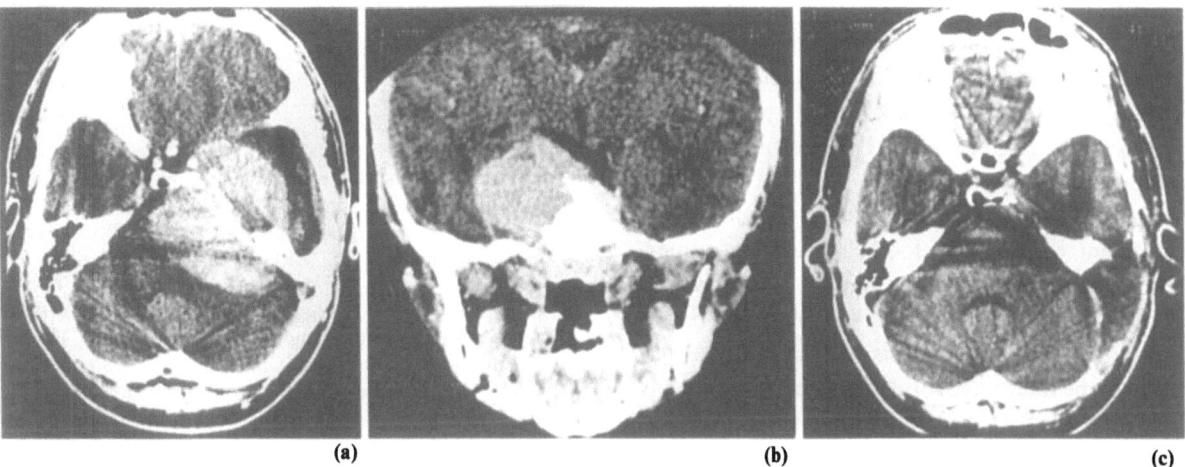

Fig. 1. Axial (a) and coronal (b) enhanced CT scan showing a large meningioma of the petroclival region extending into the left cavernous sinus and engulfing the carotid artery. The tumour was completely removed (c) through a combined retrosigmoid-subtemporal approach

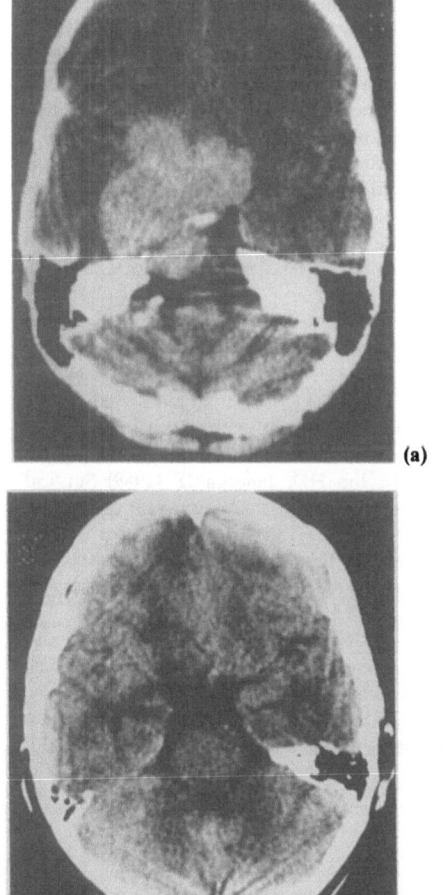

Fig. 2. Axial enhanced CT scan of an invasive pituitary adenoma with extension into the both cavernous sinus (a). Postoperative CT scan after complete tumour removal through a right subfrontal (anteromedial) approach (b)

destruction of bony structures. Histological examination revealed 3 acidophil adenomas, 4 mixed acidophil-basophil adenomas and 17 chromophobe adenomas. In 16 cases the CS was opened. The entry into the CS was performed via a subfrontal (intradural antero-medial) approach in 13 cases, a pterional (intradural anterolateral) approach in 2 cases, and a trans-ethmoidal/trans-sphenoidal (extradural medial) approach once. The adenoma was completely excised in 15 cases and subtotaly once. One patient underwent radio-therapy. Tumour recurrence was observed in one case. The average follow-up period ranged from 6 to 110 months (mean 28 months).

Discussion

The CS can be affected by different benign and malignant pathological processes[1,3,12-15]. Similar clinical symptoms such as retro-ocular pain, mild exoph-thalmos, and impairment of cranial nerves II–VI are produced independently of the causal factor[13,15]. This way, neuroradiological investigations play a important role in the diagnose of the intracavernous lesions, as well as in the pre-operative evaluation of the patients. Pre-operative angiographic studies should always be performed in order to evaluate the anatomy of the intracavernous internal carotid, the potential collateral circulation and the tumour vascularity[12]. Cerebral angiography is not unusually considered normal in intracavernous meningiomas[2]. MRI appears to be the diagnostic method of choice in the evaluation of processes involving the CS[2,5]. However, despite its excellence in demonstrating the relations between tumour and soft neurovascular structures in the region of the CS, MRI studies were in our series well complemented by CT scans with soft tissue and bone algorithms.

Preoperative tests using balloon occlusion, measurement of cerebral blood flow and intraoperative monitoring allow better patient selection and safer results[12]. Although the availability of extracranial-intracranial anastomosis and the direct reconstruction of the internal carotid artery provide a means of restoring cerebral circulation in case of carotid damage intra-operatively[1], a better result will be achieved by the intra-operative preservation of the patency of the carotid artery.

In our series, dissecting the tumour away, was the management for the intracavernous internal carotid, except when the carotid artery had already preoperatively presented with advanced narrowing or occlusion by encasing tumour. Microsurgical technique also facilitated dissection and preservation of the cranial nerves.

The operative strategy for intracavernous neoplasms depends on the nature of the tumour, its site of involvement and the clinical symptoms and signs of the patient. We believe that patients with minimal cranial nerve deficits should not undergo radical removal of a large tumour (e.g., meningioma), which has already extensively infiltrated the CS. Furthermore, we do not advocate radical removal of a malignant tumour from the CS. Dolenc *et al.* emphasize the importance of early detection of CS neoplasms, since they are easier to remove completely at an early stage[3].

Our immediate postoperative results demonstrate that: firstly, patients who underwent a radical operation with direct CS surgery showed improvement of their signs and symptoms more frequently than those patients treated by subtotal tumour removal; secondly, the operative risks in direct CS surgery remains higher than in subtotal tumour removal without CS entry. Similarly, Sekhar *et al.* suggested that for symptomatic lesions, operative results are superior to the natural course of the disease[12]. However, only further experience with a longer follow-up will be able to answer the question whether radical surgery for tumours involving the CS

is superior to conservative non-surgical treatment in the long term.

References

1. Al-Mefty O, Smith RR (1988) Surgery of the tumors invading the cavernous sinus. Surg Neurol 30: 370–381
2. Bradac GB, Riva A, Schörner W, Stura G (1987) Cavernous sinus meningiomas: An MRI study. Neuroradiology 29: 578–581
3. Dolenc VV, Kregar T, Ferluga M, Fettich M, Morina A (1987) Treatment of tumors invading the cavernous sinus. In: Dolenc DD (ed) The cavernous sinus. A multidisciplinary approach to tumours and vascular lesions. Springer, Wien New York, pp 377–391
4. Hakuba A, Suzuki T, Jin TB, Komiyoma M (1986) Surgical approaches to the cavernous sinus. Report of 52 cases. In: Proceedings of the International Symposium on Cavernous Sinus, Ljubljana, Yugoslavia, pp 302–327
5. Hirsch W, Hryshko FG, Sekhar LN, Brunberg J, Kanal E, Latchaw RE, Curtin H (1988) Comparison of MR imaging, CT, and angiography in the evaluation of the enlarged cavernous sinus. AJR 151: 1015–1023
6. Lang J (1989) Anatomy of the cavernous sinus. In: Samii M, Draf W (eds) Surgery of the skull base. An interdisciplinary approach. Springer, Berlin Heidelberg New York, pp 24–26
7. Lesoin F, Pellerin P, Clarisse J, Jomin M (1986) Direct microsurgical approach to intracavernous tumors. In: Proceedings of the International Symposium on Cavernous Sinus, Ljubljana, Yugoslavia, pp 290–300
8. Parkinson D (1965) A surgical approach to the cavernous portion of the carotid artery. Anatomical studies and case report. J Neurosurg 25: 474–483
9. Samii M, Ammirati M, Mahran A, Bini W, Sepehrnia A (1989) Surgery of petroclival meningiomas: report of 24 cases. Neurosurgery 24: 12–17
10. Samii M, Draf W (1989) Surgery of the skull base. An interdisciplinary approach. Springer, Berlin Heidelberg New York Tokyo
11. Sekhar LN, Burgess J, Akin O (1987) Anatomical study of the cavernous sinus emphasizing operative approaches and related vascular and neural reconstruction. Neurosurgery 21: 806–816
12. Sekhar LN, Sen CN, Jho HD, Janecka IP (1989) Surgical treatment of intracavernous neoplasms: a four-year experience. Neurosurgery 24: 18–30
13. Sepehrnia A, Tatagiba M, Brandis A, Samii M, Prawitz R-H (1990) Cavernous angioma of the cavernous sinus. Neurosurgery 27: 32–36
14. Trobe JD, Glaser JS, Post JD (1978) Meningiomas and aneurysms of the cavernous sinus. Neuro-ophthalmologic features. Arch Ophthalmol 96: 457–467
15. Unsöld R, Safran AB, Safran E, Hoyt WF (1980) Metastatic infiltration of nerves in the cavernous sinus. Arch Neurol 37: 59–61

Correspondence: Dr. A. Sepehrnia, Neurochirurgische Klinik, Nordstadt Krankenhaus, Haltenhoffstrasse 41, D-W-3000 Hannover 1, Federal Republic of Germany.

Acta Neurochirurgica, Suppl. 53, 127–136 (1991)
© by Springer-Verlag 1991

Pineal and Third Ventricle Tumours in the CT and MR Eras

M. Fukui, T. Matsushima, K. Fujii, S. Nishio, I. Takeshita, and T. Tashima

Department of Neurosurgery, Neurological Institute, Kyushu University, Fukuoka, Japan

Summary

We have experienced 29 cases of tumour in the pineal region and posterior third ventricle in the CT and MR eras (from 1976 to 1989). An aggressive surgical removal was performed except for germinomas and suspected germinomas. The aggressive surgical cases were 5 teratomas including one inclusion foetus, one yolk sac tumour, 3 astrocytomas, one neurocytoma, one cavernous haemangioma and one telangiectasia. The surgery was performed by either the infratentorial supracerebellar approach or the occipital transtentorial approach. There was no surgical death and the quality of postoperative survial was good in patients with benign tumours. The cases of a typical teratoma, teratoma with an arterio-venous shunt, inclusion foetus, haemorrhagic nodule of telangiectasia etc. are briefly presented. A remarkable progress in the diagnosis and surgical treatment of tumours in the pineal region in the CT and MR eras is noted in our results.

Keywords: Pineal and third ventricle tumours; diagnosis; surgical outcome.

Introduction

The history of the surgery for the pineal region started in the first quarter of this century[3,5,9] but it took a long time to reach the era, in which the surgery was done with an acceptable mortality and morbidity. In Japan the first successful removal of a pineal teratoma was reported by Nakata and Ueki in 1953[13]. In the report the mortality rate of pineal surgery at that time was recorded to be 90%.

The introduction of microneurosurgery and the development of microsurgical anatomy has greatly improved the surgery[11,14,17] of pineal tumours. The advent of CT scan and MRI has also remarkably contributed to improving the therapeutic results. Now the surgery for the pineal region can be performed with minor mortality and morbidity. There occurs a variety of tumours in and around the pineal region. We review our experiences of tumours in the pineal region in the CT and MR eras and present the results especially of surgery.

Table 1. *Incidence of Primary Tumours in the Pineal Region*
(Kyushu University Hospital, 1976–1989)

	Total: 29 cases
Germinoma	6 (21%)
Teratoma	5 (17%)
Yolk sac tumour	1 (3.4%)
Glioma	3 (10%)
Neurocytoma	1 (3.4%)
Cavernous angioma	1 (3.4%)
Unverified tumour	12 (41%)

Clinical Data and Case Presentation

The cases of tumour in the pineal region, who were treated during the period from 1976 to 1989, were 29 (Table 1). Among them germinomas and unverified tumours comprised more than 60%. The majority of the unverified tumours were considered germinomas because of their symptomatology, tumour markers, radiological findings and response to radiation therapy or chemotherapy. The verified germinomas and unverified tumours were mainly treated by irradiation.

Table 2 shows the survival rate of the verified and unverified germinomas including the cases of the suprasellar region and basal ganglia, which were mainly treated by irradiation. Out of the 22 patients 5 died in the follow-up period, but one of them, who was in complete remission, died in a traffic accident. The remission rate of germinomas over 5 years was around 80%.

Table 2. *Actuarial Survival Rate of Patients with Germinoma* (incl. unverified cases) (22 cases, 1976–1990, Kyushu Univ. Hospital)

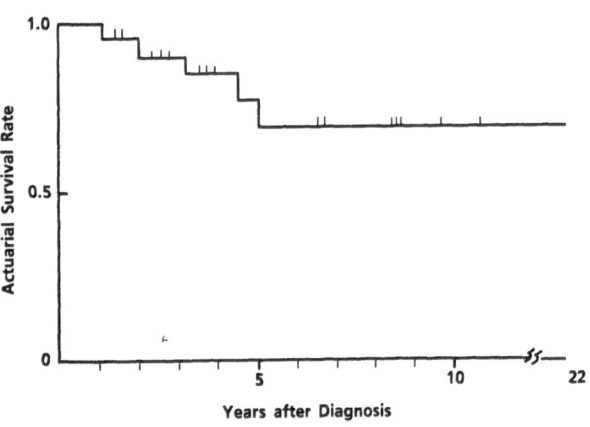

The aggressive surgical cases were thus limited to the tumours other than germinomas. Those cases are shown in Tables 3 and 4. Either the infratentorial supracerebellar approach or the occipital transtentorial approach was chosen for removal of the tumours. The surgery was performed only by the first author (M. F.). The clinical characteristics and results of surgery are briefly presented together with several case presentations.

A) Cases of Teratoma

In this group 5 cases of mature teratoma, one inclusion foetus and one yolk sac tumour are included (Table 3). The mature teratomas were all totally removed and all the patients did well postoperatively.

However, in the case of the yolk sac tumour (Case 6), surgery, radiation therapy and chemotherapy using cis-platinum could not reverse the progression of the tumour. Three cases in this group are recorded below.

1) Case of typical teratoma in the pineal region (Case 2 in the teratoma group)

A 4-year-old boy developed headache and vomiting 10 months prior to admission to us. In another hospital he was found to have a tumour in the pineal region with obstructive hydrocephalus on CT scan. After insertion of a ventriculo-peritoneal (VP) shunt for hydrocephalus, he was transferred to us for surgery of the tumour. Positive physical and neurological signs were enlarged head and Parinaud's sign. Human chorionic gonadotropin (HCG), alpha-fetoprotein (AFP) and placental alkaline phosphatase in the serum were negative. CT scan and MRI showed a large tumour (4 × 4 × 3 cm in diameter) of mixed densities or intensities in the third ventricle and pineal region (Fig. 1)

For the surgery the occipital transtentorial approach was chosen because the inion was situated low. The posterior part of the thinned splenium was incised ca. 1.5 cm in length to expose the tumour in the third ventricle and a well encapsulated tumour was totally removed. (Fig. 2) The tumour was histologically a mature teratoma. The patient did not develop any neurological deficits and was discharged in good condition (Fig. 3).

2) Case of teratoma with an arterio-venous shunt in the pineal region (Case 5 in the teratoma group)

A 24-year-old male, who had a long medical history due to a tumour in the pineal region, was admitted to us for radical surgery in July 1987. This boy was first admitted to us in 1973 at the age of 9 years. He had doubtful precocious puberty, Parinaud's sign and a large calcification in the pineal region on X-ray films. Pneumoventriculography demonstrated a large mass in the pineal region and obstructive hydrocephalus. Torkildsen's shunt was established and local radiation therapy in a dose of 40 Gy was given. At the age of 15 years he developed headache. In another hospital CT scan was taken for the first time and demonstrated a mass lesion with calcification and partial contrast enhancement in the pineal region. The tumour was considered a regrowth of a germ

Table 3. *Teratoma in the Pineal Region* (Kyushu University Hospital, 1976–1989)

Case no.	Age (yr) & sex	Histopathologic diagnosis	Surgery		Radiation, chemotherapy	Follow-up	
			Approach	Resection		Period	Status
1	2.1, M	mature teratoma (inclusion fetus)	occip. tr. tent.	Total R.	no, no	1 y 9 mos.	100
2	4.3, F	mature teratoma	occip. tr. tent.	Total R.	no, no	1 y 11 mos.	100
3	4.6, M	mature teratoma	occip. tr. tent.	Total R.	(preop.) yes, yes	2 y 11 mos.	100
4	11, F	mature teratoma	occip. tr. tent.	Total R.	no, no	1 y 5 mos.	100
5	24, M	mature teratoma	infra T. supra C.	Total R.	no, no	3 y 8 mos.	100
6	15, F	yolk sac tumour	infra T. supra C.	Partial R.	yes (preop.), yes	5 mos.	0

Status: results assessed by Karnofsky performance scale (%); occip. tr. tent.: occipital transtentorial approach; R: removal.; infra T. supra C.: infratentorial supracerebellar approach.

Table 4. *Miscellaneous Tumours in the Pineal Region* (Kyushu University Hospital, 1976–1989)

Case no.	Age (yr) & sex	Histopathologic diagnosis	Surgery		Radiation, chemotherapy	Follow-up	
			Approach	Resection		Period	Status
1	1.1, M	malignant glial tumour	occip. tr. tent.	partial R.	yes, yes	3 mos.	0
2	33, F	astrocytoma	occip. tr. tent.	partial R.	yes, no	3 mos.	0 (sudden death)
3	38, F	astrocytoma	occip. tr. tent.	partial R.	yes, no		0
			suboccip.*	subtotal R.**	yes, yes	1 y 3 mos.	
4	26, M	neurocytoma	occip. tr. tent	partial R.	no, no	3 y 3 mos.	100
5	3, F	telangiectasia	infra T. supra C.	total R.	no, no	5 y 5 mos.	100
6	22, M	cavernous angioma	infra T. supra C.	total R.	(preop.) yes, no	10 y	100

Status: results assessed by Karnofsky performance scale (%); occip. tr. tent.: occipital transtentorial approach; R: removal.
* Suboccipital craniectomy for 4th ventricle tumour.
** Subtotal removal of 4th ventricle tumour.

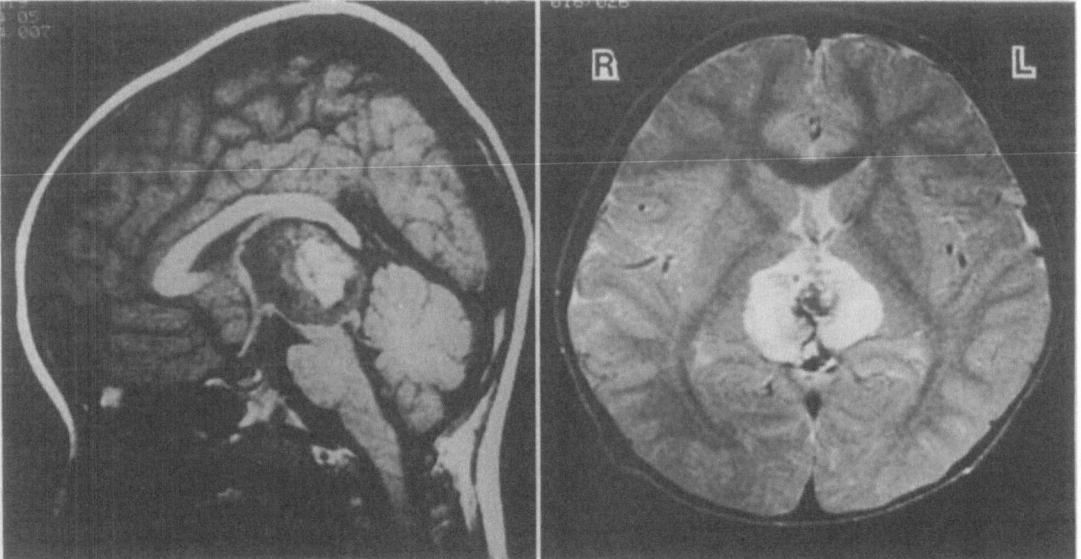

Fig. 1. MR images of a typical teratoma in the pineal region (Case 2). *Left*: a sagittal T1-weighted image (Tr 400, Te 20) and *right*: an axial T2-weighted-image (Tr 2000, Te 80)

cell tumour and irradiation was given 40 Gy to the pineal region and 36 Gy to the whole spine. He returned to his school life, and graduated at high school. At the age of 24 years he started morning headache, but did not show neurological deficits. HCG and AFP in the serum were negative. The follow-up CT scans demonstrated a gradual enlargement of the mass lesion into the right thalamus and enhancement of the wall of the mass. Because of enlargement of the mass he was admitted to us for radical surgery. MRI demonstrated a mass extending into the right thalamus with a flow void area near the midline (Fig. 4). Vertebral angiography demonstrated a mass lesion in the pineal region with a marked arterio-venous shunt (Fig. 5). The feeding arteries were both the medial posterior choroidal arteries and the draining vein (probable pineal vein) joined the great vein of Galen.

The patient was operated upon by the infratentorial supracerebellar approach. A well encapsulated vascular mass was totally removed after ligation of the draining vein (Fig. 6). Histologically the upper part of the mass consisted of a mature teratoma and the lower part of an angioma with dilated vascular cavities. The patient developed postoperative haemorrhage into the cavity after tumour removal, and underwent evacuation of the haematoma. He gradually recovered and returned to social life.

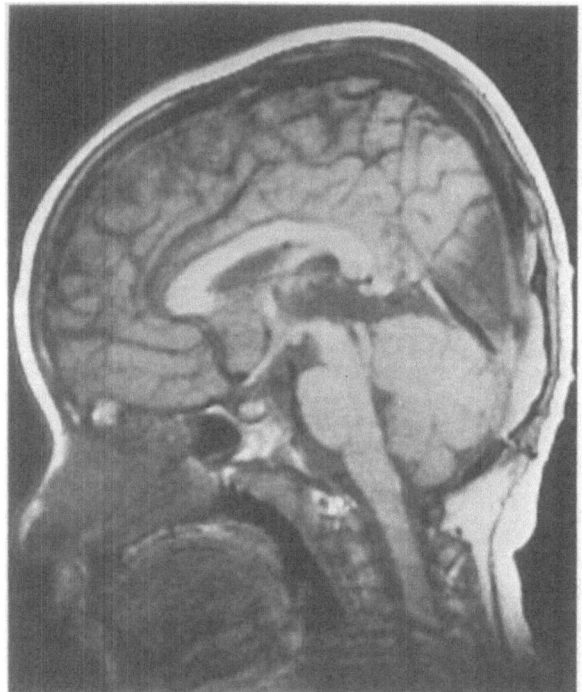

Fig. 2. Postoperative T1-weighted MR image (Tr 400, Te 20) of Case 2. The tumour was totally removed by the occipital transtentorial approach

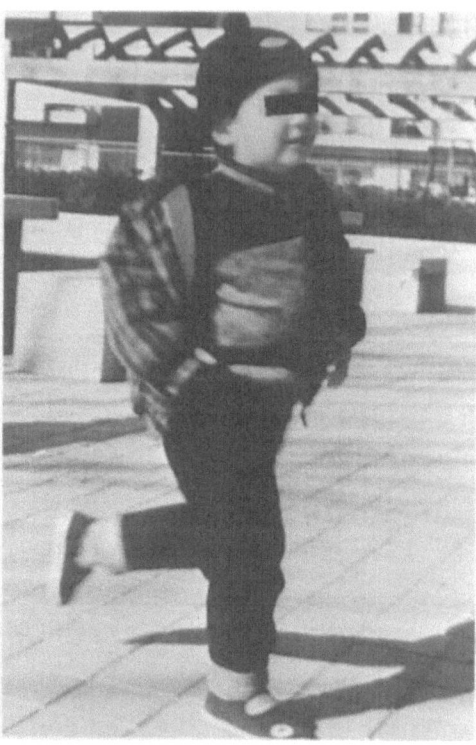

Fig. 3. The state of patient (Case 2) 2 months after surgery

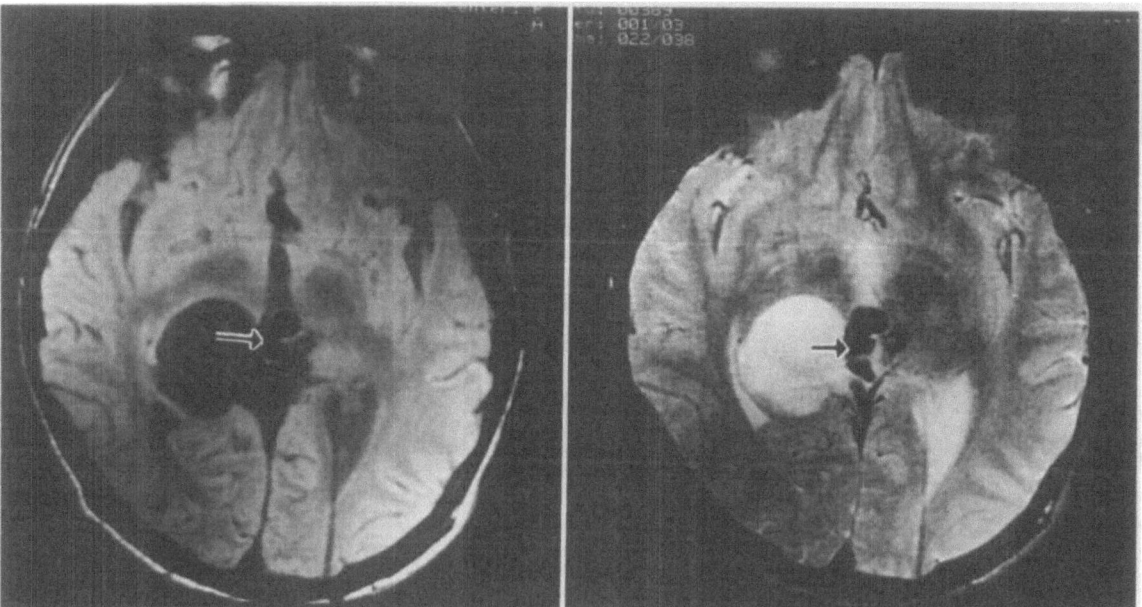

Fig. 4. MR images of a teratoma with an arterio-venous shunt (Case 5). *Left*: proton image (Tr 2000, Te 30) and *right*: T2-weighted image (Tr 2000, Te 80). Flow void signal is seen in the midline (arrow)

3) Case of an inclusion foetus in the pineal region (Case 1 in the teratoma group)

A 2-year-old boy was admitted to us with drowsiness. He was born at full term without abnormalities. At the age of 6 months he was noticed to have medial rotation of the left eye. For 2 months prior to admission he had developed vomiting. Positive neurological symptoms and signs on admission were drowsiness and Parinaud's sign. CT scan demonstrated a large mass lesion in the third ventricle with partial contrast enhancement and obstructive hydrocephalus. A ventriculo-peritoneal shunt was inserted on the day of admission. MRI showed a large cystic mass with a Gado-

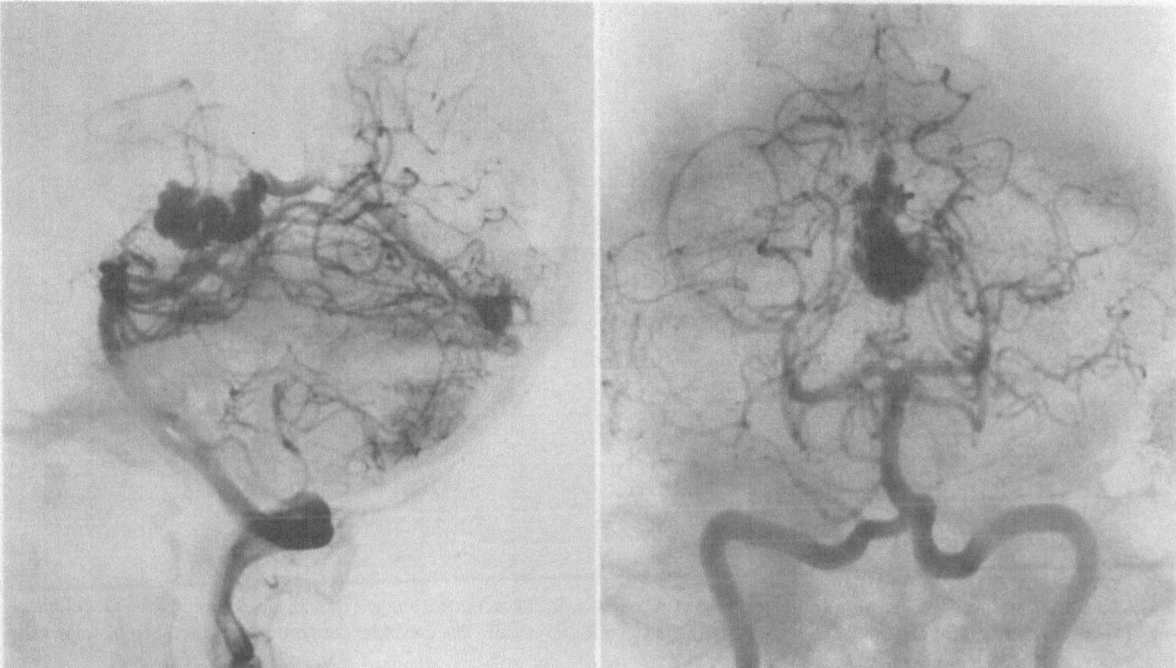

Fig. 5. Vertebral angiography showing an arterio-venous shunt in the pineal region (Case 5)

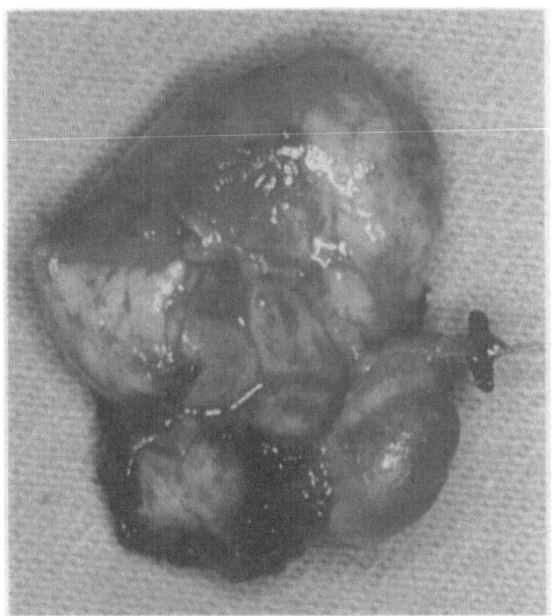

Fig. 6. A totally removed mass of Case 5. A clipped vessel is the draining vein joining the great vein of Galen

linium-enhanced solid portion in the third ventricle (Fig. 7). There was a cord-like connection between the enhanced solid mass and the wall of the cyst. The markers for germ cell tumours in the serum were negative.

Operation was performed by the left occipital transtentorial approach, because the VP shunt was placed on the right. The tumour with a large cystic portion was totally removed. In the cystic mass a solid portion attached to the cyst wall was found. Close obser-

vation of the solid mass revealed limb-like protrusions, jaw-like structure and eyes (Fig. 8). Histologically, the solid mass contained much nervous tissue in the rostral portion, spinal cord-like nervous tissue surrounded by the cartilaginous column of the axis (Fig. 9), intestine, and dermal tissue. The cord-like connection of the cyst wall contained 3 blood vessels resembling the umbilical cord and the cystic membrane was covered by columnar epithelium resembling amnion. Thus the mass was considered an inclusion foetus. The patient was discharged without surgical deficits.

B) Cases of Miscellaneous Tumours

This group includes 3 astrocytic tumours, one neurocytoma in the tectum of the midbrain, one haemorrhagic nodule of telangiectasia in the dorsomedial thalamus, and one cavernous haemangioma. All patients with glioma died in the postoperative period, but the other 3 patients survive in a good condition following surgery.

1) The case of neurocytoma in the midbrain (case 4 in the miscellaneous tumour group) was unique because the Parkinson syndrome (rigidity, tremor and akinesia) was totally improved after tumour removal. In this patient a small tumour was found in the region of the mesencephalic aqueduct (Fig. 10). Obstructive hydrocephalus was improved after VP shunt, but thereafter he developed Parkinson's syndrome. Various anti-parkinsonian drugs were not or only slightly effective. He succumbed to the bed-ridden state and finally underwent removal of the mesencephalic mass by the occipital transtentorial approach. Light and electron microscope diagnosis of the tumour was that of a neurocytoma. Postoperatively he was remarkably improved and returned to a normal life without the anti-Parkinson drugs. This case will be published in other paper.

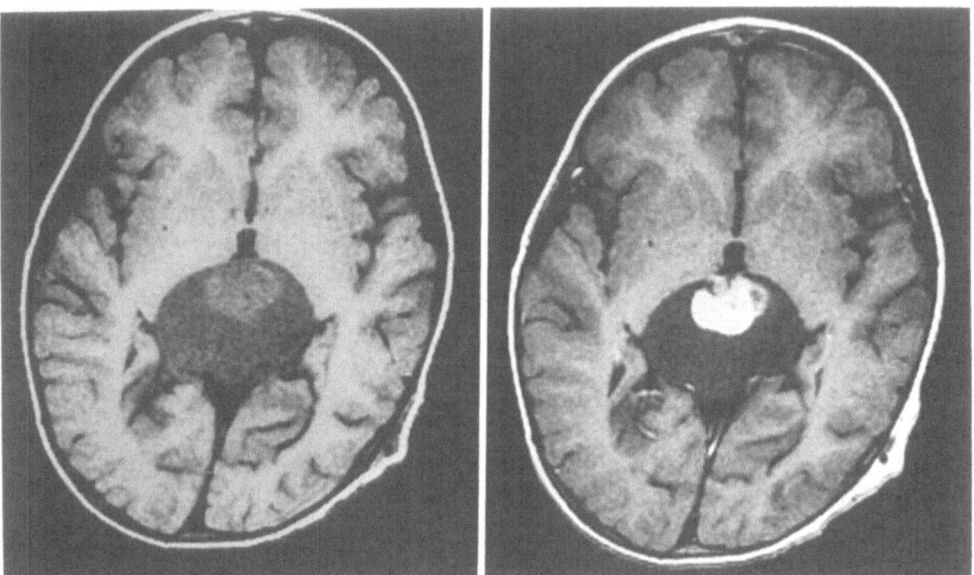

Fig. 7. MR images of an inclusion foetus in the pineal region (Case 1). *Left*: T1-weighted image (Tr 400, Te 20) and *right*: Gadolinium-enhanced T1-weighted image. An enhanced solid mass is attached to the cystic wall. The cord-like connection was found to histologically resemble the umbilical cord

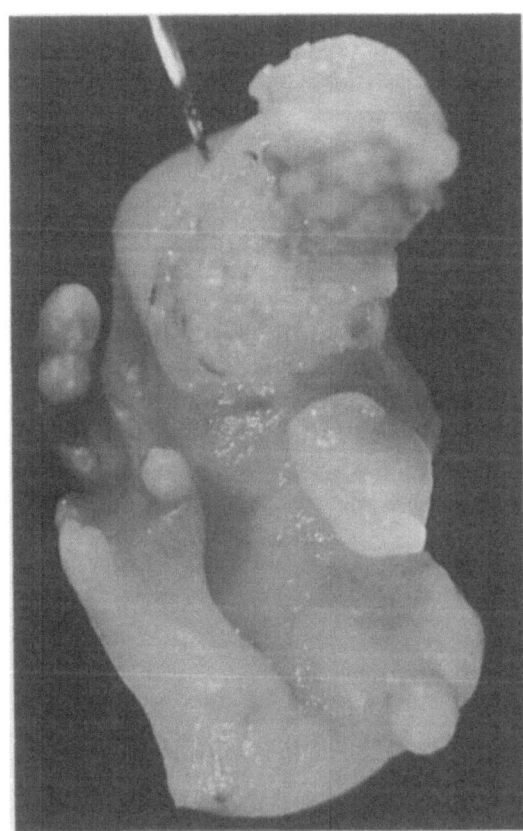

Fig. 8. Photograph of the solid mass of Case 1 showing finger-like protrusions from the body

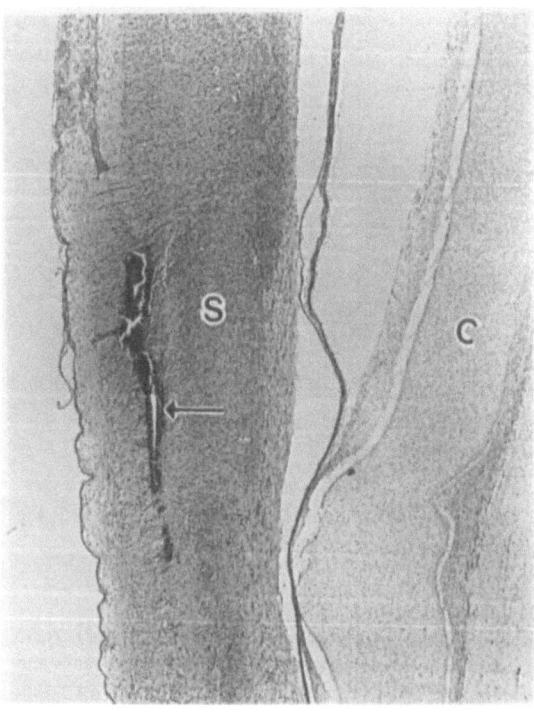

Fig. 9. Histological section of the solid mass of Case 1 showing a spinal cord-like neural tissue (*S*) with a slit covered with ependyma (arrow) and a cartilaginous column (*C*). Haematoxylin-eosin stain, 50 X

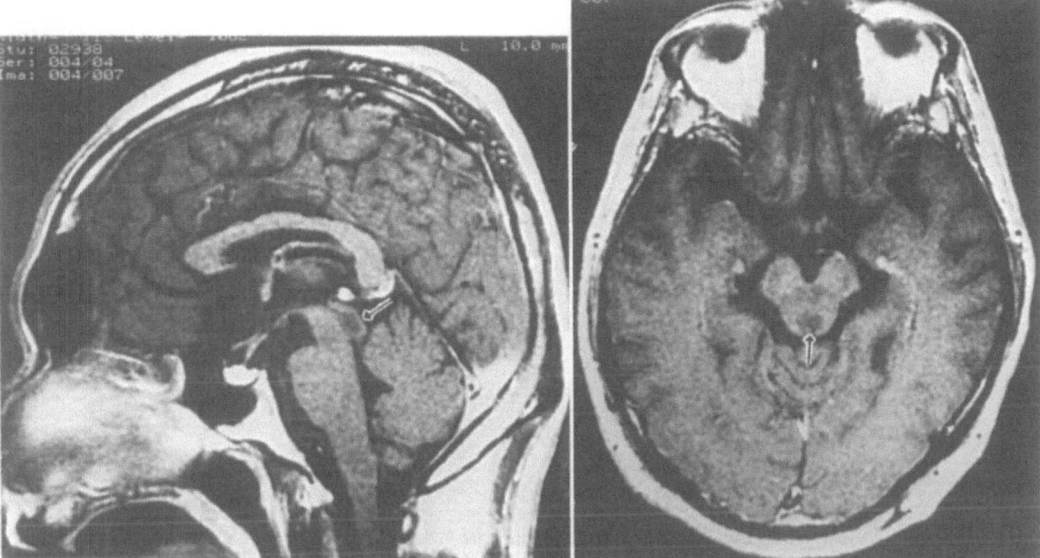

Fig. 10. MR images of neurocytoma in the tectum of the midbrain (Case 4 in the miscellaneous tumour group). *Left and right:* T1-weighted images (Tr 400, Te 20) with Gadolinium enhancement. A small non-enhancing low-intensity mass is seen in the region of the mesencephalic aqueduct (arrow)

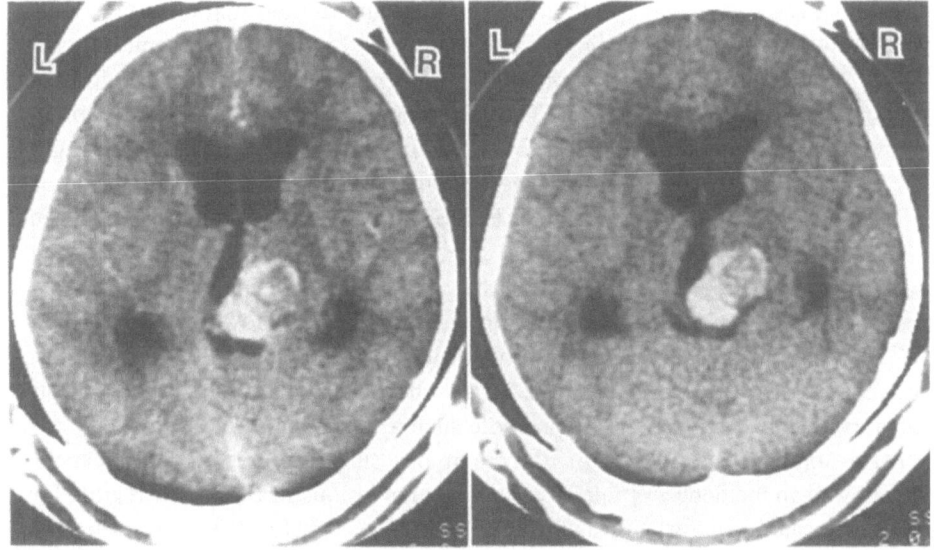

Fig. 11. CT scans of a haemorrhagic nodule in the right thalamus caused by rupture of telangiectasia (Case 5 in the miscellaneous tumour group) *Left*: enhanced CT scan, *right*: Plain CT scan

The case of cavernous haemangioma (Case 6 in the miscellaneous tumour group) was published previously[6]. In this case the tumour was erroneously suspected to be a germinoma in the pineal region by symptomatology and CT scan, and received local irradiation. However, the tumour did not respond to irradiation and angiography demonstrated abnormal tumour vessels and "blush" in the pineal region. The tumour was totally removed and the patient is doing well at present, 10 years after operation.

2) Case of telangiectasia in the dorso-medial thalamus (Case 5 in the miscellaneous tumour group)

A 3-year-old girl developed headache, vomiting and disturbance of ocular movement at the end of December 1984 and was admitted to us with Parinaud's sign on Jan. 14, 1985. CT scan demonstrated a hyperdense mass in the right dorso-medial thalamus extending into the third ventricle and obstructive hydrocephalus. Contrast CT scan did not show enhancement of the mass (Fig. 11). A VP shunt was inserted after admission. Because the mass was considered a haemorrhagic lesion, cerebral angiography was performed without demonstrating abnormal vessels or "blush".

Operation was performed by the infratentorial supracerebellar approach and a firm haemorrhagic nodule protruding from the

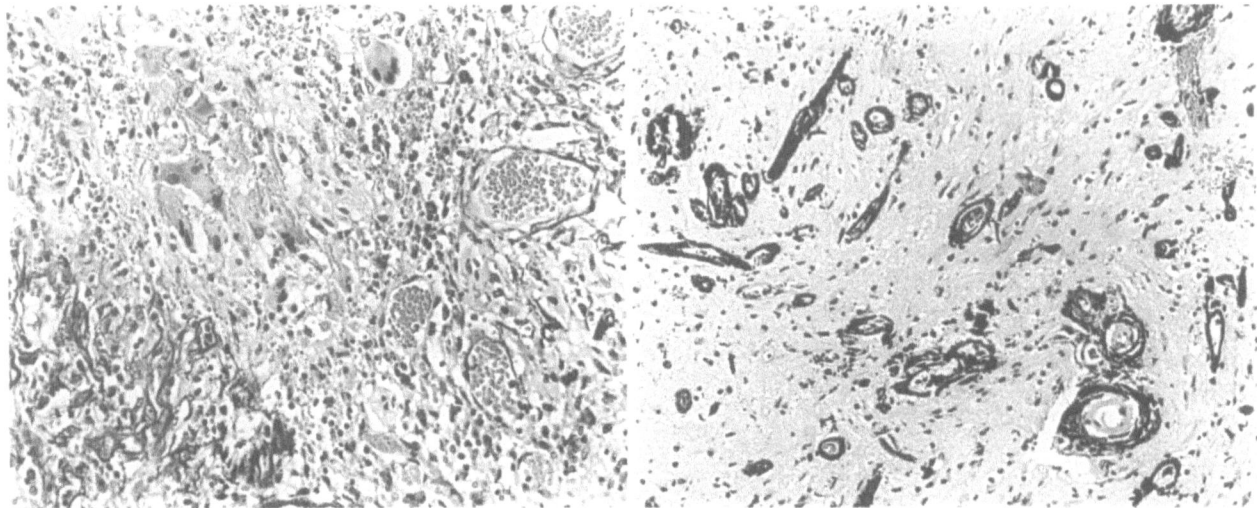

Fig. 12. Microscopic photographs of the haemorrhagic nodule in the thalamus in Case 4. *Left*: The central part of the nodule containing separate thin-walled vessels and granulomatous elements with much blood pigment and foreign body giant cells. Haematoxylin eosin stain, 200 X. *Right*: The peripheral part of nodule showing a brain with many thin-walled vessels with pseudo-calcification, which was digested by trypsin. Haematoxylin eosin stain, 160 X

right thalamus was removed. Histologically the removed mass was considered a telangiectsia with haemorrhage (Fig. 12). Postoperatively she developed bilateral moderate hearing loss of the central type (auditory brain stem response was normal.), which improved slightly in the follow-up period. At present, 5 years after surgery, she is going to school without any recurrence of bleeding.

Discussion

It is well known that various kinds of tumour occur in the pineal region and the most common tumour in this region is a germinoma[4,8,21]. The germinoma is highly radiosensitive and the 15-year-survival rate of the patients with germinoma after radiation therapy is reported to be 84.5%[12]. The brain tumour registry in Japan from 1969 through 1983 showed an incidence of verified germinoma in 33% and unverified tumour in 40% out of 996 tumours in the pineal region[2]. In our series 22 tumours in the pineal region were verified and unverified germinomas. The 5-year-survival rate of the patients with germinoma and unverified tumour (probable germinoma) after radiation therapy was around 80% in our series, and, therefore, the high incidence of germinoma in the unverified tumours is suggested.

Based on such data we have treated patients with germinoma or probable germinoma mainly by irradiation without surgical intervention, and recently by irradiation and/or chemotherapy using cis-platinum etc. For the differential diagnosis symptomatology, radiological findings and tumour markers are helpful, and those patients with probable germinoma are submitted to a diagnostic irradiation to a dose of 20 Gy. The germinomas respond well to irradiation in such a low dose. If there is any contradictory point against germinoma, direct surgical intervention is indicated. Except for suspected germinomas we have performed aggressive surgery. There is a strong suggestion that all tumours in the pineal region should be surgically verified[10,15,18]. However, we have a conservative attitude for the suspected germinomas. Progress in the chemical and radiological diagnosis may promote such a tendency in the future.

As shown in our surgical cases we have experienced various benign lesions in the pineal region, for which direct surgery was useful. We used either the infratentorial supracerebellar approach or the occipital transtentorial approach for removal of tumours. In the early cases we used the infratentorial approach more frequently, because the intra-operative orientation of the midline could be secured and separation of a tumour from the major veins situated above could be more easily carried out. However, there is a risk of venous air embolism with a patient in the semi-sitting position. Also in a case with a low-situated inion, which is sometimes encountered in a child, the infratentorial approach is not desirable. Therefore, in the recent cases we have used the supratentorial approach more frequently. Large teratomas were successfully removed by this approach when the posterior part of the splenium, which was usually thinned by compression of the tumour, was sectioned for 2 cm in length. No surgical deficit by sectioning the posterior part of the splenium was experienced. We had no surgical mortality in our cases and all the patients without a malignant tumour survived. The postoperative quality of life is satisfactory in most of the surviving patients.

In our surgical experience several interesting cases are included. A teratoma with a radiologically demonstrated arteriovenous shunt was not reported in the literature. This case was misdiagnosed as a germinoma before introduction of CT scan. MRI was very useful to detect a flow void signal in the tumour and suggested an angiomatous portion in the tumour. We should know that a variety of abnormal components may be possible in combination with a teratoma. An inclusion foetus in the pineal region was also unique. The main part of the mass was cystic, and a small solid mass was attached to the cystic wall. The former was later considered an amnion and the latter a foetus, though not complete in shape. Without close macroscopic observation of the removed mass, the diagnosis could have easily been missed. Preoperative diagnosis of inclusion foetus was not possible, but the MRI features well corresponded to the structure of the mass. As far as we know only one surgical case of inclusion foetus in the third ventricle was reported in the literature[1]. Probably the MRI of our case is the first, which demonstrated an intracranial inclusion foetus.

A cavernous haemangioma in the pineal region is also very rare[6]. Clinical features and CT findings of our case resembled those of germinoma, but response of the tumour to irradiation and angiographic findings differed from those of germinoma. At that time MRI was not in use. At present, MRI is useful for differentiation of an angioma from a germinoma. We shall not now make such a misdiagnosis in the future.

A surgical case of telangiectasia in the thalamus is rare and, as far as we know, only a few surgical cases are reported in the literature[7,16,20]. In our case the lesion was angiographically occult and operation was carried out with a tentative diagnosis of haemorrhage from a cryptic angioma. Removal of an angioma in the unilateral dorso-medial thalamus in our case was considered useful to prevent rebleeding. However, hearing impairment of the central type occurred due to the surgery. It was probably due to damage to the lateral lemniscus fed by the medial posterior choroidal artery. At surgery in the pineal region we must more or less manipulate the artery. In cases of teratoma we sacrificed the distal portion of this artery in the third ventricle without resulting in any neurological deficits. However, the mesencephalic portion of the artery should be carefully preserved.

As reported in the excellent surgical results of other authors[15,18,19] we have passed the pessimistic era of direct surgery for the pineal region. Now we are in the era, in which we can have a correct judgement for treatment in nearly all of the tumours in the pineal region. All of the lesions in the pineal region should be treated according to their topographical and biological characteristics.

References

1. Afshar F, King TT, Berry CL (1982) Intraventricular fetus-in fetu. Case report. J Neurosurg 56: 845–849
2. Brain tumor registry of Japan (1990) Vol. 7. The committee of brain tumor registry of Japan
3. Dandy WE (1933) Benign tumor in the third ventricle of the brain. Charles C Thomas, Springfield, Ill, 88pp
4. DeGirolami U, Schmidek H (1973) Clinicopathological study of 53 tumors of the pineal region. J Neurosurg 39: 455–462
5. Foerster O (1928) Das operative Vorgehen bei Tumoren der Vierhügelgegend. Wien Klin Wochenschr 41: 986–990
6. Fukui M, Matsuoka S, Hasuo K, Numaguchi Y, Kitamura K (1983) Cavernous hemangioma in the pineal region. Surg Neurol 20: 209–215
7. Hayashi T, Fukui M, Shyojima K, Utsunomiya H, Kawasaki K (1985) Giant cerebellar hemangioma in an infant. Child's Nerv Syst 1: 230–233
8. Jenkins RDT, Simpson WJK, Keen CW (1978) Pineal and suprasellar germinomas. Results of radiation treatment. J Neurosurg 48: 99–107
9. Krause F (1926) Operative Freilegung der Vierhügel nebst Beobachtungen über Hirndruck und Dekompression. Zbl Chir 53: 2812–2819
10. Lapras C, Patet JD, Mottolese C, Lapras Ch Jr (1987) Direct surgery for pineal tumors; Occipital transtentorial approach. In: Kageyama N, et al (eds) Intracranial tumors in infancy and childhood. Progress in experimental tumor research: Vol. 30 Homburger F (ed). Karger, Basel, pp 268–280
11. Lazar ML, Clark K (1974) Direct surgical management of mass in the region of the vein of Galen. Surg Neurol 2: 17–21
12. Matsutani M, Takakura K, Sano K (1990) Long-term follow-up of patients with primary intracranial germinomas. Neurosurgeons (Proceedings of the 9th Japanese Congress of Neurological Surgeons) 9: 134–140
13. Nakata M, Ueki Y (1953) Successful removal of a pineal tumor (Case report). Acta Med Biol 1: 45–50
14. Pendl G (1985) Pineal and midbrain lesions. Springer, Wien New York
15. Pendl G (1990) Surgery for lesions in the third ventricle and midbrain. Neurosurgeons (Proceedings of the 9th Japanese Congress of Neurological Surgeons) 9: 127–133
16. Pozzati E, Gaist G Galassi E, Tognetti F (1982) Giant cerebral telangiectasis in an infant. Child's Brain 9: 114–120
17. Stein BM (1971) The infratentorial supracerebellar approach to pineal lesions. J Neurosurg 35: 197–201

18. Stein BM (1979) Surgical treatment of pineal tumours. Clin Neurosurg 26: 490–510

19. Tanaka R (1989) Occipital transtentorial approach in lateral semiprone position to pineal region tumors. Neurosurgeons (Proceedings of the 8th Japanese Congress of Neurological Surgeons) 8: 124–132

20. Vaquero J, Manrique M, Oya S, Cabezudo JM, Bravo G (1980) Calcified telangiectatic hamartomas of the brain. Surg Neurol 13: 453–457

21. Wara WM, Jenkin RDT, Evans A, et al (1979) Tumors of the pineal and suprasellar region. Childrens cancer study treatment results 1960–1975. Cancer 43: 698–701

Correspondence: M. Fukui, M. D., Department of Neurosurgery, Neurological Institute, Kyushu University, Fukuoka 812, Japan.

Acta Neurochirurgica, Suppl. 53, 137–143 (1991)

Microsurgery of Intrinsic Midbrain Lesions

G. Pendl[1] and P. Vorkapic[2]

[1] Department of Neurosurgery, University of Graz, Austria, [2] Department of Neurosurgery, University of Vienna, Austria

Summary

The advanced tools of neuro-imaging provide sufficient details for an appropriate open microsurgical approach to those lesions, which are well circumscribed even as intrinsic lesions of the midbrain. 30 reported cases with only 3 postoperative death related to surgery but otherwise no morbidity except in one case, demonstrate the safety of modern microsurgical techniques, provided the case has been well selected for surgery and the appropriate approach is choosen well. A clear histological diagnosis also is the foundation for the additional methods of postoperative treatment.

Keywords: Brain tumour; cavernoma; midbrain lesions; microsurgery; brain stem.

Introduction

The optimal management of brain stem lesions is a widely discussed matter and open surgery is not always considered to be the treatment of choice and furthermore there seems to be no standard therapy. Although advances in imaging technology provide excellent localization with clear topographical characteristics even stereotactic biopsy is considered as a non-routine procedure. But constant advances in microsurgery have provided enough experience in these deep seated lesions, that it is possible to approach them under certain morphological and topographical conditions. Especially the region of the midbrain seems to be an area for rewarding outcome by direct surgical excision of various lesions with almost no further morbidity and low mortality.

Case Material

In the period between 1973 and July 1989, 46 patients of all age groups with space occupying lesions within the midbrain were observed. 16 patients

were not considered to be subjects for surgical exploration either of apparently benign lesions with a long standing history and low morbidity without life threatening conditions, poor condition with entirely intrinsic diffuse growth or where consent was not given. Since these 16 patients are a very heterogenous group with varied pathological conditions, clinical onset and course, they are not able to serve as a control group and will not be discussed further.

Only 12 of these 30 surgical cases (Table 1, Fig. 1) exhibited signs and symptoms related to raised intracranial pressure, with headache, nausea, vomiting, and lethargy. It is noteworthy that neither Weber's syndrome, Benedict's syndrome, nor the Sylvian aqueduct syndrome in its full clinical appearance were observed in any of these patients. The conditions of 5 patients with acutely increased local pressure on the midbrain showed rapid clinical deterioration with loss of consciousness and decerebration, and they were immediately taken to surgery, although 4 of them were initially treated with placement of a ventriculo-atrial shunt (cases 3, 5, 10 and 22). The presenting signs and symptoms showed that:

a) the presence of hydrocephalus could not be correlated with the size or location of the lesion;

b) conjugate eye movement disorders were present with lesions at or near the tectal plate;

c) lesions within or near the cerebral peduncle in most cases caused hemiparesis or hemiplegia from disturbance of the corticospinal tract;

d) cerebellar signs such as ataxia and vertigo were present with lesions near the upper portion of the midbrain relating to involvement of the tracts of the brachium conjunctivum;

Table 1. *Clinical Data in 30 Patients who Had Direct Microsurgical Removal of Lesions Within the Midbrain*

Case number	Age/sex	Histological finding[a]	Localization[b]	Signs and symptoms	Surgical approach[c]	Additional therapy	Survival or length of postoperative follow-up	Karnofsky rating Preop	Postop
1	11 yr/F	PA	L cerebral peduncle	hydrocephalus, hemiplegia, Parinaud's syndrome acute decerebration	IT	preoperative radiotherapy, torkildsen	16 yr, alive with mild deficit	40 (10)	90
2	9 yr/M	EB	M-posterior 3rd V	hydrocephalus, Parinaud's syndrome	IS	preoperative radiotherapy, Torkildsen	1½ yr, death from disease	80	90 (1 yr)
3	3 yr/F	M B	M-posterior 3rd V	oculomotor disorder, acute decerebration	IS	postoperative radiotherapy, VA shunt	15 mo, death from disease	(10)	(50)
4	16 yr/M	H	interpeduncular cistern	gelastic epilepsy, precocious puberty	RST	none	5 yr, alive with deficits, no further follow-up	40	60
5	2 yr/M	MB	vermis-M-posterior 3rd V	hydrocephalus, hemiplegia	IT	preoperative VA shunt	2 mo, death, postoperative, related to surgery		
6	5 yr/M	A II	4th V-M	Parinaud's syndrome vertigo, ataxia, 7th nerve palsy	IT	postoperative radiotherapy	2 yr, alive with deficits, no further follow-up	40	60
7	57 yr/F	C/haemorrhages	R M	hemiparesis, Parinaud's syndrome, other oculomotor disorders, vertigo, ataxia, 5th, 6th nerve signs, acute decerebration	IS	preoperative VS shunt	8 yr, alive with mild deficits	40	90
8	31 yr/F	MA/haemorrhage	R M	Parinaud's syndrome, oculomotor disorder, 7th nerve palsy	IT	none	8 yr, alive with mild deficits	70	90
9	17 mo/M	EI	4th V-L M	hydrocephalus	IT	postoperative radiotherapy,	2 yr, death from disease		

No.	Age/Sex	Histology	Location	Clinical presentation	Approach	Treatment	Follow-up		
10	14 yr/F	C/haemorrhage	R M	subacute decerebration with occlusive hydrocephalus hemiparesis	IS	VA shunt preoperative VA shunt	6 yr, alive and well	20	100
11	52 yr/F	GB	R M	hemiparesis	IT	postoperative radiotherapy	2 yr and 9 mo, death from disease	40	80 (2 yr)
12	68 yr/F	M	L M	chronic intracranial pressure, oculomotor disorder, vertigo	IS	intraoperative Torkildsen	11 days, death, postoperative, related to surgery	40	
13	16 yr/M	PA	M	hydrocephalus, vertigo ataxia, acute decerebration	IT	partial resection, prior VA shunt	5 yr, alive and well	40	100
14	13 yr/M	PA	quadrigeminal plate	hydrocephalus, vertigo, ataxia	IS	pre-operative VA shunt	3 mo, alive with deficits, no further follow-up	90	90
15	5 yr/M	A II–III	L M	hemiplegia, oculomotor disorders	IT	radiotherapy	2 mo, alive with deficits, no further follow-up	50	80
16	17 yr/M	PA	M	chronic intracranial pressure, oculomotor disorders	IT	postoperative VA shunt	5 yr, alive with oculomotor disorders	50	70
17	68 yr/M	cystic M	R M	extrapyramidal motor disorder	IS	none	4 wk, death from pneumonia	50	(70)
18	18 mo/F	PNET	M	ataxia	IT	radiotherapy and chemotherapy	9 mo, death from disease		
19	53 yr/M	M	R M	oculomotor disorders, cephalalgia	RST	radiotherapy	6 mo, mild oculomotor disorder, death from disease	80	(100)
20	42 yr/F	M	R peduncle	hemiparesis	RST	2 mo previous frontal metastasis, lobectomy for lung tumour planned	3 yr, alive deteriorating during last 5 mo	90	90 (2 yr)

Table 1 (continued)

Case number	Age/sex	Histological finding[a]	Localization[b]	Signs and symptoms	Surgical approach[c]	Additional therapy	Survival or length of postoperative follow-up	Karnofsky rating Preop	Postop
21	6 yr/M	PA	L M	hemiparesis	IT	preoperative radiotherapy, postoperative VA shunt	2 yr and 8 mo, well with mild deficits	70	90
22	9 yr/M	PA	R M	hemiparesis	IT	preoperative radiotherapy, VA shunt	2 yr, alive with progression	70	90
23	3 yr/M	C/haematoma	L peduncle and upper pons	acute hemiparesis	LST	resection of a second cavernoma right frontal lobe, 9 mo postop.	2 yr, alive with progression	70	80
24	17 yr/F	C/haemorrhage	lower M	acute onset of vertigo and ataxia, cephalgia	IT	none	1 yr and 8 mo, alive with progression	40	80
25	27 yr/M	G	right M-sylvian fissure	progressive temporal lobe epilepsy	RST	none	1 yr and 7 mo, no further episodes	80	100
26	19 yr/M	A III	M P	ataxia, oculomotor disorders	LST	10 yr preop. radiotherapy, postoperative chemotherapy	14 mo, death from disease	90	(100)
27	18 yr/M	G	M Th	hemitremor, hemiparesis	RST		20 mo	100	100
28	14 yr/M	G	M	hydroceph., oculomotor disorder	IT	preoperative VA shunt, postoperative radiosurgery	18 mo	100	80
29	58 yr/M	A	AQU	hydroceph., bilateral spasticity	IT	intraoperative catheterization of aqueduct	11 mo	80	100
30	13 yr/F	C	M P	hemiparesis, ataxia	IT	preoperative radiotherapy	11 mo	80	80

[a] PA, pilocytic astrocytoma; EB, ependymoblastoma; MB, medulloblastoma; H, harmatoma; A, astrocytoma; C, cavernoma; MA, microangioma; E, ependymoma; GB, glioblastoma; M, metastasis; PNET, primitive neuroectodermal; G, ganglioglioma.
[b] L, left; R, right; M, midbrain; V, ventricle; P, pons; Th, thalmus; AQU, aqueduct.
[c] IT, infratentorial transcerebellar; IS, infratentorial supracerebellar; RST, right subtemporal transtentorial.

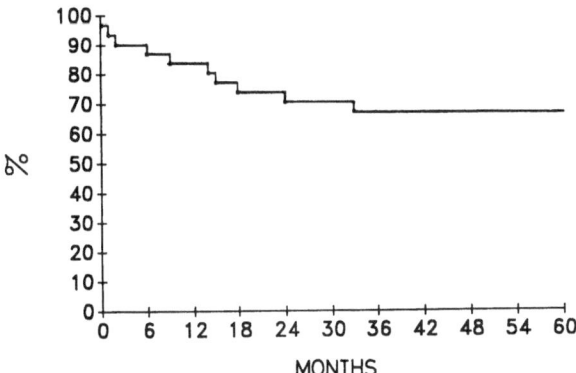

Fig. 1. Survival statistic of 30 surgically treated midbrain lesions (Kaplan-Meier)

e) only 1 patient harbouring a ganglioglioma extending toward the hippocampal gyrus exhibited temporal lobe epilepsy (case 25);

f) a coarse rhythmic tremor produced by involvement of the contralateral red nucleus was observed in one patient (case 17), a mild hemitremor in another case of a ganglioglioma in the midbrain extending towards the thalamus; and

g) lesions at the base of the midbrain or near the interpeduncular cistern produced homolateral or bilateral third nerve disturbance.

In 7 patients, ataxia was related to disturbance of coordination by compression or damage to the cerebellar tracts. Hemiparesis or hemiplegia occurred from involvement of corticospinal tracts; in 8 of 9 patients there was a surprising improvement after surgery. The prognosis for 3 of 5 patients with Parinaud's syndrome was good.

Localization of lesions in the era before CT scanning was primarily accomplished by scintigraphy and ventriculography (cases 1 to 4). In all subsequent patients, CT scanning was possible and provided sufficient information for evaluating the size and topographic features of the lesions. Magnetic resonance imaging (MRI) scans were performed in all patients after case 20, giving more detail for choosing the appropriate surgical approach and providing information about the histological and structural pattern of the lesion. Angiography did not help to establish either localization or tentative diagnosis even in patients with vascular pathological lesions (cavernomas).

The surgical approach was determined exclusively by topographical criteria, not by the tentative pathological characteristics of the lesion; for lateral extension, the subtemporal transtentorial approach proved to be the most appropriate (cases 4, 19, 20, 23, 25, 26 and 27). In most patients the approach was by an infratentorial route. The supracerebellar approach was only possible in those patients in whom lesions were limited entirely to the midbrain. A transcerebellar resection of the tumour was necessary in 9 patients (cases 5, 6, 9, 18, 21, 24, 28, 29 and 30), since the tumour extended toward the cerebellum and pons. The gliomatous lesions were intrinsic growths except for the cavernomas (with haemorrhage or haematomas), the metastatic tumours, and gangliogliomas, which fungated out of the right midbrain into the ambient cistern and toward the median aspect of the temporal lobe or toward the thalamus. In all patients delineation of the tumour from normal tissue was well visualized, as seen on CT scans, and even better on MRI scans. Radical extirpation of all lesions was not possible. Pre-operative neurological deficits diminished in all patients who survived except in one patient, in whom ataxia and oculomotor disorder only occurred postoperatively (case 28). In general, postoperative morbidity was of short duration and in most patients did not preclude satisfactory recovery.

Three deaths were related to the surgical procedure. One paediatric patient died 2 months after surgery, following a second haemorrhage into the tumour cavity (case 5). A second postoperative death occurred in an adult patient with metastasis who remained in a vegetative state postoperatively and died from a secondary haemorrhage into the tumour cavity on day 11 after surgery (case 12). Two years after a lobectomy for lung cancer, a 68-year-old patient died of pneumonia 4 weeks after resection of a midbrain metastasis following an initial excellent recovery (case 17).

Shunting procedures were necessary in many patients. Exceptions included 1 patient with a hamartoma in the interpenduncular cistern (case 4), 1 with an astrocytoma Grade ll (case 6) and 1 with a glioma (case 11) treated by radiotherapy postoperatively, 3 with metastatic tumours (case 17, 19 and 20), 2 with cavernomas (case 23 and 24), and 1 with a ganglioglioma (case 25). In 4 patients acute decerebration necessitated emergency ventriculoatrial shunt placement immediately after admission. In these patients subsequent surgery for the lesion itself was performed 7 days (case 10), 10 days (case 5), and 1 month later (cases 3 and 22). Shunt placement by a Torkildsen procedure was performed intra-operatively in 3 patients (cases 1, 2 and 12), in 1 patient with a pilocytic astrocytoma in the aqueduct a catheter was placed through the aqueduct during surgery (case 29).

Discussion

Tumour localization and the histological nature of the lesion within the brain stem seem to be the most important factors concerning postoperative morbidity and mortality. Walker and Storrs[8] presenting 10 cases of intrinsic brain stem gliomas had poor outcome in the lesions within the pons, with death at surgery in one case and survival with only a few months even if only open biopsy was possible, on the other hand in the one case of a tumour within the midbrain with radical extirpation they had an excellent outcome and in 4 cases of gliomas within the medulla oblongata they had 3 excellent results.

Usually the authors do not differentiate between prognosis concerning the growth of the lesion within the various levels of the brain stem. We consider the lower pons as the most dangerous area to be approached by open surgical procedures, a more favourable outcome can be expected in lesions within the medulla oblongata and even more in the midbrain area[3]. We do not agree with many authors who state that the more complex neuroanatomy of the brain stem and the great risk of injury to vital neurological function has discouraged the same aggressive approach to intrinsic lesions of the midbrain[4,7] and therefore, stereotactic CT-guided biopsy for diagnosis of these lesions is recommended[1,2].

Computed tomographic scans in combination with magnetic resonance imaging, the latter being superior to the first, afford good localisation of the lesion encountered, not only of their topographic peculiarities but also in most cases of their histological nature. This is in contrast to Smith et al.[6], who reported on 34 paediatric brain stem tumours, where only in 9 cases a biopsy was performed but all received radiotherapy; surgical excision was not discussed at all.

Compared with our own experiences and in relation to the literature we consider lesions within the midbrain as most rewarding lesions for direct surgical attack without stereotactic biopsy, if the patient is in a good and stable neurological and medical condition, and the lesion shows well delineated borders either solid or cystic.

No indication for surgery we find in patients with a short history and in poor neurological condition, and the lesion is diffuse with no echancement or in cases with partially or totally calcified processes with

stable mild symptoms. The alternative in these cases might be stereotactic biopsy. The need for a histological diagnosis for appropriate management of patients with brain stem lesion might be achieved by stereotatic biopsy. If possible we prefer open biopsy with the possibility of radical or subtotal resection of the lesion. In radiosensitive lesions a partial resection or debulking of the mass might improve the possibilities of further treatment by reducing the tumour burden. Also a clear tissue diagnosis will avoid empirical radiation therapy especially in the young age group with possible benign lesions.

Cavernomas will have the only chance of cure by open surgical approach and radical removal, stereotactic biopsy has no place in these cases. Radiation therapy and even radiosurgery has no effect on these lesions; they are a considerable problem if not resected totally.

Concerning the surgical approach we consider the vascular architecture surrounding the midbrain as the guideline for the proper exposure. Here the subtemporal transtentorial approach offers good access to the cerebral peduncle and also a lesion can be followed well toward the pons if there is a growth pattern in this direction. An infratentorial supracerebellar approach and occasionally an infratentorial transcerebellar approach is the ideal access for the more dorsally located lesions within the midbrain.

Surgical excision and even total removal might be easier with exophytic parts of the lesion or cystic components, but as Hoffman et al.[5] have demostrated there is a clinically and pathologically distinct group of benign brain stem gliomas that can be treated successfully by subtotal surgical excision even without these preliminaries. This group of tumours usually shows a long history and fungates into the fourth ventricle or extends out into the cerebellopontine angles, in CT scan they are radiodense with bright enhancement, histologically they prove grade l or ll astrcytomas or gangliogliomas. This same group of tumours is present within the midbrain, especially in the younger age group, where also only a subtotal surgical excision had extremely successful results with survival rate in our own series of more than 5 years without clinical or CT/MRI evidence of further tumour growth.

References

1. Chhang W, Kak VK, Banerjee AK, Rajwanshi A (1990) Stereotaxic biopsy of brain-stem tumours in children. Child's Nerv Syst 6: 409–411
2. Coffey RJ, Lunsford LD (1985) Stereotactic surgery for mass

lesions of the midbrain and pons. Neurosurgery 17: 12–18

3. Epstein F, Wisoff J (1987) Intra-axial tumours of the cervicomedullary junction. J Neurosurg 67: 483–487

4. Heffez DS, Zinreich SJ, Long DM (1990) Surgical resection of intrinsic brain stem lesions: an overview. Neurosurgery 27: 789–798

5. Hoffman HJ, Becker L, Craven MA (1980) A clinically and pathologically distinct group of benign brain stem gliomas. Neurosurgery 7: 243–247

6. Smith RR, Zimmerman RA, Packer RJ, Bilaniuk LT, Sutton LN, Goldberg HI, Grossman, RI, Schut L (1990) Pediatric brainstem glioma. Postradiation clinical and MR follow-up. Neurorad 32: 265–271

7. Stronik AR, Hoffman HJ, Hendrick EB, Humphreys RP, Davidson G (1987) Transependymal benign dorsally exophytic brain stem gliomas in childhood: Diagnosis and treatment recommendations. Neurosurgery 20: 439–444

8. Walker ML, Storrs BB (1985) Surgical therapy for intrinsic brain stem gliomas. Concepts pediat Neurosurg, Vol 5. Karger, Basel, pp 178–186

Correspondence: Prof. G. Pendl, M.D., Department of Neurosurgery, University of Graz Medical School, Auenbruggerplatz 29, A-8036 Graz, Austria.

Acta Neurochirurgica, Suppl. 53, 144–147 (1991)

Three-Quarter Prone Approach to the Pineal-Tentorial Region. Report of Seven Cases

J. Brotchi, M. Levivier, C. Raftopoulos, O. Dewitte, B. Pirotte, and J. Noterman

Department of Neurosurgery, Erasme Hospital, Free University of Brussels, Brussels, Belgium

Summary

We report our preliminary results (seven cases) with a three-quarter prone approach to the pineal-tentorial region using an opening beneath the midline. The technique we have used eliminates the risk of air embolism because the head is just over the right atrium, the table remaining in an horizontal plane. Using the natural effect of gravity, it is no more necessary to use retraction on the occipital lobe. So, hemianopsia is eliminated. We confirm the results of other teams who have used this approach which seems to us to be the best way to treat any lesion in the pineal-tentorial area.

Keywords: Pineal region tumours; three-quarter prone occipital transtentorial approach; midbrain tumours; tentorial tumours.

Introduction

The difficulty in approaching the pineal region and the dissatisfaction with surgical techniques described can be verified with the number of operative plans that have been proposed to reach this area: transcallosal[4], occipital transtentorial[5,11,12], infratentorial supracerebellar approaches[7,9,14,15] and sitting[5], prone[13], Concorde[6] positions. This emphasizes the surgeon's dissatisfaction with the surgical techniques described.

Recently, a three-quarter prone position with the bone flap placed beneath the midline has been described[1,3,8]. We have decided to test this approach and we report our preliminary results on seven cases.

Surgical Technique

The patient is placed in a position between the three-quarter prone position and the right lateral decubitus with the right arm slipping off the end of the operating table and supported by a pillow. Fixed in a Mayfield head holder, the head is rotated to a 30 degrees angle with the floor, with a moderate flexion to avoid any venous compression. The operating table is maintained horizontally and may be rotated during surgery if one desires more or less head

rotation with the floor. Finally, the head is tilted towards the upper shoulder by elevating the vertex 30 degrees from the horizontal (Fig. 1).

This position gives an excellent view over the tentorium and the tentorial hiatus and allows the right hemisphere to fall away from the midline while the falx cerebri supports the left hemisphere. A 10 cm (6 to 8 in children) unilateral bone flap, 2 cm superior to the torcula, is made just over the midline, giving an excellent view over the area. The dura is opened in a conventional horseshoe fashion, basing the horseshoe on the superior sagittal sinus with preservation of the parasagittal draining veins which are not numerous in this area. The patient is premedicated with steroids the day before operation and receives Mannitol and Furosemide at the beginning of surgery. Spinal drainage is used after dura opening, providing a very good operative corridor. Brain retraction is not always necessary as the right hemisphere falls away by gravity. The tentorial hiatus is approached and, to provide greater room, the tentorium may be divided 2 mm lateral to the straight sinus and parallel to it. This gives an excellent view over the superior vermis, the quadrigeminal plate, the vein of Galen, the splenium and the posterior third of the corpus callosum. If necessary, one may divide the inferior longitudinal sinus and cut the falx to have a complete view over the opposite side. Under the microscope, one may attack

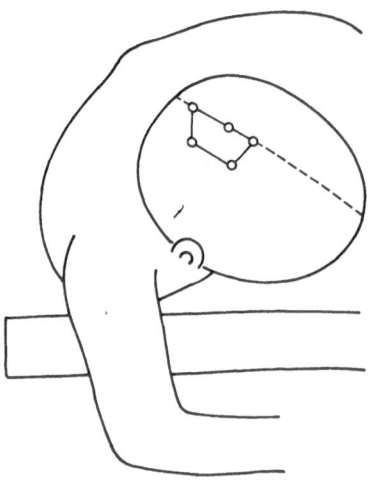

Fig. 1. Patient's position

Table 1

Cases	Sex	Age	Pathology	Location	Surgery	Follow-up
1.	F	6	Giant aneurysm	Posterior choroidal arteries	Complete removal with trapping	Asymptomatic
2.	M	40	Mycotic aneurysm	Posterior cerebral art. P2-P3 junction	Complete removal with trapping	Asymptomatic
3.	F	41	Arachnoid cyst	Quadrigeminal cistern area	Large resection and opening into quadrigeminal cistern	Asymptomatic
4.	M	46	Huge arachnoid cyst	Corpus callosum, pineal and upper brain stem	Large resection and opening into 3rd ventricle	Asymptomatic
5.	M	46	AVM	Superior vermis	Gross total excision of the angioma	Asymptomatic
6.	M	56	Melanoma metastasis	Superior quadrigeminal plate	Total resection	No post-operative deficit. After 8 months, death from multiple brain metastases.
7.	M	5	Glioma (astrocytoma II)	Pulvinar, pineal and vermis	Subtotal resection	No post-operative deficit. Moderate disability post-radiotherapy and chemotherapy.

all the lesions of this area with the help of bipolar coagulation, the Cavitron or the laser. After completion of the operative procedure, the dura is closed as watertight as possible. The bone flap is replaced and wired in position. The scalp is closed in the two-layers.

Results

Our preliminary results concern seven cases: 2 tumours, 2 aneurysms, 2 arachnoid cysts, 1 arterio-venous malformation (AVM) (Table 1). The most important clinical fact is the absence of any post-operative visual field deficit. We encountered no problem related to superficial parasagittal veins nor to deep venous drainage. In case 7, we explored the posterior fossa through opening of the tentorium and the third ventricle after cutting the corpus callosum 2 cm prior to the splenium. In vascular pathology, we had a rapid control of the arterial feeders. We may say that this position is very comfortable for the surgeon and the assistant (Fig. 2).

Discussion

Using the supracerebellar infratentorial approach, one must coagulate the veins draining the cerebellar hemisphere to reach the pineal region. This might result in cerebellar venous infarction[9]. The advantages of the occipital transtentorial approach over the supracerebellar infratentorial approach have been described by surgeons using both approaches[12]. But, by using the sitting position, one may encounter two main problems: air embolism, and hemianopsia due to occipital lobe retraction. By putting the operating table in an horizontal plane, we have no more risk than during supine surgery[16]. We like to use lumbar CSF drainage rather than tapping the lateral ventricle. This provides good surgical access by helping the right hemisphere to fall away with gravity. No aggressive brain retraction is necessary to reach the pineal region. This is the reason why hemianopsia may be avoided. We see no advantage in making a bony opening accross the midline to the opposite side and at the level of the transverse sinus[3]. With the head slightly tilted to the upper shoulder (30° from the horizontal), the superior border of the operative field is effaced. The surgical approach we have used is more comfortable than the Concorde or the sitting position. Furthermore, it is the shortest way to approach the pineal region. The assitant's help is not limited. We confirm the general paucity of significant parasagittal veins in the posterior third of the sagittal sinus[8]. The

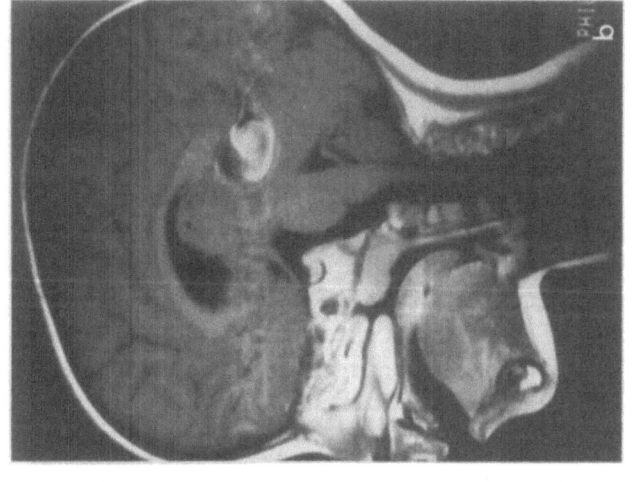

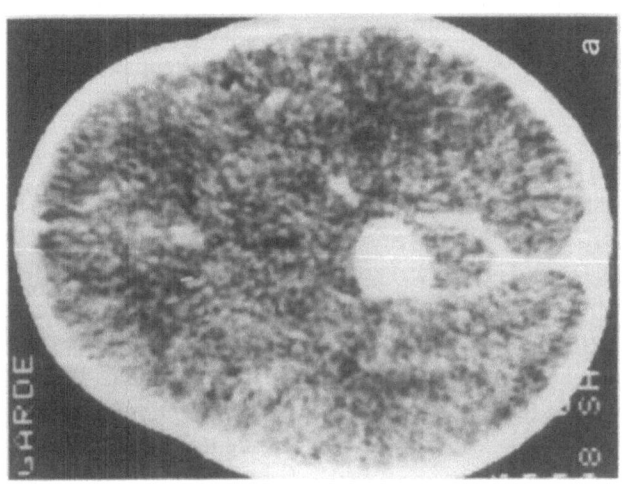

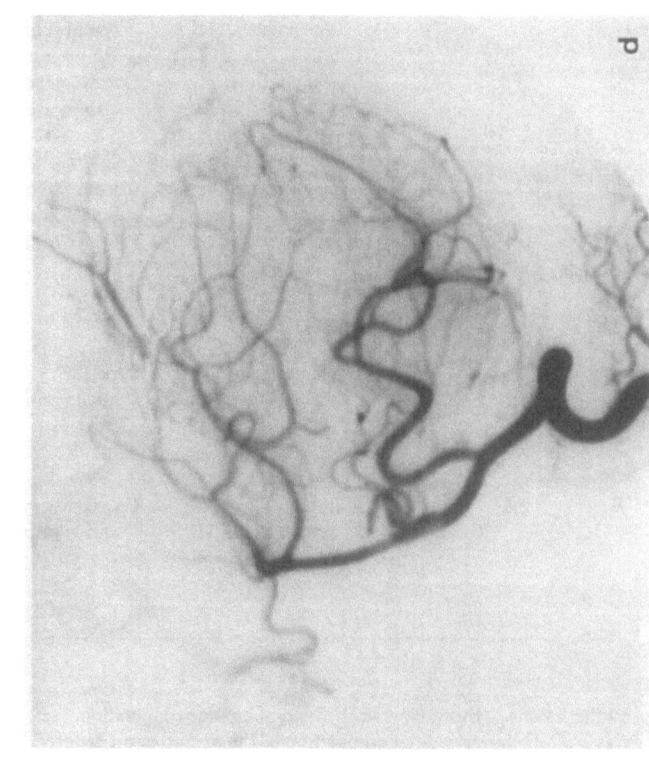

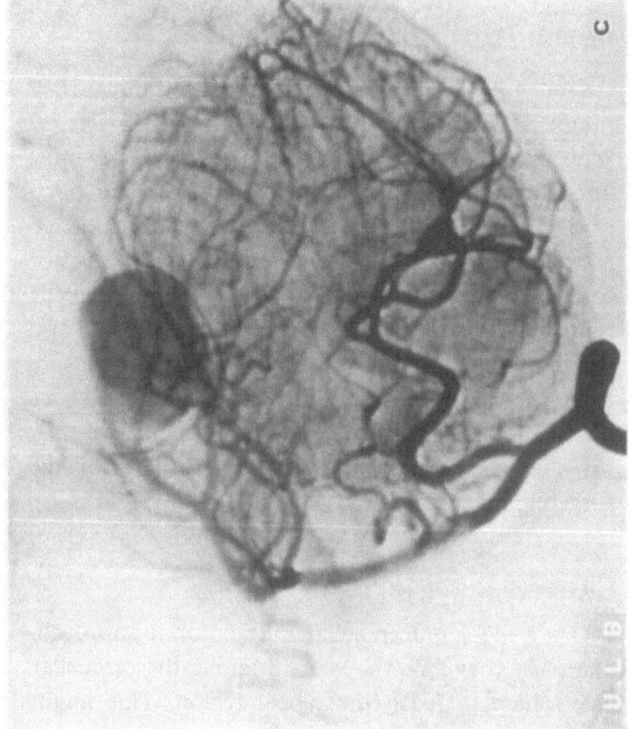

Fig. 2. Case 1, a) CT Scan demonstrating a homogeneously contrast-enhancing lesion of the midline. b) Sagittal T1-weighted MRI with gadolinium-enhanced lesion situated at the upper vermian area. The characteristics are in favour of a partially thrombosed giant aneurysm. c) Vertebral angiography showing a distal giant aneurysm. d) Postoperative vertebral angiogram

tentorial opening inferiorly parallel to the straight sinus is easy, providing an excellent view of the superior vermis, the quadrigeminal plate and the perimesencephalic cistern on the other side. Access to the posterior part of the third ventricle is possible by retraction of the splenium. The internal cerebral veins, the basilar veins of Rosenthal are frequently displaced by the tumour mass. Usually, one can work around them[8]. We never had to divide them but if necessary one could coagulate and divide one or two of these vessels[8] without harmful effects[2]. So far, our limited experience with this approach is encouraging and we are decided to continue using it.

References

1. Ausman JI, Malik GM, Dujovny M, Mann R (1988) Three-quarter prone approach to the pineal-tentorial region. Surg Neurol 29: 298–306
2. Caron JP, Nick J, Contamin F, Singer B, Comoy J, Keravel Y (1977) Tolerance de la ligature et de la thrombose aseptique des veines cérébrales profondes chez l'homme. Ann Med Interne (Paris) 12: 899–906
3. Clark WK (1987) Occipital transtentorial approach. In: Apuzzo MLJ (ed) Surgery of the third ventricle. William & Wilkins, Baltimore, pp 591–610
4. Dandy WE (1921) An operation for the removal of pineal tumors. Surg Gynecol Obstet 33: 113–119
5. Jamieson KG (1971) Excision of pineal tumors. J Neurosurg 35: 550–553
6. Kobayashi S, Sugita K, Tanaka Y, Kyoshima K (1983) Infra-tentorial approach to the pineal region in the prone position: Concorde position. J Neurosurg 58: 141–143
7. Krause F (1926) Operative Freilegung der Vierhügel nebst Beobachtungen über Hirndruck and Dekompression. Zentralbl Chir 53: 2812–2819
8. McComb JG, Apuzzo MLJ (1987) Posterior intrahemispheric retrocallosal and transcallosal approaches. In: Apuzzo MLJ (ed) Surgery of the third ventricle. William & Wilkins, Baltimore, pp 611–641
9. Page LK (1977) The infratentorial supracerebellar exposure of tumors in the pineal area. Neurosurgery 1: 36–40
10. Pendl G (1985) Microsurgical approaches to the pineal and midbrain region. In: Pendl G (ed) Pineal and midbrain lesions, Springer, New York, Wien pp 103–116
11. Poppen JL (1966) The right occipital approach to a pinealoma. J Neurosurg 25: 706–710
12. Reid NS, Clark WK (1978) Comparison of the infratentorial and transtentorial approaches to the pineal region. Neurosurgery 3: 1–8
13. Sano K (1983) Pineal region tumors: problems in pathology treatment. Clin Neurosurg 30: 59–91
14. Stein BM (1971) The infratentorial supracerebellar approach to pineal lesions. J Neurosurg 35: 197–202
15. Stein BM (1982) Supracerebellar approach for pineal region neoplasms. In: Schmidek HH, Sweet WH (eds) Operative neurosurgical techniques. Indications, methods and results, vol 1. Grune & Stratton, New York, pp 599–607
16. Stone JL, Cybulski GR, Crowell RM, Moody RA (1990) The lateral position-dependant occipital approach-to pineal and medial occipito-parietal lesions. Acta Neurochir (Wien) 102: 133–136

Correspondence: Prof. J. Brotchi, Department of Neurosurgery, Erasme Hospital, Free University of Brussels, route de Lennik 808, B-1070 Brussels, Belgium.

Acta Neurochirurgica, Suppl. 53, 148–158 (1991)

Direct Surgery for Brainstem Tumours

A. Bricolo, S. Turazzi, L. Cristofori, and A. Talacchi

Department of Neurosurgery, University Hospital, Verona, Italy

Summary

Updating a previous report, the authors offer a review of 45 patients between age 2 and 63 treated by direct surgical excision for brainstem tumours of various description. Since 1986 all candidate patients were examined by NMR imaging in addition to CT scanning, sometimes with the further addition of digital-subtraction vertebral angiography. By Epstein and McLeary's criteria, 24 of the tumours were focal, 12 were cervicomedullary and 9 were diffuse. The most frequent histological diagnosis was glioma (36 cases between low-grade astrocytoma, anaplastic astrocytoma and glioblastoma); the balance was provided by cavernoma (6 cases), haemangioblastoma (2 cases), and lipoma (2 cases). Gross total resection was achieved in 28 patients, namely all those with ependymoma or vascular tumours and 14 of 17 with low-grade astrocytoma. Resection was subtotal in 16 cases and confined to a generous biopsy in one. There was no operative mortality, but 2 deaths occurred in the early postoperative period. At discharge, neurological status was unchanged or improved in 35 cases. At 3-month followup examination, 12 patients were improved, 27 were unchanged and 3 were worsened. By January 1990 (6 to 72 months postoperatively) 27 of the first 40 patients treated were alive: 13 had resumed normal life, 6 were self-sufficient and 8 were disable. The authors conclude that present-day microsurgical resection of intra-axial brainstem tumours is associated with low mortality and morbidity and affords favourable results-for which they credit high-quality NMR imaging, efficient microsurgery, adequate anesthesia, and competent postoperative intensive care.

Keywords: Brainstem; glioma; intrinsic tumour; microneurosurgery.

Introduction

Formerly off-limits to neurosurgical intervention, intrinsic brainstem tumours are still regarded with a good deal of perplexity, much conflict originating from the clash of inherited tenets and the apertures offered by new diagnostic and surgical technics[3,8,13]. Tumours located in the brainstem were considered for a long time a homogeneous nosologic category, not amenable to surgical aggression and treated empiri- cally by blindfold radiotherapy (sometimes associated with antitubercular treatment), with altogether disappointing results[2,9,16,23,24]. Thus, most of the published series of cases lack histological verification and are therefore of no use.

Direct surgical aggression of these lesions has been viewed by some as plain looking for trouble[15,22]; others have conceded that it may play a marginal role in terms of evacuating cyst formations, removing exophytic parts of the tumour, or collecting tissue specimens for histological examination[4,21,23,28]. The result of this still prevalent attitude is that whereas the longevity of patients with tumours of the posterior cranial fossa has been sizably improved, prognosis remains definitely poor for those with intrinsic tumours of the brainstem. None of the treatments proposed or tried in the past escapes being labeled as mere palliation; in essence, patients are allowed to follow a downward course of progressive, inexorable neurologic deterioration. With only a few patients mysteriously surviving for a long time after diagnosis, most die within one year[16,18].

The direct surgical aggression of tumours located in the brainstem is discouraged by the fundamental objection that any manipulation, however delicate, of so vital an area of the central nervous system will only invite major morbidity – to say nothing of a mortality formerly up to 60% – or at any rate entailing unacceptably high risks. This resistance is only just beginning to slacken as important surgical results appear in the literature[3,10,11,12,13,18,19,20,26,27]. Progress in neuroimaging, the use of the operative microscope in connection with microsurgical technics, the use of ultrasound aspiration and laser surgery, refinements in neuro-anesthesia, and the increasing availability of neurosurgical intensive care units are affording a more anatomical (hence safer) approach to the brainstem with less and less risk in terms of survival and function.

In 1980 Hoffmann and his associates[14] were the first to affirm the value of direct surgery in a minority of brainstem gliomas which they called "benign" in that they were not·infiltrating and showed exophytosis into the fourth ventricle. Later, several other workers reported the successful removal of brainstem gliomas[13,17,19,25,26,27]; and in 1986 Epstein and McLeary[10] published a fundamental contribution concerning the radical excision of intrinsic brainstem gliomas; this gave decisive impulse to further work along the same lines. For our part, we presented our own initial experience with the removal of brainstem tumours in 1987 at the annual meeting of the Italian Neurosurgical Society[6], amounting to 11 cases at the time; by now, our caseload has been considerably amplified and long-term results have become available for older cases; at this point we definitely agree with the view expressed by other neurosurgical groups, that many brainstem tumours can be removed radically or apparently so not only without aggravating the neurological picture but in fact with considerable amelioration sometimes amounting to permanent cure, as we shall try to illustrate in this present paper.

Patients and Methods

Our aggregated experience with direct brainstem surgery, started in 1984, now totals 45 patients treated by extensive or possibly radical tumour excision. Our series consists of 25 males and 20 females between 2 and 63 years of age (mean age 30). Thirty per cent of our cases were in the pediatric age group (under 16). All were operated on by the same surgeon (A. B.) and by the same technic.

All patients had been diagnosed tentatively or finally as being brainstem tumour elsewhere and were referred to our Department for an assessment of operability. Only 3 patients had been radiated; one had undergone stereotaxic biopsy and radiotherapy, and one carried a ventriculo-peritoneal shunt.

Clinically they presented with a history of progressive neurological deterioration with involvement of the intermediate and lower cranial nerves, hemiparesis or quadriparesis, and spasticity. At the time of surgery the majority (65%) were moderately or severely disabled.

Tumour Classification

For purposes of surgical planning the presenting tumours were classified as suggested by Epstein and McLeary[10] into three subgroups, namely focal, cervicomedullary (Fig. 1) and diffuse. In our first 8 cases, classification was based on the returns of enhanced CT scanning; later it was determined also, indeed chiefly, on nuclear magnetic resonance (NMR) imaging. The series so classified

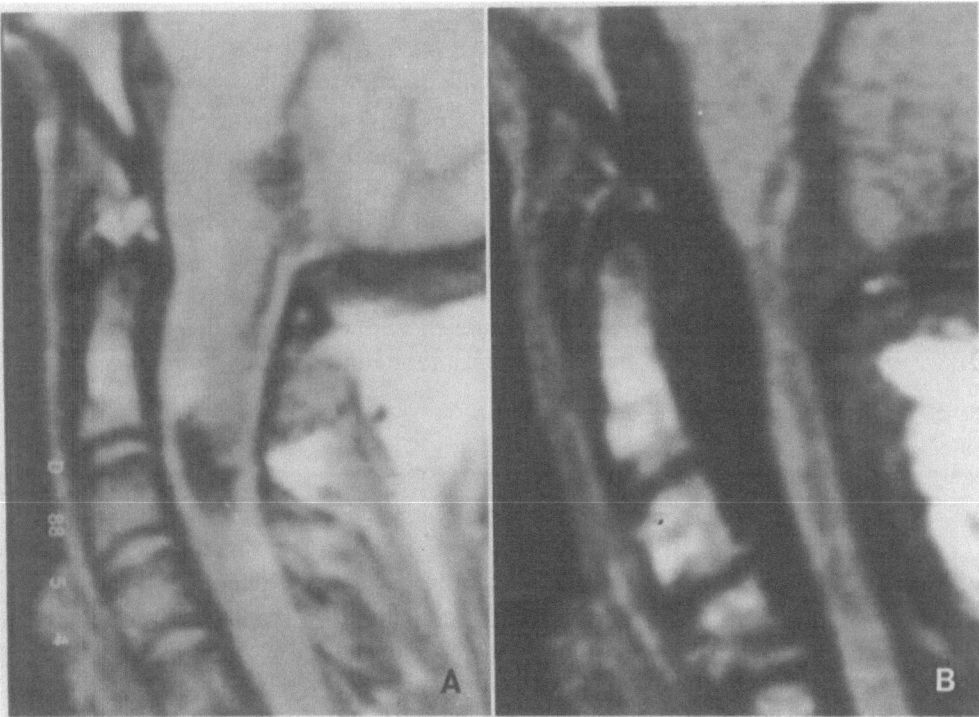

Fig. 1. Sagittal magnetic resonance T_1-weighted imaging in a patient with a cervicomedullary astrocytoma. On the preoperative image (A) the intraaxial tumour enlarging the rostral spinal cord and the medulla can be seen. Two years postoperatively (B) there is a morphological rearrangement with no signs of recurrence

comprises 24 focal tumours, 12 tumours of the cervicomedullary junction, and 9 diffuse tumours. The anatomical sites and extent of these 45 resected tumours are displayed in Table 1.

Surgical Technic

Currently the excellent multiplanar imaging capability of NMR technology, in addition to enhanced CT scanning and when necessary digital angiography, affords accurate preoperative localization of brainstem tumours. From a detailed analysis of the information so obtained in each case we proceeded to choosing the surgical approach most likely to afford good surgical exposure without undue risk of injuring nervous and vascular structures along the way or adjacent to the tumour mass. Table 2 particularizes the various approaches that were used and the types of tumours so approached.

Table 1. *Neuroimaging Classification and Anatomical Location of Brainstem Tumours in 45 Patients*

No of cases	Subgroup	Location
24	*Focal*	
	15 intraaxial	6 midbrain
		6 pons
		3 medulla
	9 with exophytosis	1 midbrain – temporal fossa
		3 pons – p.c. angle
		5 pons – IV ventricle
12	*Cervicomedullary*	
	10 intraaxial	10 cervicomedullary junction
	2 with exophytosis	2 cerebellomedullary cisterns
9	*Diffuse*	
	7 intraaxial	7 brainstem
	2 with exophytosis	2 pons and cerebellomedullary cisterns

Table 2. *Surgical Approaches and Location of the Tumour*

No of cases	Surgical approach	Location of tumour
18	Suboccipital craniectomy and cervical laminectomy	12 cervicomedullary junction
		3 focal in the medulla
		3 diffuse
18	Suboccipital craniotomy via the fourth ventricle	6 exophytic into IV ventricle
		5 focal in the pons
		1 focal in the midbrain
		6 diffuse
3	Suboccipital retromastoid craniotomy via the c.p. angle	2 exophytic into c.p. angle
		1 exophytic into brachium pontis
5	Suboccipital craniotomy via the infratentorial supracerebellar route	5 focal in the lamina quadrigemina
1	Fronto-pterional craniotomy via subtemporal route	1 midbrain exophytic

All operations but one were done with the patient in a semisitting position with suitable anesthesiological arrangements; rigorous microsurgical technology was used throughout. After reaching the tumour area and removing exophytic formations if any, a short incision was made in the brainstem surface nearest to the tumour. In 23 cases the tumour was exposed through an incision made into the floor of the fourth ventricle; for midline or paramedian tumours the incision was made along the median sulcus to afford entry without injury to the facial collicula. In the 3 patients with medullary tumours (Figs. 2, 3, 4 and 5) the incision was again on the midline, astride the obex, and the tumour was exposed after careful splaying of the gracilis and cuneate funiculli and of the trigone of the hypoglossal nerve. In the great majority of cases, lifting the cerebellar tonsils and vermis was enough to give good exposure of the floor of the fourth ventricle; in only 4 cases, adequate exposure required a short additional cut into the inferior vermis and tela choroidea. The 12 cervicomedullary tumours were exposed through a midline myelotomy of the cervical spinal cord, extended to and beyond the obex; then the tumour formation was removed by the same technic used for intrinsic medullary tumours.

Once exposed, glial tumours were removed piecemeal by mechanical or ultrasonic aspiration or bipolar coagulation and cutting, care being taken to remain consistently inside the tumour. At the start of mass debulking we collected enough specimens to afford state and definitive histological examination. Obviously, immediate information about the pathology and degree of malignancy of the tumour on hand is of value in regard to the greater or lesser need to strive for radical excision. In all cases, at any rate, debulking was maintained rigorously within the tumours tissue, and it was suspended whenever the boundaries with normal tissue became poorly defined.

Results

Pathology

The most common histological diagnosis in our series was glioma (36 of 45 cases) with a prevalence of benign forms (21 between astrocytoma I–II and ependymoma) as against 15 malignants. Concerning the relationship between subgroups of the adopted classification and the types of pathology identified at surgery (Table 3), we may note a definite prevalence (7 of 9 cases) of malignant gliomas in the subgroup of diffuse tumours, and conversely the prevalence of benign forms in the other two subgroups.

Extent of Removal

Radical tumour excision, as adjudged intraoperatively by the certainty of having reached healthy tissue boundaries around the tumour, was achieved in 28 of our 45 patients (62%). Removal was incomplete in 16 cases (36%), albeit extensive in proportion to the tumour mass; in these cases, debulking was suspended because of technical difficulties or operational wariness before achieving gross total removal. In a single case surgery amounted to nothing more than an

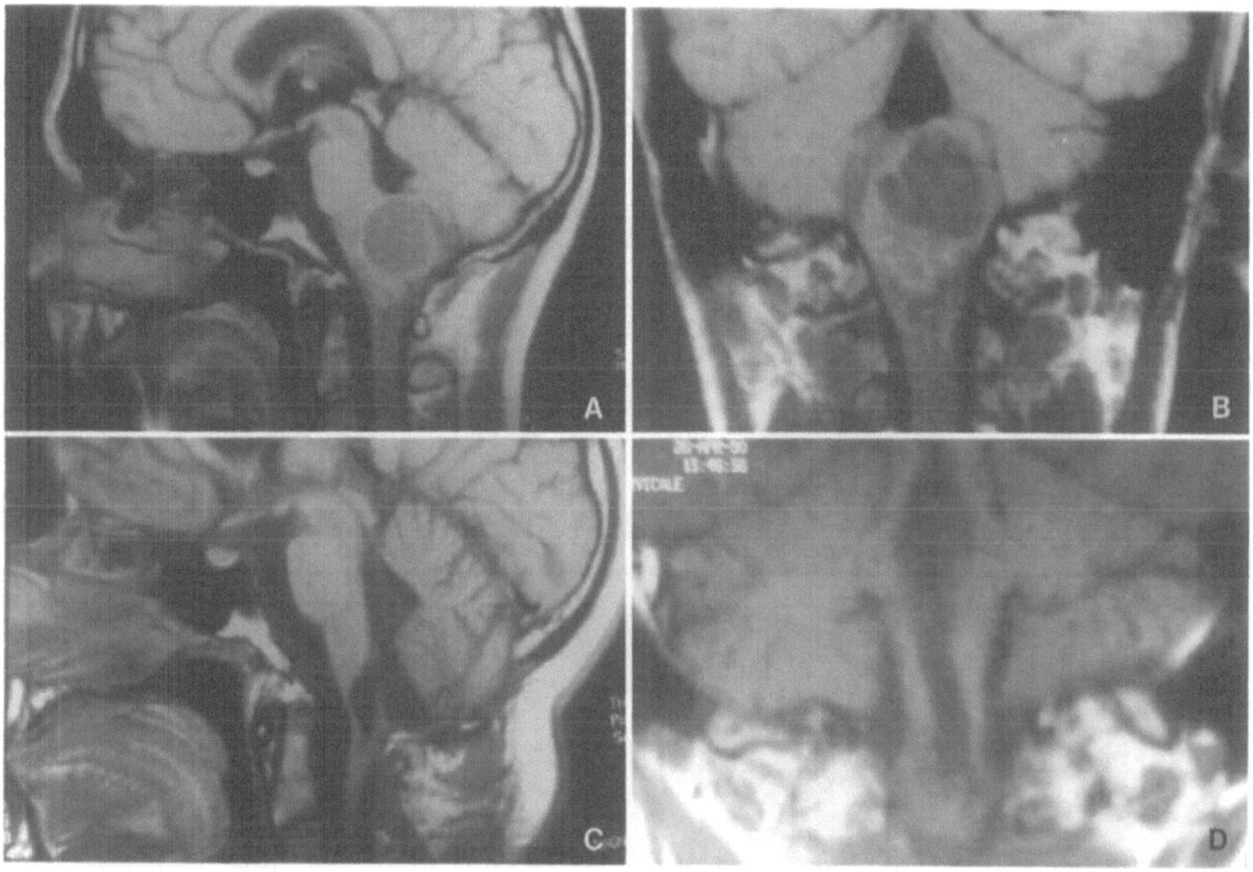

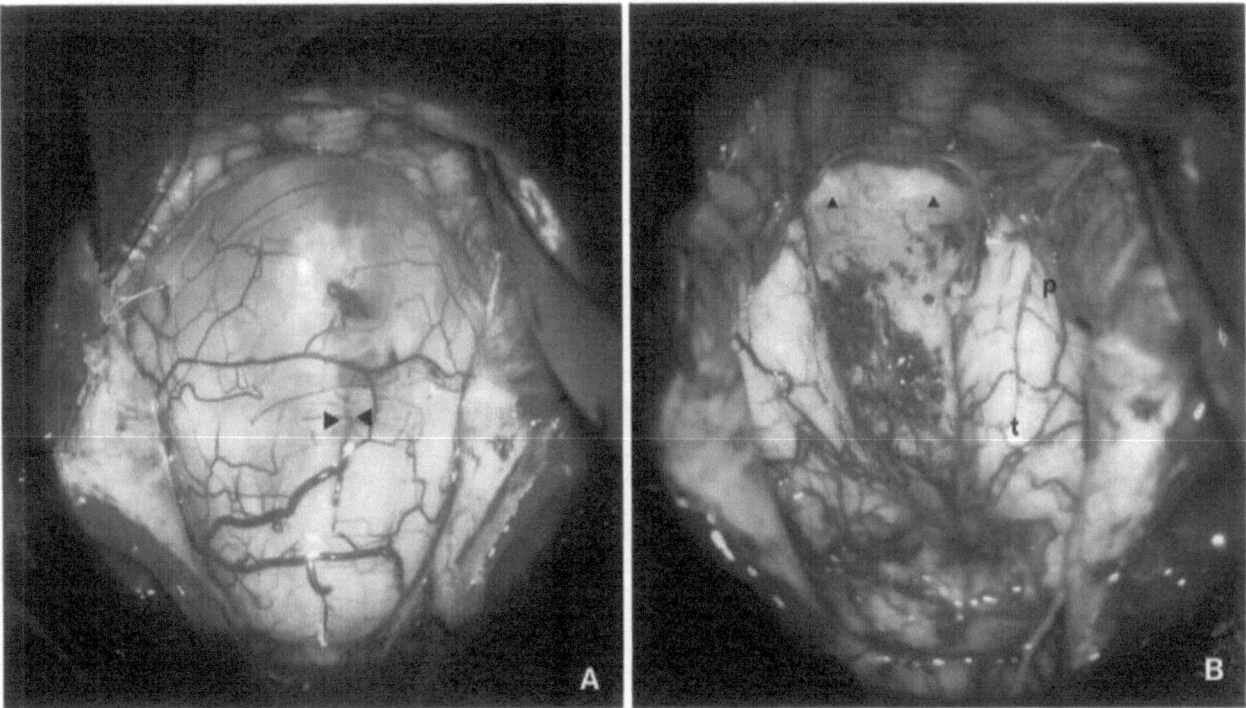

Fig. 2. Sagittal and coronal magnetic resonance images (T$_1$-weighted) of a patient with a medullary focal ependymoma, before surgery (A and B) and 4 months later (C and D). The tumour was completely removed and the patient resumed normal life

Fig. 3. Operative photographs of the same patient as in preceding figure. At the opening of the dura (A) a tremendous expansion of the medulla oblongata can be seen. After the tumour excision (B) the medulla is collapsed. (*Large arrows* = posterior median fissure; *small arrows* = striae medullares on the floor of the fourth ventricle; *p* = PICA, *t* = cuneate and cinereus tubercles)

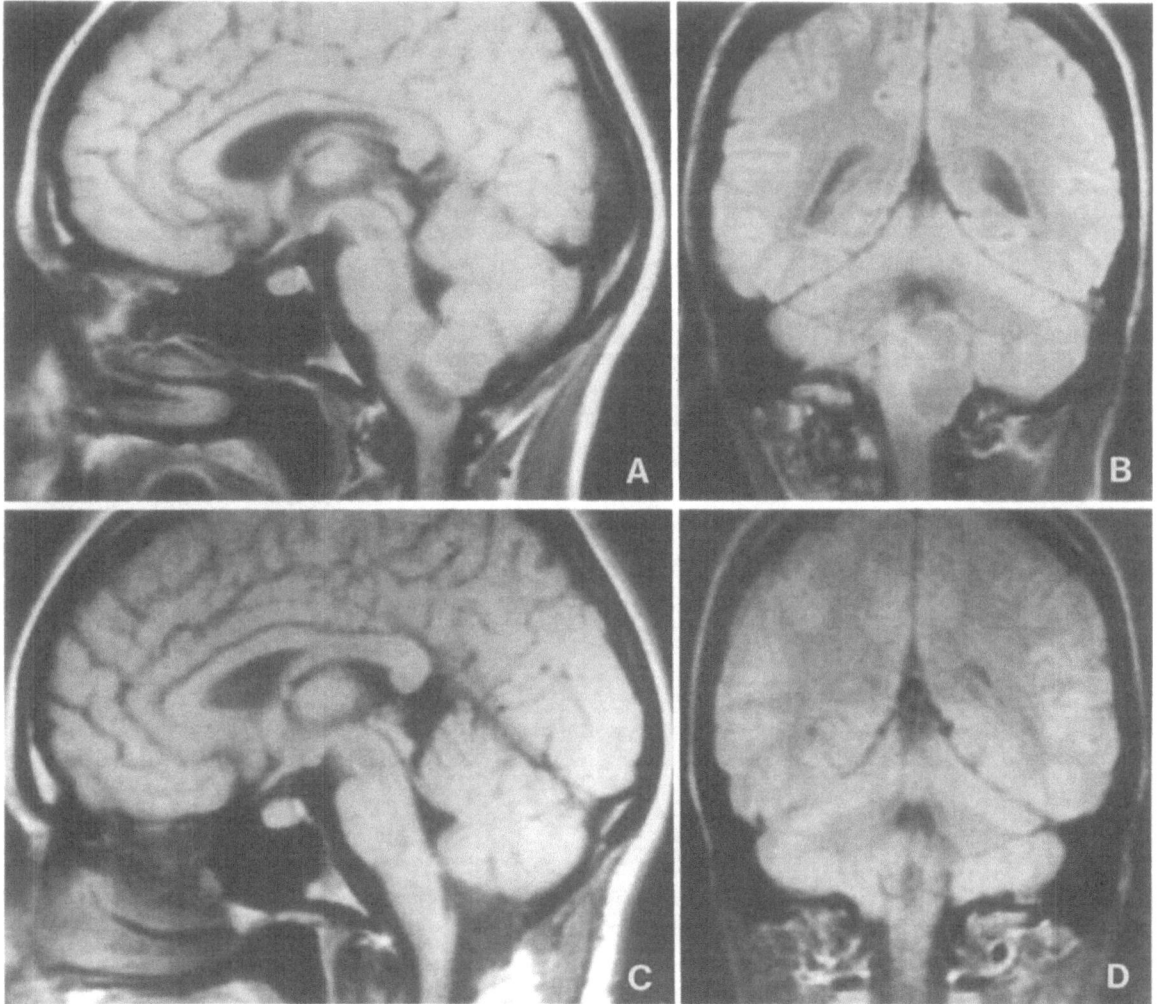

Fig. 4. Preoperative (A and B) and postoperative (C and D) magnetic resonance images in a patient with a medullary ependymoma

Table 3. *Neuroimaging Classification and Pathology of the 45 Brainstem Tumours in Present Series*

Tumour classification	No of cases	Pathology				
		Astro I, II	Malignant glioma	Ependymoma	Vascular	Lipoma
Focal	24	10	4	3	6	1
Cervicomedullary	12	5	4	1	1	1
Diffuse	9	2	7	–	–	–
Total	45	17	15	4	7*	2

* Cavernoma 5, angioreticuloma 2.

extended biopsy (Tables 4 and 5). In nearly all cases the surgeon's appraisal of the degree of removal achieved found confirmation in neuroimaging returns elicited about 3 months after surgery.

Radical exeresis proved possible in 79% of focal tumours and 75% of cervicomedullary junction

tumours. In terms of histological types, in addition to all ependymomas and vascular tumours (Figs. 6 and 7), 82% of our low-grade astrocytomas were removed radically. Conversely, subtotal removal was practically the rule for diffuse tumours (8 of 9 cases) and malignant tumours (11 of 15 cases).

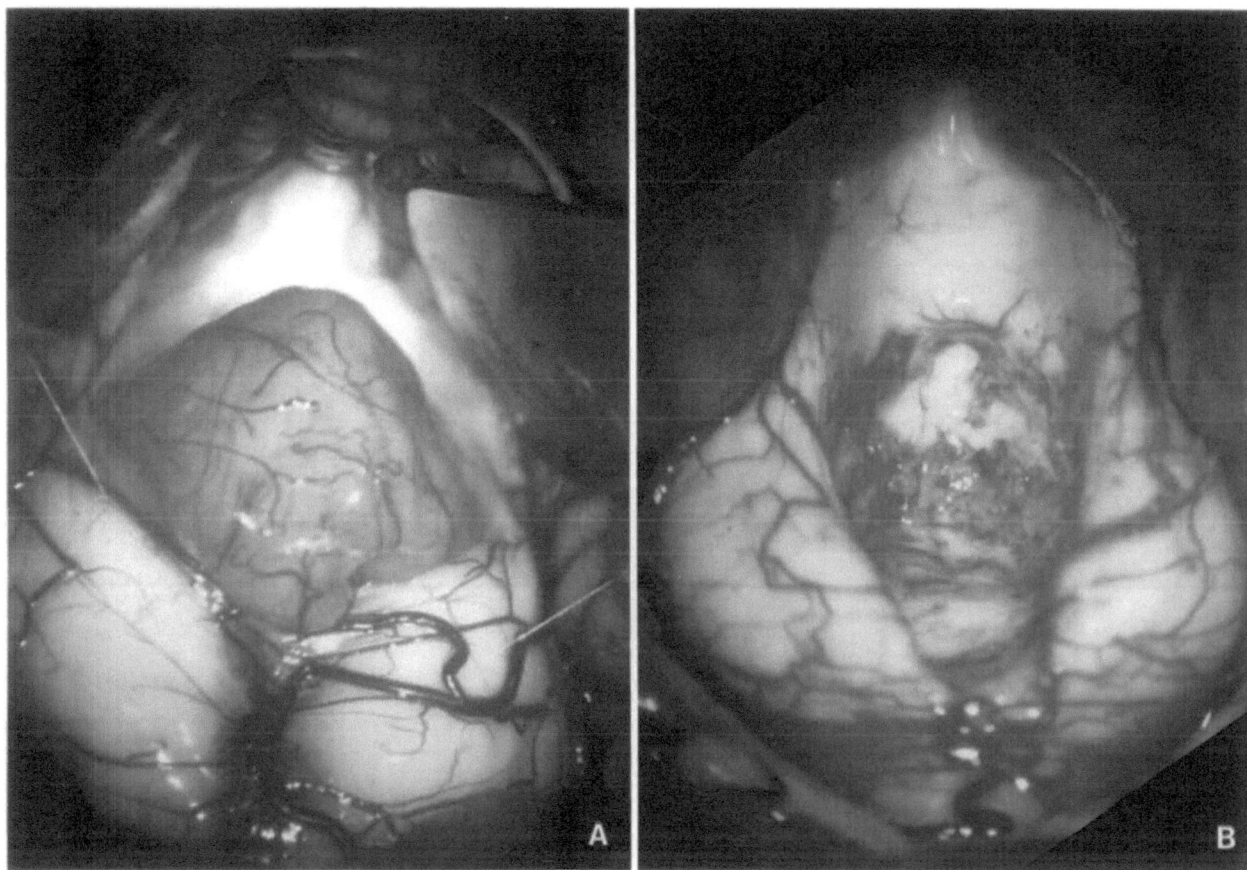

Fig. 5. Operative photographs of the same patient as in Fig. 4 that show the lower brainstem with the ependymoma exophiting from the medulla in the obex region (A). The tumour was totally removed (B) by opening the posterior median fissure

Table 4. *Extent of Surgical Removal Related to Tumour Subgroups*

Surgical removal	No of cases	Type of tumour		
		Focal	Cervicomedullary	Diffuse
Complete	28 (62%)	19 (79%)	9 (75%)	–
Subtotal	16 (36%)	5 (21%)	3 (25%)	8 (89%)
Partial	1	–	–	1
Total	45	24	12	9

Table 5. *Extent of Surgical Removal Related to Pathology*

Surgical removal	No of cases	Pathology				
		Astro I, II	Malignant glioma	Ependymoma	Vascular	Lipoma
Complete	28 (62%)	14 (82%)	3 (20%)	4 (100%)	7 (100%)	–
Subtotal	16 (36%)	3 (18%)	11 (73%)	–	–	2 (100%)
Partial	1	–	1	–	–	–
Total	45	17	15	4	7	2

Postoperative Course

There was no intraoperative mortality; two patients died in the early postoperative period and another died before the 3-month recheck. Immediately after surgery all the patients were removed to our Neuro-surgical Intensive Care Unit, where they remained for periods of 2 days to 3 weeks. All showed an initial clinical and neurological aggravation of varying severity; some required assisted respiration with

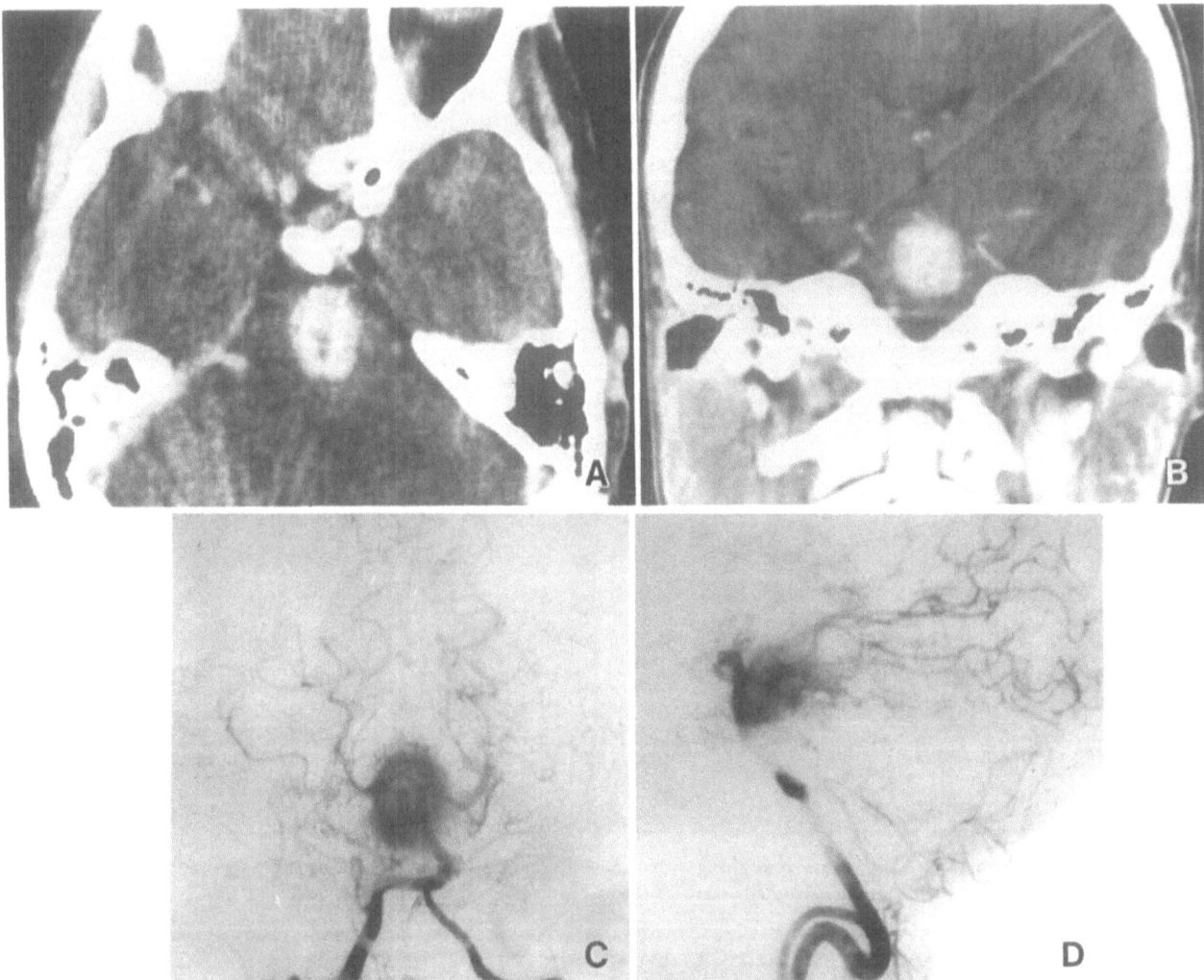

Fig. 6. Contrast enhanced CT scan in axial (A) and coronal views (B) showing an intraaxial midbrain angioreticuloma. Anteroposterior (C) and lateral (D) vertebral angiograms document its conspicuous vascularization

Table 6. *Neurological Status Three Months After Surgery Related to Pathology*

	No of cases	Pathology				
		Astro I, II	Malignant glioma	Ependymoma	Vascular	Lipoma
Improved	12	5	2	2	2	1
Unchanged	27	11	10	2	3	1
Worsened	3	1	1	–	1	–
Dead	3	–	2	–	1	–
Total	45	17	15	4	7	2

nasotracheal intubation for more than one week. All patients, at any rate, were hooked to an apnea alarm, since respiratory arrest may occur suddenly during sleep – a iatrogenic Ondine's curse.

Aside from general aggravation and the onset of 6th and 7th nerve palsies and pyramidal defect (none inherently life-threatening), the main problem was represented by difficulties in swallowing and raising sputum, with the risk of aspiration pneumonia. Sedulous and dedicated intensive care, such as is required for these patients presenting with major motor and respiratory problems but otherwise fully

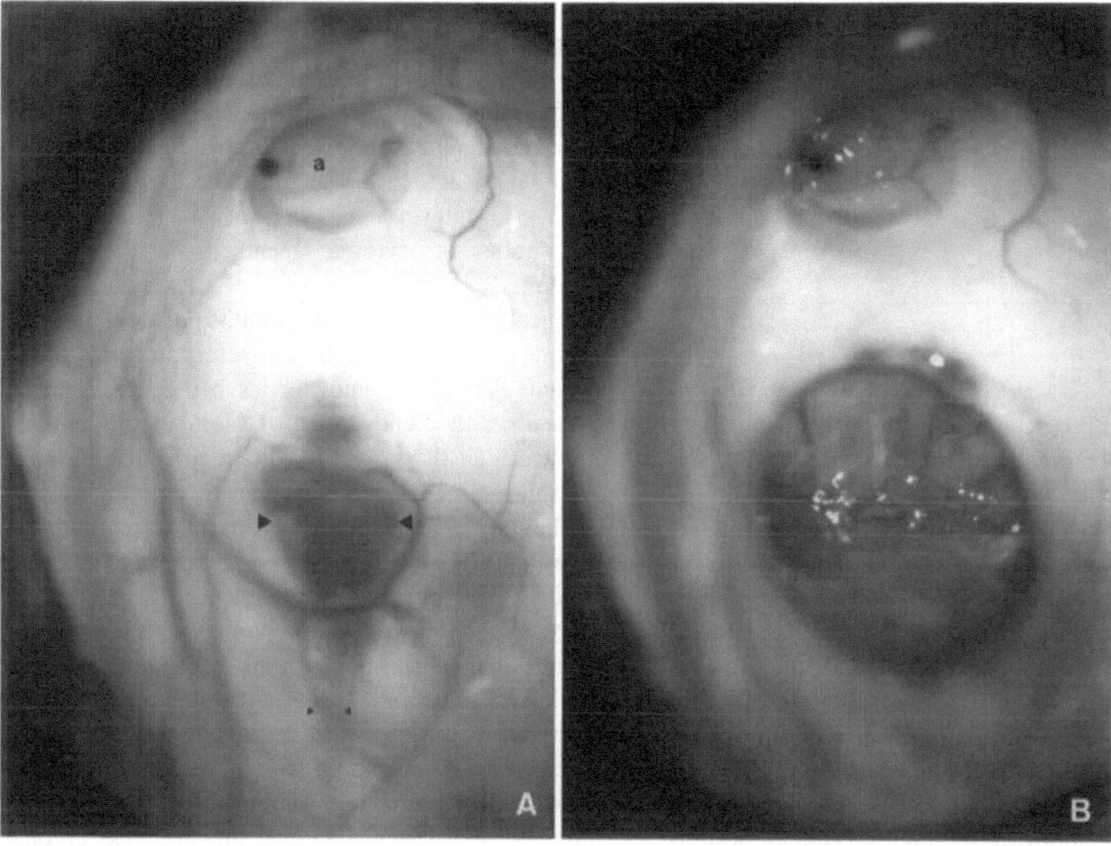

Fig. 7. Operative photographs showing the upper part of the floor of the fourth ventricle berfore (A) and after (B) the complete removal of the tumour in the same patient as in figure 6 (*a* = cerebral acqueduct; *large arrows* = discoloration of the floor due to the tumour: *small arrows* = median sulcus)

awake, made it possible to get over this critical period and open the way to subsequent gradual recovery. This was materially slower in patients that were severely disabled at the time of surgery, generally more expeditious in the others. Withal at 3 months postoperative the neurologic status was conspicuously better than preoperatively in 12 cases; it was unchanged in 27 cases, and further deteriorated in 3 (Table 6).

Our medium-term results were in keeping both with the anatomical sites and with the histological types of treated tumours. Patients with diffuse tumours (for the most part highly malignant) showed little change in their tendency to neurological deterioration, with the single exception of one patient who had a diffuse tumour enlarging the whole brainstem and was again able to eat without difficulty after extensive debulking of the tumour mass. In the group of focal, predominantly nonmalignant tumours, only 3 patients deteriorated importantly after surgery; all the others benefited considerably from surgery in terms of better

and more stable neurologic conditions. Intra-axial cervicomedullary tumours gave contrasting results. Six of 12 (5 benign astrocytomas and 1 ependymoma) made excellent neurologic recoveries; the remainder (4 malignant gliomas, 1 angioreticuloma and 1 lipoma) showed no appreciable improvement.

Follow-up

In January 1990, at 6 to 72-month removes from surgery, we reviewed the first 40 cases of our series in order to make a provisional assessment of the long-term results of aggressive surgery such as we have been doing since 1984. Thirteen patients (32.5%) were reported dead, most of them (9 cases) after surgery for malignant glioma. All patients with ependymoma or lipoma survived, and so did 12 of 14 with low-grade astrocytoma. The functional status of our 27 survivors (Table 7) was satisfactory, especially considering their preoperative conditions: 13 patients had resumed normal living and 6 were self-sufficient.

Table 7. *Follow-up as of January 1990 (6 to 72 months) of First 40 Patients*

Quality of life	No of cases
Return to school/work	13 (32%)
Independent	6 (15%)
Dependent	8 (20%)
Dead	13 (32%)
Total	40

Conclusions

Despite progress made in the diagnosis and treatment of brainstem tumours, prognosis remains poor; in fact, none of the therapeutic innovations in this field has been found univocally adequate or above criticism. There is no general consensus as to the real therapeutic advantages that can be extracted from histological diagnosis obtained stereotaxically or intraoperatively as opposed to the diagnostic information afforded by CT scanning, digital angiography or NMR imaging – all of which prove more richly contributory as time goes by[1,2,5,8,9,13,24]. Even the real effectiveness of radiotherapy and chemotherapy in modifying the biology of these lesions is challenged[8,16]; and direct surgery is still regarded with suspicion.

Yet, in the general climate of pessimism and impotence that surrounds this pathology, some innovation have emerged in recent years that may promote a more rational approach to the therapeutic problem – and this is where we offer our own contribution in terms of first-hand surgical experience.

To begin with, it is by now a recognized fact that brainstem tumours do not constitute a homogeneous nosologic family amenable to empiric (nonspecific) treatment based on radiation and corticosteroids with or without associated chemotherapy[2,9,10,13,14,26]. These tumours, formely thrown into the same basket merely because they affect a vital and highly functional area of the central nervous system and therefore make surgery a high-risk enterprise, actually differ by their histopathological, radiological and clinical characteristics. Along with highly malignant and rapidly evolutive forms we find neatly circumscribed benign tumours most amenable to radical extirpation with a good chance of obtaining clinical improvement or even a permanent cure. Most of these tumours are gliomas; but differential diagnosis must consider vascular tumours, ependymoma, lipoma, and others. This broad gamut of pathological events, easily discrimi-

nated by modern neuro-imaging technics, offer the possibility of choosing the therapeutic procedures most likely to avail in each individual case.

In such a picture a more aggressive policy such as we have followed in this series, aimed at removing tumour tissue as radically as possible, seems to improve the longevity of patients with low-grade astrocytoma, ependymoma or vascular tumours[10,11,12,13,14,17,18,20,26,27]. In our caseload the surgical result assessed at 3 months postoperative and in our recent review was satisfactory in terms of the extent of tumour removal (this being radical in all patients with ependymoma or vascular tumours and in nearly all those with low-grade gliomas); in terms of anatomical physiognomy, focal tumours with or without exophytosis and those located at the cervicomedullary junction gave the best results.

Of special interest are the intrinsic glial tumours, largely represented by astrocytomas with a moderate degree of anaplasia and showing an essentially benign biological behaviour. Many patients of this description survived with a degree of neurologic deficit compactible with an acceptable style of life; in such cases, control NMR imaging demonstrated the complete absence of tumour tissue or the presence of only minor residues. For these patients we did not prescribe radiotherapy except in cases where symptoms indicated disease progression.

Malignant gliomas were relatively rare in our series and occurred mostly in adult patients. Obviously, surgery cannot accomplish much in the presence of massive tumoural infiltration and a markedly enlarged brainstem.

Several authors have upheld the prognostic importance of the location of brainstem gliomas[2,5,10,15,25]. In the series of Riegel et al.[23] there was a high incidence of glioblastoma multiforme in bulbar localizations; according to Epstein and Wisoff[11], Hoffman et al.[14] and Stroink et al.[25,26], tumours located at the cervicomedullary junction are for the most part low-grade astrocytomas, often with the benign characteristics of tumours of the spinal cord – of which they may constitute an extension. This interpretation, however, is not cofirmed by the data of Edwards and Prados[8] or by our own.

While one could hardly recommend direct surgery for "diffuse" gliomas that enlarge the brainstem, surgery itself affords the only opportunity for appraising the possibilities of identifying and removing tumour tissue without damaging nerve structures (Fig. 8). The statement that accurate selection of

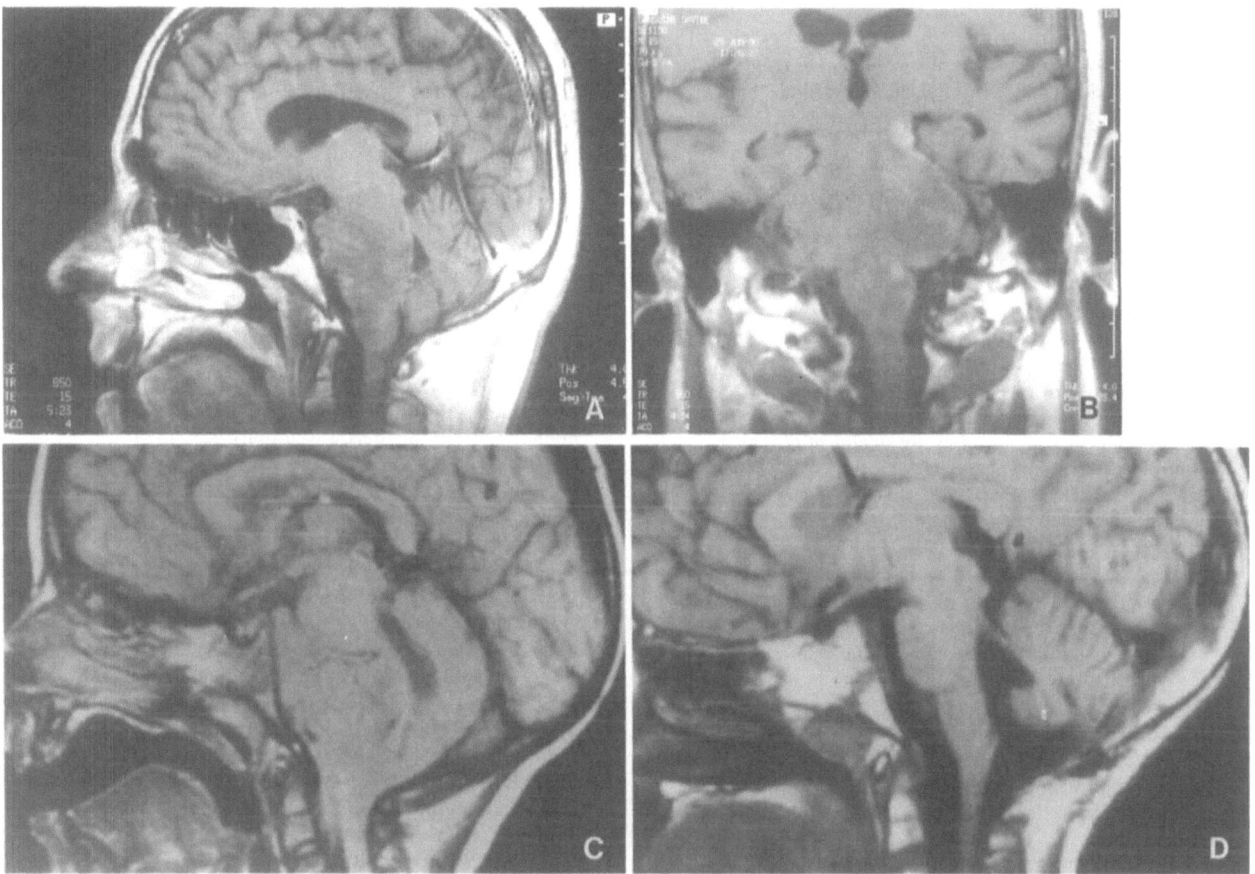

Fig. 8. Sagittal (A) and coronal (B) magnetic resonance T-weighted images after infusion of Gadolinium in a patient with a "diffuse" brainstem glioma. A global and homogeneous enlargement of the brainstem can be seen. This patient was not operated on. T_1-weighted sagittal magnetic resonance images showing another "diffuse" brainstem glioma preoperatively (C) and 3 years after its complete removal (D). The tumour was fungating from the left brachium pontis into the fourth ventricle and into cerebello-pontine angle, and was diffluent in the basilar cisterns

candidate patients for surgery constitutes the crucial problem to solve may lose some of its cogency if surgery is associated with a relatively low risk; be that as it may, experience in this area remains limited.

Surgery seems to be of definite value when the tumour is located at the cervicomedullary junction and when neuroradiological imaging plus a slow clinical course suggest a focal, noninvasive tumour formation[2,10,11]. Such tumours can indeed be removed completely or nearly so with acceptably low mortality and morbidity. The classical tenet, that the growth of brainstem gliomas is characteristically infiltrative and vigorously proliferative, and so causes the enlargement inaccurately called brainstem hypertrophy, is probably true only in a minority of cases[10,13,14,26]. The expanding mass of a slow-growing glioma usually dislocates the normal nerve structures without invading them; also, the mass tends to occur at some

place near the surface of the brainstem. Once the tumour is surgically penetrated and debulked, the reduced mass can be excised without undue distraction of the surrounding nerve pathways. When the boundaries between tumour tissue and normal white matter are well marked, the tumour can be removed completely; and with a correct neurosurgical technic the risk of creating new neurologic deficits remains acceptably low. While we are far from claiming that the prognosis of brainstem tumours should be viewed with optimism, we like to conclude that direct surgery, carefully planned and meticulously executed, represents a valid and worthwhile form of treatment. In that respect, the factors most contributory to safety and a successful outcome are NMR imaging, microsurgery with the use of newly developed instruments, and flawless intensive care assistance in the early postoperative period.

Acknowledgements

The Authors wish to thank the nursing staff of the Neurosurgical Intensive Care Unit for their invaluable cooperation.

This work was supported in part by N. H. Marastoni Foundation.

References

1. Abernathey CD, Camacho A, Kelly PJ (1989) Stereotaxic suboccipital transcerebellar biopsy of pontine mass lesion. J Neurosurg 70: 195–200

2. Albright AL, Guthkelch AN, Packer RJ, Price RA, Rourke LB (1986) Prognostic factors in pediatric brain-stem gliomas. J Neurosurg 65: 751–755

3. Albright AL, Schlabassi RJ (1985) Use of the cavitron ultrasonic aspirator and evoked potentials for treatment of thalamic and brain-stem tumours in children. Neurosurgery 17: 564–568

4. Alvisi C, Cerisoli M, Maccheroni ME (1985) Long terms results of surgically treated brain-stem gliomas. Acta Neurochir (Wien) 76: 12–17

5. Berger MS, Edwards MSB, La Masters D, Davis RL, Wilson CB (1983) Pediatric brain stem tumors: radiographic, pathological, and clinical correlations. Neurosurgery 12: 298–302

6. Bricolo A, Turazzi S (1987) Esperienza nella chirurgia dei gliomai del tronco cerebrale. In: Attualità in neurochirurgia. Monduzzi Ed, Bologna, pp 45–50

7. Bricolo A, Turazzi S, Cristofori L, Gerosa MA, Grosslercher JC, Mazza C, Talacchi A, Vitale M (1988) Direct surgery for intrinsic brain-stem gliomas. In: Proceedings of XI Congress of European Society for Pediatric Neurosurgery, Naples, Sept. 25–28, p 26

8. Edwards MSB, Prados M (1987) Current management of brainstem gliomas. Pediat Neurosci 13: 309–315

9. Edwards MSB, Wara WM, Urtasun RC, Prados M, Levin VA, Fulton D, Wilson CB, Hannigan J, Silver P (1989) Iperfractionated radiation therapy for brain-stem glioma: a phase I–II trail. J Neurosurg 70: 691–700

10. Epstein F, McLeary EL, (1986) Intrinsic brain-stem tumors of childhood: surgical indications. J Neurosurg 64: 11–15

11. Epstein F, Wisoff J (1987) Intra-axial tumors of the cervico-medullary junction. J Neurosurg 67: 483–487

12. Fahlbusch R, Strauss C, Huk W, Rockelein G, Kompf D, Ruprecht KW (1990) Surgical removal of pontomesencephalic cavernous hemangiomas. Neurosurgery 26: 11–15

13. Gui G, Jan M, Guegan Y (1989) Les lésions chirurgicales du tronc cérébral. Neurochirurgie B [Suppl] 7

14. Hoffman HJ, Becker L, Craven MA (1980) A clinically and pathologically distinct group of benign brain stem gliomas. Neurosurgery 7: 243–248

15. Hood TW, Gebarski SS, McKeever P, Venes HL (1986) Stereotaxic biopsy of intrinsic lesions of the brain stem. J Neurosurg 65: 172–176

16. Jenkin RDT, Boesel C, Ertel I, Evans A, Hittle R, Ortega J, Sposto R., Wara W, Wilson C, Anderson J, Leikin S, Hammond D (1987) Brain-stem tumors in childhood: a prospective randomized trial of irradiation with and without adjuvant CCNU, VCR, and prednisone. A report of the Children's Cancer Study Group. J Neurosurg 66: 227–233

17. Jooma R, Torrens MJ, Bradshow J, Brownell B (1985) Subependymomas of the fourth ventricle. Surgical treatment in 12 cases. J Neurosurg 62: 508–512

18. Kashiwagi S, van Loveren HR, Tew JM, Wiot JG, Weil ST, Lukin RA (1990) Diagnosis and treatment of vascular brain-stem malformations. J Neurosurg 72: 27–34

19. Konovalov A, Atieh J (1988) The surgical treatment of primary brain stem tumors. In: Schimidek HH, Sweet WH (eds) Operative Neurosurgical techniques, Ed 2. Grune & Stratton, New York, pp 709–737

20. Konovalov A, Spallone A, Makhmudov UB, Kukhlajeva JA, Orezova VI (1990) Surgical management of hematomas of the brain stem. J Neurosurg 73: 181–186

21. Lassiter KRL, Alexander EJ, Davis CH Jr, Kelly DL Jr (1971) Surgical treatment of brain stem gliomas. J Neurosurg 34: 719–724

22. Matson DD (1969) Neurosurgery of infancy and childhood, 2nd ed. Springfield Ill, ChC Thomas, 410 pp

23. Riegel DH, Scarff TB, Woodford JE (1979) Biopsy of pediotric brainstem tumors. Child's Brain 5: 329–340

24. Strange P, Wohlert L (1982) Primary brain stem tumors. Acta Neurochir (Wien) 62: 219–232

25. Stroink AR, Harold JH, Hoffman HJ, Hendrick EB, Humphreys RP (1986) Diagnosis and management of pediatric brain stem gliomas. J Neurosurg 65: 745–750

26. Stroink AR, Hoffman HJ, Hendrick EB, Humphreys RP, Davidson G (1987) Transependymal benign dorsally exophytic brain stem gliomas in childhood: diagnosis and treatment recommendations. Neurosurgery 20: 439–444

27. Tomita T (1986) Surgical management of cerebellar peduncle lesions in children. Neurosurgery 18: 568–575

28. Villani R, Gaini SM, Tomei G (1975) Follow-up study of brainstem tumors in children. Child's Brain 1: 126–135

Correspondence: Prof. A. Bricolo, Department of Neurosurgery, University Hospital, Piazzale Stefani 1, 37126 Verona Italy.

Acta Neurochirurgica, Suppl. 53, 159–165 (1991)
© by Springer-Verlag 1991

Modifications of Temporal Approaches:
Anatomical Aspects of a Microneurosurgical Approach

E. Knosp[1], M. Tschabitscher[2], Ch. Matula[1], and W. Th. Koos[1]

Departments of [1]Neurosurgery and [2]Anatomy, Vienna Medical School, Wien, Austria

Summary

All subtemporal approaches have in common the risk of temporal lobe damage. To reduce the retraction of the temporal lobe we combine two synergistic modifications of temporal approaches to reach the prepontine space. The first is the temporary resection of the zygomatic arch which allowes to bring the temporalis muscle more caudally and subsequently allowes an anterior subtemporal approach with only minimal temporal lobe retraction. The second modification is the resection of the apex of the petrous bone after incision of the tentorium. This provides an excellent view into the posterior fossa between the trigeminal nerve medially, the internal carotid artery caudally and the internal auditory canal laterally. The anatomical aspects of a microneurosurgical approach regarding these modifications are reported and discussed.

Keywords: Zygomatic approach; microneurosurgery; anatomy.

Introduction

The frontotemporal approach is the most commonly used for the surgery of aneurysms in the anterior circulation as well as for sellar and parasellar processes. Access to the posterior fossa, however, is only possible within a limited space.

The subtemporal approach as described by Drake[7] allows for direct access from a more lateral direction to structures behind the dorsum sellae.

For better access to the posterior fossa a number of modifications of the frontotemporal approach have been proposed, e.g. extradural resection of the lesser sphenoid wing with splitting of the Silvian fissure in the classical pterional approach[36,37], or partial resection of the temporal lobe[29,34,30]. Modifications of the subtemporal approach [7,6,22] include splitting of the tentorium[29,3,13], fenestration of the tentorium[9,10] or temporary splitting of the zygomatic arch. This modification may also include resection of the lateral

orbital rim[16,5,1,23] and has been presented as an approach to the basilar aneurysms[24] as well as for tumours[30,10].

The combination of a subtemporal approach and lateral suboccipital craniotomy is another possibility[18,3,34,27] to reach pathologies involving the middle and posterior cranial fossa.

A very interesting and helpful modification to gain better access to the posterior fossa has been proposed by Samii[26] and is described in detail by us[12]. After incision of the tentorium the apex of the petrous pyramid will be exposed and partly resected. This gives additional space to reach the prepontine space between the trigeminal nerve and the facial nerve. Sugita[33] uses this modification for aneurysms of the basilar trunk. Kawase[9] developed a similar modification to clip basilar artery aneurysms.

This study focuses on two aspects of frontotemporal and temporal approaches: How to avoid temporal lobe damage and how to gain better access to the posterior fossa when using temporal approaches.

Our concept to avoid "temporal lobe problems" is rather to "go into the skull base" than to retract the temporal lobe. With temporary resection of the zygomatic arch together with resection of the petrous apex we combine two modifications of temporal approaches with synergetic effects. In this paper the anatomical aspects of this microneurosurgical approach will be presented.

Material and Methods

Dissections were carried out in formalin fixed and unfixed cadaver specimens mostly in an elderly population group, which represents the majority of specimen available for anatomical studies. For special investigations we performed arterial as well as venous injections with coloured latex.

Special investigations of the petrous bone were performed on dry temporal bones as well as on skull bases with all dural envelopes.

Serial sections in a slice thickness of 2 mm were performed in horicontal plane as well as in sagittal plane and perpendicular to the petrous ridge.

To study the approach, the skulls were positioned in a three-pin head holder, identical to operative conditions. Craniotomies were performed as for standard neurosurgical approaches. For modification, however, the approach was enlarged to study the topography of the surrounding structures. Intradural preparation was performed with a ZEISS OP Mi-6 using microsurgical techniques as well as instrumentation. Photographs were taken in each case.

Anatomical Aspects

In standard frontotemporal (pterional) approaches the frontal branch of the *facial nerve* will not be severed, when the scalp dissection is carried out interfascial as proposed by Yasargil[37,39]. The facial nerve crosses the zygomatic arch in the middle between the lateral canthus and the tragus, so subperiostal dissection is recommended when the zygomatic arch is dissected.

The *temporalis muscle* is covered by two fasciae with the middle temporal vein in between. It originates from the temporal fossa and from the deep fascia. The deep fascia inserts at the zygomatic arch, which explains temporalis muscle fibers also originating from the arch. The temporalis muscle inserts on the coronoid process of the mandible. The vascular supply is provided mainly by the deep temporal arteries originating from the maxillary artery. Usually there are two branches (anterior and posterior) which strictly follow the sutures of the greater sphenoid wing (sphenozygomatic and sphenosquamosal suture). A minor arterial supply of the temporal muscle (middle temporal artery) originates from the superficial temporal artery and pierces the fasciae. Parallel and medial to the deep temporal arteries the deep temporal nerves reach the muscle. They branch from the mandibular nerve immediately below the foramen ovale and run directly adjacent to the periost of the fossa infratemporalis. When they bend around the infratemporal crest they are embedded in a sulcus with a bony spurr on the side (Fig. 1). These spurrs together with the course along the sutures make it easier to identify the neurovascular pedicle.

Zygomatic Arch Resection:

At the lateral side of the zygomatic arch the deep temporal fascia inserts and gives origin to a small

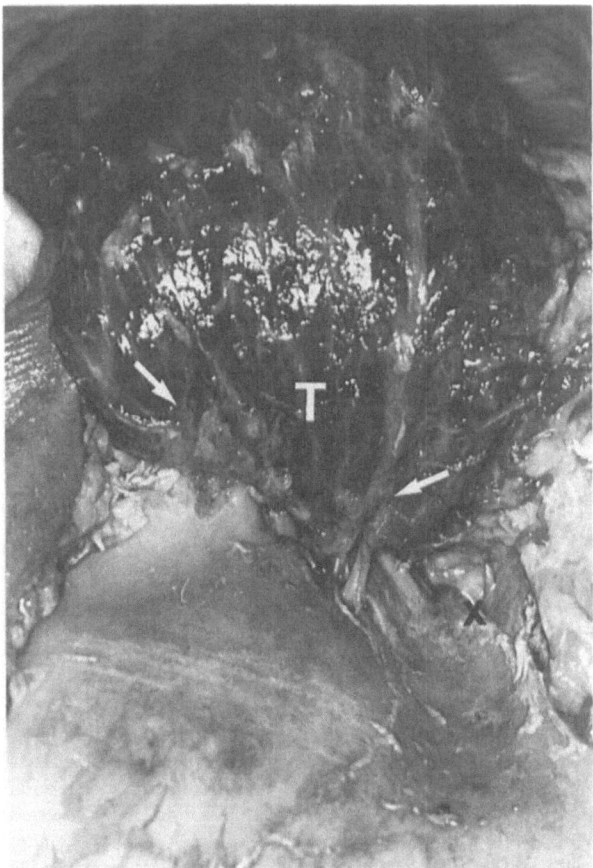

Fig. 1. After the zygomatic arch has been temporary transsected, the temporalis muscle (*T*) can be flected caudally as far as to the infratemporal crest. Here the neurovascular pedicles run into the muscle (arrows)

portion of temporalis muscle fibers which have to be cut together with the fascia. At the inferior rim of the arch the masseter muscle originates and is left in place except for placement of burrholes and cutlines. Then the zygomatic arch is transsected in V-shaped cutlines flected caudally with the masseter muscle attached to it. This allows to bring the temporalis muscle further caudally and makes bone resection along the floor of the middle cranial fossa possible without temporal lobe retraction. Bone resection may be carried out as far as to the round and oval foramen, if desired. After opening of the dura an anterior subtemporal approach can be performed with minimal temporal lobe retraction. For better access into the posterior fossa we propose the following modification: incision of the tentorium and resection of the apex of the petrous bone.

The *trochlear nerve* (IV) surrounds the brainstem in the ambient cistern, where it is fixed by arachnoid. The distance between the free margin of the tentorium and IV is 2 mm[1-3,6]. So elevation of temporal lobe together with arachnoid of the ambient cystern will bring the IV into vision from beneath the tentorium. The dural entry of the trochlear nerve is located in the so called "Wannenregion" in 80% of cases and in the anterior petroclinoid fold in 20% of the cases[14]. The distance between cranial nerves V and IV measures 6.6 mm and is almost equal to the distance V and VII (7 mm[14]).

The *superior petrosal sinus* runs along the superior petrosal ridge and in most cases the connection to the cavernous sinus is above the porus of the trigeminal nerve. In 2.5% of cases considered, the superior petrosal sinus bifúrcates to enter the cavernous sinus above and below the V[4]. Usually the superior petrosal vein drains into the superior petrosal sinus 5–7 mm laterally to the trigeminal nerve[4]. Only rarely does the vein run caudally or mediocaudally to the trigeminal nerve. At least during the fetal period this vein and the superior petrosal sinus drain laterally into the sigmoid sinus[11].

The course of the *petrosal nerves* is almost parallel to the petrous ridge. They become subdural, as they leave their bony canals. The smaller petrosal nerve comes from the tympanic cavity and leaves the skull on the medial side of the mandibular nerve (spheno-petrosal fissure). Two millimeters dorsal[20] the greater petrosal nerve takes it's course from the geniculate ganglion to the foramen lacerum. Usually the ganglion and the canal segment of the greater petrosal nerve are covered by bone. In 15% the bone is missing[25]. In these cases injury to the facial nerve may happen when the dura is elevated. The course of the greater petrosal nerve markes the course of the internal carotid artery (ICA) in the horizontal segment, thus serving as an excellent landmark for the intrapetrous ICA. The petrosal nerves are accompanied by branches of the middle meningeal artery supplying the tympanic cavity (sup. tympanic art.) and the geniculate ganglion (petrosal artery). The distance from the middle meningeal artery to the petrosal nerves is 8 mm[20].

Immediately caudal and dorsal to the greater petrosal nerve there is the bony canal of the *Eustachian tube* (Figs. 2 and 3). The canal itself consists of two semicanals with the tensor tympany muscle in the cranial half. The course of the Eustachian tube is also parallel to the petrous ridge and to the carotid canal. It's angulation from laterocranial to mediocaudal is different to the ICA canal but it serves as another important landmark for the carotid canal with the ICA always dorsal to it. A thin bone lamella separates the tensor tympany muscle from the carotid canal. It may be missing also in rare cases[21].

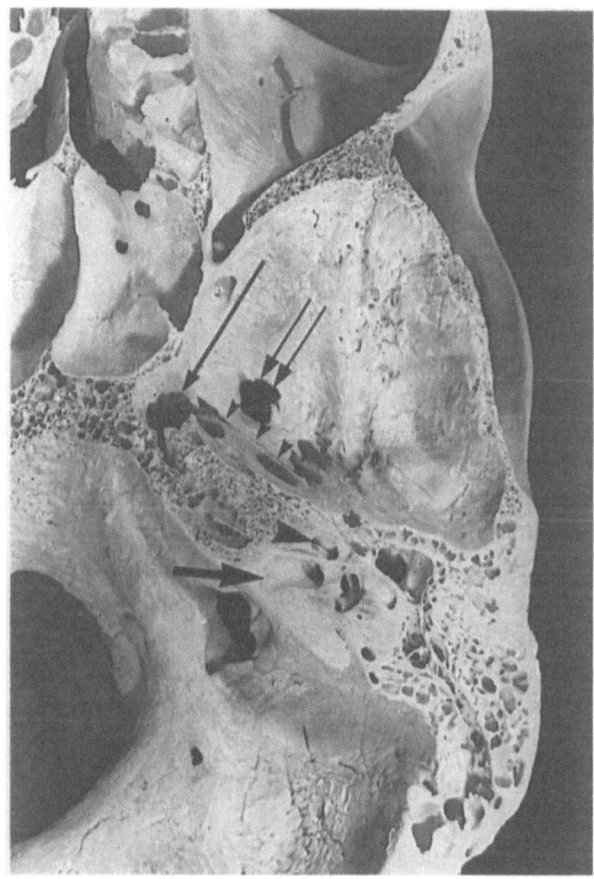

Fig. 2. Horizontal section of a dry skull in the level of the internal auditory canal (large arrow). Anterior to the fundus of the canal the basal turn of the cochlea is opened (large arrowhead). Immediately lateral to the cochlea the beginning of the facial nerve canal can be seen. In the middle cranial fossa the bony landmarks can be seen: the entrance of the internal carotid artery into the cavernous sinus (long arrow), the oval foramen (double arrow) and the foramen spinae just lateral to it. Dorsal to the oval foramen the course of the greater petrosal nerve and the Eustachian tube is marked by small arrowheads

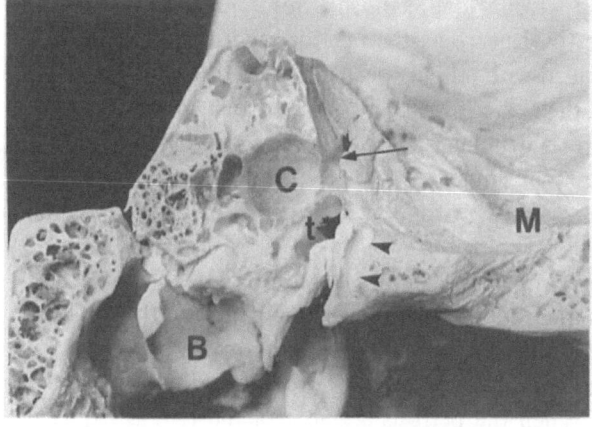

Fig. 3. Section perpendicular to the petrousridge. The intimate relationship between the carotid canal (C) the Eustachian tube (t), the greater petrosal nerve (arrow) and the middle meningeal artery (arrowheads) is evident. Middle cranial fossa (M); jugular bulb (B)

The *ICA canal* in it's lateral part borders to the *cochlea* with only a thin bone lamella in between. The level of the basal turn of the cochlea is few mm above the floor of the internal auditory canal. When bone resection at the entrance of the internal auditory canal is limited to the superior and anterior circumference of the internal auditory canal, the cochlea will not be damaged (Fig. 2). Bone resection should not be carried out to the fundus of the internal auditory canal.

In anterior subtemporal approaches dissection is carried out perpendicular to the petrous ridge. The course of the middle meningeal artery guides to the foramen spinae with the oval foramen immediately medial to it. A few millimeters dorsal, the petrosal nerves cross the approach parallel to the petrous ridge. The same holds true with the Eustachian tube between the middle meningeal artery and the carotid canal. With these landmarks the carotid canal can be approached with certitude in the "triangle" between the trigeminal nerve medially, the greater petrosal nerve and/or the Eustachian tube anteriorly and the petrous ridge dorsally.

Incision of the Tentorium and Resection of the Petrous Apex

The transsection of the tentorium starts after identification of the trochlear nerve and is carried out into Meckel's cave, thus exposing the trigeminal nerve. A semicircular duraflap is created to expose the petrous apex (Fig. 4 a). Before drilling starts, the surgical landmarks have to be recognized with certainty. The middle meningeal artery leads to the foramen spinae just lateral to the foramen ovale with the V/3 and Gasserian ganglion as the medial border, the petrous ridge as the superior border and the greater petrosal nerve as the inferior landmark. The apex is drilled with a high speed diamond drill until the dura of the posterior aspect of the petrous bone is reached. When drilling is carried out inferiorly, the inferior petrosal sinus can be opened. The petrous bone may be resected as far as to the internal auditory canal thus exposing the cranial nerves seven and eight. Bone resection at the internal auditory canal should not carried out to the fundus, but limited to the anterior and superior rim of the canal, in order not to damage the cochlea (Fig. 2).

When the petrous segment of the ICA is exposed we also have the caudal limit of this approach. If exposure of the ICA is intended for proximal vessel control, additional bone resection has to be done anterior to the artery thus opening the Eustachian tube. The approach to the posterior fossa is then limited by the trigeminal nerve medially, the ICA caudally and VII and VIII laterally.

Discussion

It makes a great difference in the selection of an approach whether the pathological process is a space occupying lesion or a vascular malformation. Space occupying lesions cause anatomical changes as they displace parts of the brain, cranial nerves and vessels. In such cases the approach is mainly designed to the fact that the tumour itself can be used for it's own removal. In many cases complete or partial damage of cranial nerves preexist, so one may also calculate to "sacrifice" it, if recovery is unlikely. Such "favorable" circumstances are, however, usually absent in vascular processes, such as basilar tip aneurysms. Here the approach is mostly determined by the "normal" anatomy, which means that the individual anatomy playes a much more important role, e.g. the length of the supraclinoid ICA, the size and course of the posterior communicating artery and the development of the posterior clinoid process[28,38,12]. The drawback in all subtemporal approaches is the temporal lobe, be it intraoperatively or postoperatively by swelling, intracerebral haemorrhage or development of epilepsy. To reduce this "temporal lobe risk" we propose to use two modifications together as they have a synergistic effect: to transsect the zygomatic arch temporaryly, and in addition to that to resect the apex of the petrous bone after incision of the tentorium.

As the upper rim of zygomatic arch markes the bottom of the middle cranial fossa, an anterior subtemporal approach can not be performed without temporal lobe retraction, if the zygomatic arch is intact and the temporalis muscle flected over it. After temporary resection of the zygomatic arch, as recommended[24,19,23,31,32], the approach can be performed with minimal retraction. Bone resection is not limited to the zygomatic arch but may include resection of the lateral orbital rim[5,1,23]. But zygomatic arch resection is not without additional risk. The more caudal the resection is carried out, the more attention should be payed to the facial nerve and the temporalis muscle. To avoid paresis of the frontalis branch of the facial nerve, an interfascial dissection should be carried out[39]. When freeing the zygomatic arch,

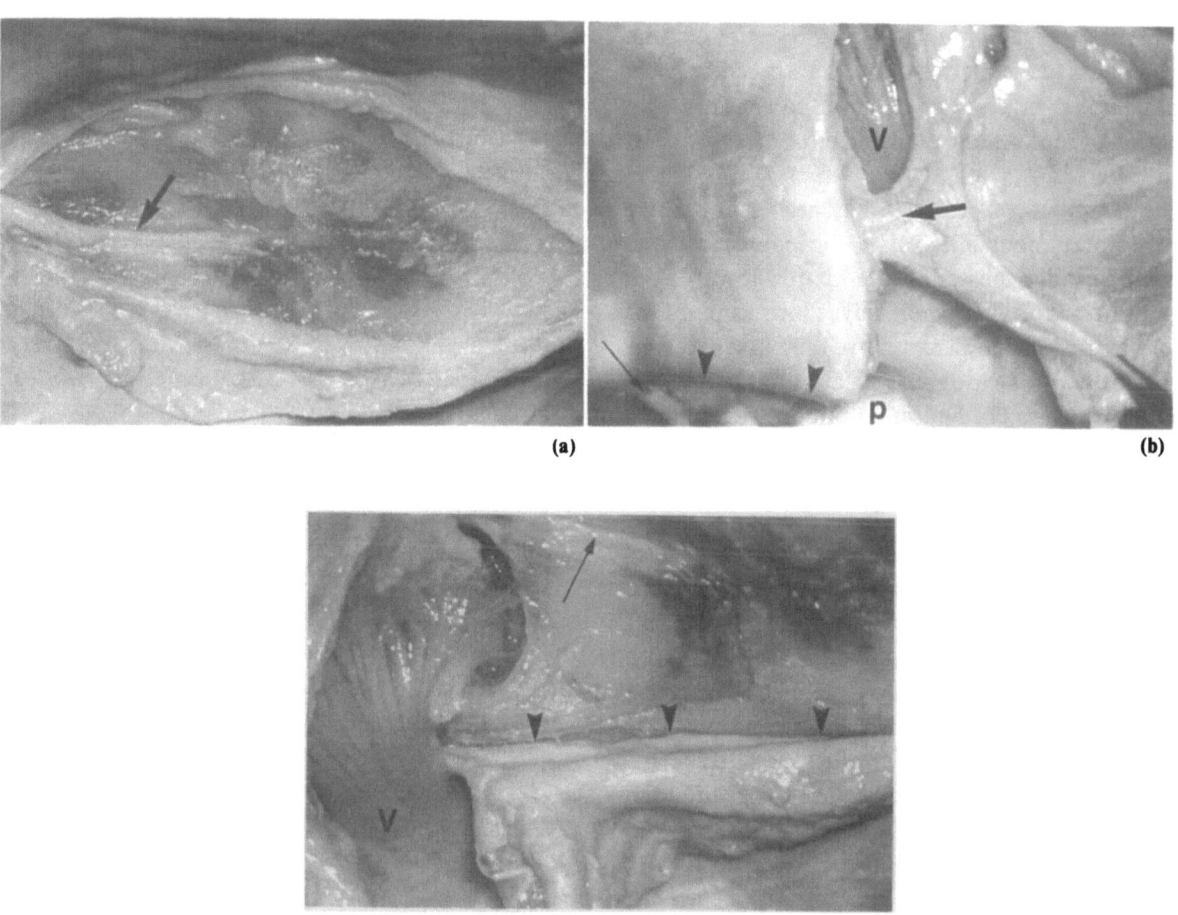

(a)

(b)

(c)

Fig. 4. Opening of the dura of the middle cranial fossa for removal of the petrous apex: a) the course of the greater petrosal nerve from it's hiatus towards medial serves as the first landmark for the internal carotid canal. b) Incision of the tentorium starts at the free margin of the tentorium (arrowheads) and is carried out after identification of the trochlear nerve (small arrow) into Meckel's cave (V). The superior petrosal sinus (arrow) has to be divided. Pons (p). c) Bone resection starts at the petrous apex between the trigeminal nerve (V) medially the petrous ridge (arrowheads) superiorly and the greater petrosal nerve (arrow)

dissection has to be done subperiostally. Facial nerve monitoring may also be helpful.

Temporalis muscle atrophy causes cosmetic as well as functional disturbances. Damage of the muscle occurs, when flecting the sometimes bulky muscle too vigorously or when coagulating a teared muscle artery. Most authors using this approach do not mention this problem except Pitelli et al.[24], who report temporalis muscle atrophy in their cases. Trigeminal motor nerve involvement by a tumour, however, may cover this fact. Complete transsection of the temporalis muscle and upward flection as described by Al Mefty[2] must result in total atrophy and is not recommended. Our investigations may help to recognize the neurovascular pedicles with their course parallel to the sphenozygomatic and sphenosquamosal sutures. The bony spurrs

at the infratemporal crest will also provide a good localizer.

The resection of the zygomatic arch allows a more anterior approach, e.g. to aneurysms of the basilar bifurcation than the classical subtemporal approach does. This brings both posterior cerebral arteries into view. It also enables the surgeon easily to change to a more lateral view to dissect the perforators, thus combining the advantages of the pterional[37] and the subtemporal approaches[6]. The relation of aneurysm to the level of the dorsum sellae seems not to be that important, as high bifurcations can be approached better compared to the pterional as well as to the subtemporal approach[19]. In our opinion there is no necessity for resection of the anterior part of the temporal lobe as described[34,30,8]. Together with the incision of the tentorium and the resection of the petrous apex these modifications give excellent view to low basilar bifurcations and even to aneurysms of the basilar trunk as low as the inferior anterior cerebellor artery[33].

The petrous apex resection has been reported by Samii[26] for tumour removal in the posterior fossa. This modification creates a large window towards the prepontine space which not only allows clipping of aneuryms[33,9] but allows to remove tumours involving the petroclival and clival area as far as to the internal auditory canal[12]. The limitation of bone resection at the petrous ápex is given by the trigeminal nerve medially, by the ICA inferiorly and by the internal auditory canal laterally. When trigeminal nerve damage is complete preoperatively or the nerve can not be saved intraoperatively the window into posterior fossa increases significantly towards medial. Then the trochlear and oculomotor nerves are the superior and the abducent nerve the medial borders.

Hearing loss by cochlea damage is a serious problem in petrous bone resection[33,10]. When bone resection is limited to the superior aspect of the internal auditory canal and not carried out to the fundus along the anterior wall, no damage will occur to the cochlea.

Rhinorrhea, caused by opening of the Eustachian tube can be avoided by covering the tube with a piece of muscle. The same should be done to cover the pneumatized petrous apex.

In most cases of petrous apex resection, transsection of the greater petrosal nerve is necessary. This results in diminished lacrimation. When tearing the nerve near the geniculate ganglion, which is more likely when the bony cover is missing[25] a facial nerve paralysis can result, so transsection is recommended.

References

1. Al-Mefty O (1987) Supraorbital-pterional approach to scull base lesions. Neurosurgery 21: 474–477
2. Al-Mefty O (1986) Skull base: Zygomatic approach. Neurosurgery 19: 674–675; comment to Ref. Pitelli.
3. Bonnal J, Louis R, Combalbert A (1964) L'abord temporal transtentorial de l'angle ponto-cerebelleux et du clivus. Neuro-Chirurgie 10: 3–12
4. Boskovic M, Savic V, Josifov J (1963) Über die Sinus petrosi und ihre Zuflüsse. Gegenbaurs Morphol Jahrb 104: 420–429
5. Dolenc VV, Skrap M, Sustersic J, Surbec M, Morina A (1987) A transcavernous-transsellar approach to the basilar tips aneurysms. Br J Neurosurg 1: 251–159
6. Drake CHG (1973) Management of aneurysms of posterior circulation. In: Youmans JR (ed) Neurological surgery, Vol 2. WB Saunders Co, Philadelphia, pp 787–806
7. Drake CHG (1965) Surgical treatment of ruptured aneurysms

8. of the basilar artery. Experience with 14 cases. J Neurosurg 23: 457–473
8. Heros RC (1988) Zygomaticotemporal approach to the basis cranii and basilar artery. Neurosurgery 23: 22, comment to Ref. Neil-Dwyer
9. Kawase T, Toya S, Shiobara R, Mine T (1985) Trans-petrosal approach for aneurysms of the lower basilar artery. J Neurosurg 63: 857–861
10. Kawase T, Toya S, Shiobara R, Kimura C, Nakajima H (1987) Skull base approaches for meningeomas invading the cavernous sinus. In: Dolenc VV (ed) The cavernous sinus. Springer, Wien New York, pp 346–354
11. Knosp E, Müller G, Perneczky A (1987) Anatomical remarks on the fetal cavernous sinus and on the veins of the middle cranial fossa. In: Dolenc VV (ed) The cavernous sinus. Springer, Wien New York, pp 104–116
12. Knosp E, Samii M (1991) Approaches to the clivus. Springer, Berlin Heidelberg New York Tokyo (in preparation)
13. Krayenbühl H, Yaşargil MG (1975) Chondromas. Progr neurol Surg (Karger, Basel) 6: 435–463
14. Lang J (1981) Klinische Anatomie des Kopfes. Springer, Berlin Heidelberg New York
15. Lanz T, Wachsmuth W (1979) Praktische Anatomie. Band 1, Teil 1. Lang J, Wachsmuth W (ed). Springer, Berlin Heidelberg New York
16. McDermott MW, Durity FA, Rootman J, Woodhurst WB (1990) Combined frontotemporal–orbitozygomatic approach for tumors of the sphenoid wing and orbit. Neurosurgery 26: 107–116
17. Muren C, Wadin K, Wilbrand HF (1990) The cochlea and the carotid canal. Acta Radiol 31: 33–35
18. Naffziger HC (1928) Brain surgery with special reference to exposure of the brainstem and posterior fossa. Surg Gynecol Obstet 46: 240–48
19. Neil-Dwyer G, Sharr M, Haskell R, Currie D and Hosseini M (1988) Zygomaticotemporal approach to the basis cranii and basilar artery. Neurosurgery 23: 20–22
20. Parisier SC (1977) The middle cranial fossa approach to the internal auditory canal—an anatomical study stressing critical distances between surgical landmarks. Laryngoscope [Suppl] 4, 87: 1–20
21. Paullus WP, Paid TG, Rhoton AL (1977) Microsurgical exposure of the petrous portion of the carotid artery. J Neurosurg 47: 713–26
22. Peerless SJ, Drake CHC (1982) Aneurysms of the posterior circulation. In: Youmans JR (ed) Neurological surgery. Saunders WB, Philadelphia, pp 1715–1764
23. Perneczky A, Knosp E, Matula CH (1988) Cavernous sinus surgery. Approach through the lateral wall. Acta Neurochir (Wien) 92: 76–82
24. Pitelli SD, Almeida GG, Nakagawa EJ, Marchese AJ, Cabral ND (1986) Basilar aneurysm surgery: The sub-temporal approach with section of the zygomatic arch. Neurosurgery 18: 125–128
25. Rhoton AL, Pulec JL, Hall MG, Boyd AS (1968) Absence of bone over the geniculate ganglion. J Neurosurg 28: 48–53
26. Samii M (1986) Neurosurgical aspects of processes at the tentorial margin. In: Samii M (ed) Surgery in and around the brainstem and third ventricle. Springer, Berlin Heidelberg New York, pp 416–443
27. Samii M, Ammirati M, Mahram A, Bini W, Sepekirnia A (1989) Surgery of petroclival meningeomas: Report of 24 cases. Neurosurgery 24: 12–17
28. Samson DS, Hodosh RM, Clark WR (1978) Microsurgical evoluation of the pterional approach to aneurysms of the distal basilar circulation. Neurosurgery 3: 135–141

29. Schisano G, Tovi D (1962) Clivus chordomas. Neurochirurgia 5: 99–120
30. Sekhar LN, Schramm VL, Jr, Jones NF, Yonas H, Horton J, Latchaw RE, Curtin H (1986) Operative exposure and management of the petrous and upper cervical internal carotid artery. Neurosurgery 19: 967–982
31. Shimizu H, Suzuki I, Ishijima B (1989) Zygomatic approach for resection of mesial temporal epileptic focus. Neurosurgery 25: 798–801
32. Shiokawa Y, Saito I, Aoki N, Mizutani H (1989) Zygomatic temporopolar approach for basilar artery aneurysms. Neurosurgery 25: 793–797
33. Sugita K, Kobayashi S, Takeae T, Tada T, Tanaka Y (1987) Aneurysms of the basilar trunk. J Neurosurg 66: 500–506
34. Symon L (1982) Surgical approaches to the tentorial hiatus. In: Advances and technical standards in neurosurgery, Vol 9. Krayenbühl H et al (eds) Springer, Wien New York, pp 70–112
35. Todd NW, Martin WS (1988) Relationship of eustachian tube bony landmarks and temporal bone pneumatization. Ann Otol Rhinol Laryngol 97: 277–280
36. Yaşargil MG, Fox JL, Ray MW (1975) The operative approach to aneurysms of the anterior communicating artery. In: Krayenbühl H et al (eds) Advances and technical standards in neurosurgery, Vol 2. Springer, Wien New York, pp 113–170
37. Yaşargil MG, Antic J, Laciga R, Jain KK, Hodosch RM, Smith RD (1976A) Microsurgical pterional approach to aneurysms of the basilar bifurcation. Surg Neurol 6: 83–91
38. Yaşargil MG (1984) Microneurosurgery, Vol II. Thieme, Stuttgart New York
39. Yaşargil MG, Reichman MW, Kubik ST (1987) Preservation of the fronto-temporal branch of the facial nerve using the interfascial temporalis flap for pterional craniotomy (technical article). J Neurosurg 67: 463–467

Correspondence: E. Knosp, M. D., Department of Neurosurgery, Vienna Medical School, Währinger Gürtel 18–20, A-1090 Wien, Austria

Acta Neurochirurgica, Suppl. 53, 166–170 (1991)
© by Springer-Verlag 1991

The Petrosal Approach: Indications, Technique, and Results

O. Al-Mefty[1], S. Ayoubi[2], and R. R. Smith[3]

[1] Division of Neurological Surgery, Loyola University Medical Center, Chicago, Illinois, U.S.A., [2] Hurstwood Park Neurological Center, Haywards Heath, U.K., [3] Department of Neurosurgery, University of Mississippi Medical Center, Jackson, Mississippi, U.S.A.,

Summary

Surgical access to the clivus and petrous apex remains a formidable challenge. Intradural tumours at the clivus and petroclival area are superbly exposed via the petrosal approach described here. To date, we have operated on 33 patients having benign tumours using this approach. Total removal was achieved in all patients except 3 with meningiomas. There was no mortality, morbidity included 1 patient with hemiparesis and several with cranial nerve deficits.

Keywords: Petrosal approach; clivus; brain tumour; meningioma.

Introduction

The petrosal approach is used for intradural tumours located in the clival and petroclival areas. It allows access to tumours extending from the suprasellar area and the cavernous sinus to as caudal as the foramen magnum. This approach is centered on the petrous ridge, analogous to the pterional approach, which is centered on the sphenoid ridge. This approach has evolved over the years. As early as 1904, Fraenkel and Hunt[5] described a suboccipital-translabyrinthine approach to a cerebellopontine angle (CPA) tumour. Bailey[4] used a combined supratentorial-infratentorial approach through a single bone flap with sectioning of the sigmoid sinus, which was reunited at the time of closure. Morrison and King[9] used a subtemporal and translabyrinthine approach, preserving the sigmoid sinus. Hakuba and his colleagues[6] preserved the labyrinth and used this approach for removing a clival meningioma. Our early experience using this approach for clival meningiomas[2] was very encouraging, inducing us to use it for a variety of intradural lesions at the clival and petroclival areas. Those cases are reported here.

Operative Technique

Positioning and Monitoring

The patient is placed supine on the operating table. The ipsilateral shoulder is elevated by placing a folded towel underneath it. The head and trunk are elevated 20° to 30°; the head is turned and tilted to the opposite side, inclined toward the floor, and fixed in a Mayfield headrest (Fig. 1).

Brain stem auditory evoked potentials and median nerve somatosensory evoked potentials are recorded bilaterally. An electromyogram (EMG) is recorded from several facial muscle groups to locate the facial nerve and monitor its function on the operative side. Other cranial nerves are monitored as required.

Bone Removal

A reverse question mark incision is made, extending from the zygoma, circling above the ear, and descending 1 cm behind the mastoid process. The skin flap is raised to the level of the external auditory meatus. A large triangular pericranial flap is elevated, with its base at the base of the skin flap. This will be used at the time of closure to cover the drilled temporal bone. The temporal muscle is retracted anteriorly. The insertion of the sternomastoid muscle is detached from the mastoid bone and the muscle is retracted postero-inferiorly. At this stage, the mastoid and the temporal squama and the occipital bones are exposed. Located at the junction of the lambdoidal, occipital mastoid, and parietal mastoid sutures, the asterion is the key landmark in this area.

Four burr holes are drilled. The first one is made just medial and inferior to the asterion; this opens into

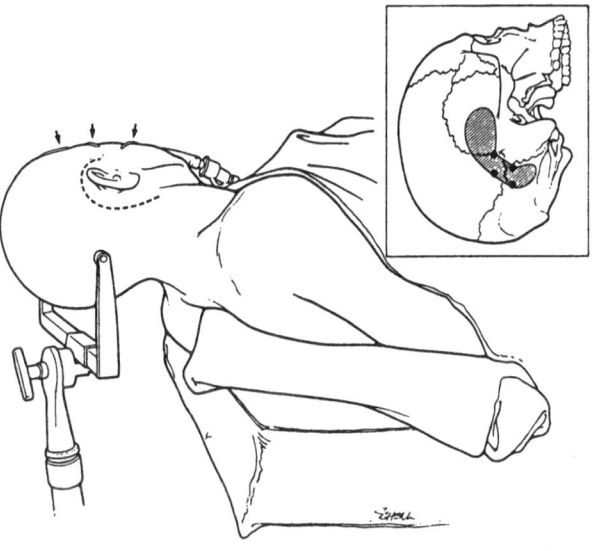

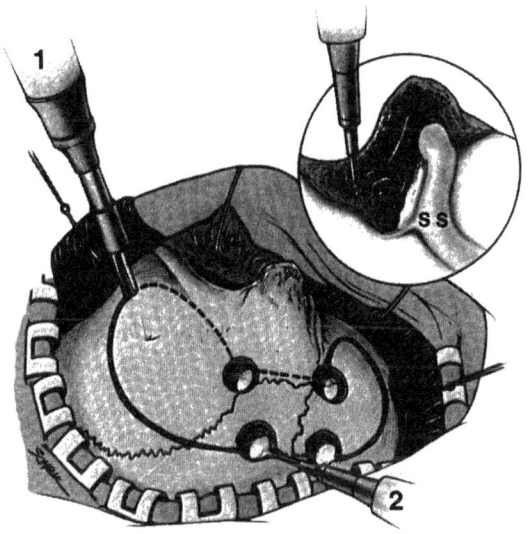

Fig. 1. Artist's illustration of patient's position and the skin incision for a right-sided petrosal approach. EMG needle electrodes (arrows) are inserted in muscle group innervated by the facial nerve. *Inset*: Skull model depicting position of the burr holes and outlining the bone flap. (Reproduced with permission from Al-Mefty O, Schenk MP, Smith RR (in press) Petroclival meningiomas. In: Wilkins RH, Rengachary SS (eds) Neurosurgical operative atlas. Williams & Wilkins, Baltimore)

Fig. 2. Artist's illustration (*right side*): Surgeon's view: the temporal (*TM*) and sternomastoid muscles (*SM*) are elevated and retracted. A pericranial triangular flap (*F*) is elevated and saved for later covering of the drilled surface of the temporal bone. The position of the burr holes flanking the transverse sigmoid sinus is outlined. A craniotome with foot attachment (*1*) is used to make the bony cut in the temporal and posterior fossae, while a drill (*2*) is used to cross over the sinus. *Inset*: The bone flap has been removed, the dura of the temporal and posterior fossa are exposed, the right sigmoid sinus (*SS*) is skeletonized, and the petrous bone has been extensively drilled. The anatomical landmarks in the temporal bone (the facial canal and the semicircular canals) are demonstrated. (Reproduced with permission from Al-Mefty O, Schenk MP, Smith RR (in press) Petroclival meningiomas. In: Wilkins RH, Rengachary SS (eds) Neurosurgical operative atlas. Williams & Wilkins, Baltimore)

the posterior fossa below the transverse sigmoid sinus junction. The second hole is made at the squamal and mastoid junctions of the temporal bone, along the projection of the superior temporal line. This opens into the supratentorial compartment. These two holes flank the sigmoid sinus. The third and fourth holes are made medial to the latter two holes on each side of the transverse sinus.

With the foot attachment of a craniotome, the temporal bone and a portion of the occipital bone above the tentorium are incised between the supratentorial burr hole. The occipital bone below the tentorium is incised between the infratemporal burr holes. The foot attachment of the craniotome is not used to cross the sinus. The bone over the sinus is carefully drilled until the sinus is exposed between each of the burr holes flanking the sinus (Fig. 2). The single bone flap is then elevated and carefully separated from the sinus and the dura. The bone severely adheres to the sinus at the transverse sigmoid junction.

A complete mastoidectomy is performed, using a diamond drill when working near vital structures. The sigmoid sinus is skeletonized down to the jugular bulb, exposing the dura on both sides of the sinus. The dura

anterior to the sigmoid sinus is exposed only enough to open and close the dura. The sinodural angle of Citelli, which identifies the position of the superior petrosal sinus, is exposed. The superficial mastoid cells behind the posterior wall of the external ear canal, as well as the deep retrofacial air cells, are resected to identify but not open the facial canal and the lateral and posterior semicircular canals. Drilling is continued along the pyramid to thin the petrous bone towards its apex. Open air cells are obliterated with bone wax.

Opening the Dura and Incising the Tentorium

The supratentorial dura is opened on the floor of the temporal fossa. The posterior fossa dura anterior to the sigmoid sinus is opened along the anterior margin of the sinus, and the incision is extended toward the supratentorial incision. The superior

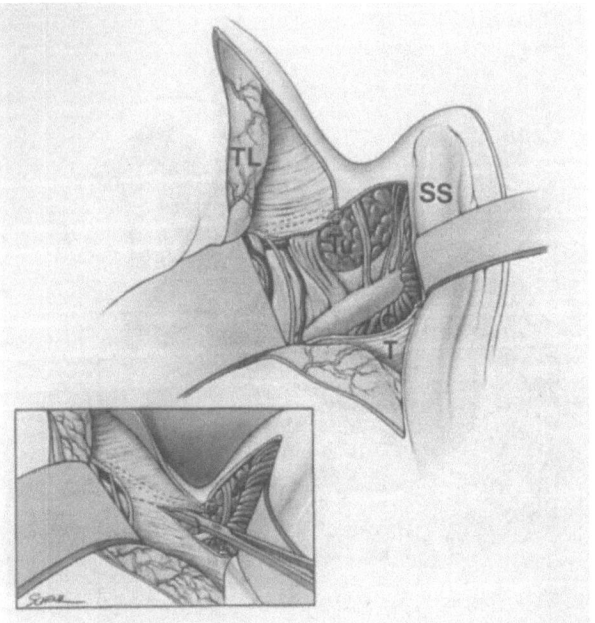

Fig. 3. Artist's illustration (*right side*): Surgeon's view demonstrating exposure of the tumour via a pre-sigmoid sinus avenue. The sigmoid sinus (*SS*) and cerebellum (*c*) are retracted medially while the temporal lobe (*TL*) is retracted superiorly. The tentorium (*T*) is incised along the pyramid through the incisura. The brain stem, cranial nerves (III–XI), and tumour (*Tu*) are visualized. *Inset*: Demonstration of tentorial sectioning along the pyramid toward the incisura. (Reproduced with permission from Al-Mefty O, Schenk MP, Smith RR (in press) Petroclival meningiomas. In: Wilkins RH, Rengachary SS (eds) Neurosurgical operative atlas. Williams & Wilkins, Baltimore)

petrosal sinus is clipped or coagulated and divided. The vein of Labbé is dissected off the cortical surface and preserved. The temporal lobe is gently retracted so that no tension will be placed on the dissected vein. The trochlear nerve is identified as the tentorium is incised parallel to the pyramid (Fig. 3 Inset). This incision is extended through the incisura, incising the tentorial notch at a point behind the area where the fourth nerve pierces the notch. When the tentorium is incised, the operative field opens to allow wide exposure of the upper pole of the tumour and the anterior and lateral aspects of the brain stem (Fig. 3). The trigeminal nerve rootlets, which are frequently stretched by the tumour, are identified under the tentorium. A retractor is placed anteriorly, retracting medially the sigmoid sinus, the cerebellum, and the cut edge of the tentorium. The arachnoid and cerebellomedullary cisterns are then opened, and cerebrospinal fluid (CSF) is drained to obtain further relaxation.

Tumour Resection

The tumour's insertion on the pyramid is coagulated, and the meningeal feeders over the tentorium are divided, reducing the blood supply to the tumour. In some cases, the petrous tip (anterior to the internal auditory meatus and medial to the carotid canal) is drilled away, facilitating tumour removal, particularly of the attachment of a meningioma. The seventh and eighth cranial nerves are usually posterior to a small tumour but may be engulfed by larger tumours. A suitable area on the surface of the tumour is coagulated and the arachnoid over the tumour is opened. The tumour is then debulked using suction, bipolar coagulation and microscissors, a laser or a Cavitron Ultrasonic Surgical Aspirator (CUSA, Cooper Medical Devices, Mountain View, California). This should be done carefully because the anterior (AICA) and posterior inferior (PICA) cerebellar arteries or the cranial nerves may be embedded in the tumour.

Dissection must be maintained within the arachnoid plane to preserve vital neurovascular structures. The tumour capsule is dissected from surrounding structures within this plane. Cranial nerves and the basilar artery and its branches may be encased in the tumour, demanding meticulous dissection.

Alternating the visual field between the supra- and infratentorial routes allows careful dissection of all cranial nerves and the brain stem. The abducens nerve is dissected from the tumour and is followed distally. With the assistance of stimulation and EMG recording to locate the facial nerve, the seventh and eighth nerves are dissected free. The lower cranial nerves are gently dissected from the inferior pole of the tumour to avoid hypotension and bradycardia from vagal stimulation. The basilar artery is usually displaced to the opposite side. The artery and its branches are carefully dissected from the tumour. Once the tumour is removed, its site of insertion is extensively vaporized with the laser. Extensions of the tumour into the internal auditory meatus or the jugular foramen are handled by drilling the bone to fully expose and remove the tumour.

Closure

The temporal and presigmoid dura is closed watertight. The triangular pericranial flap raised at the start of surgery is turned over the drilled surface of the petrous bone to avoid CSF leakage, and secured with fibrin glue. The temporal muscle is rotated over the defect and sutured to the sternomastoid muscle and the soft tissues and skin are closed in layers.

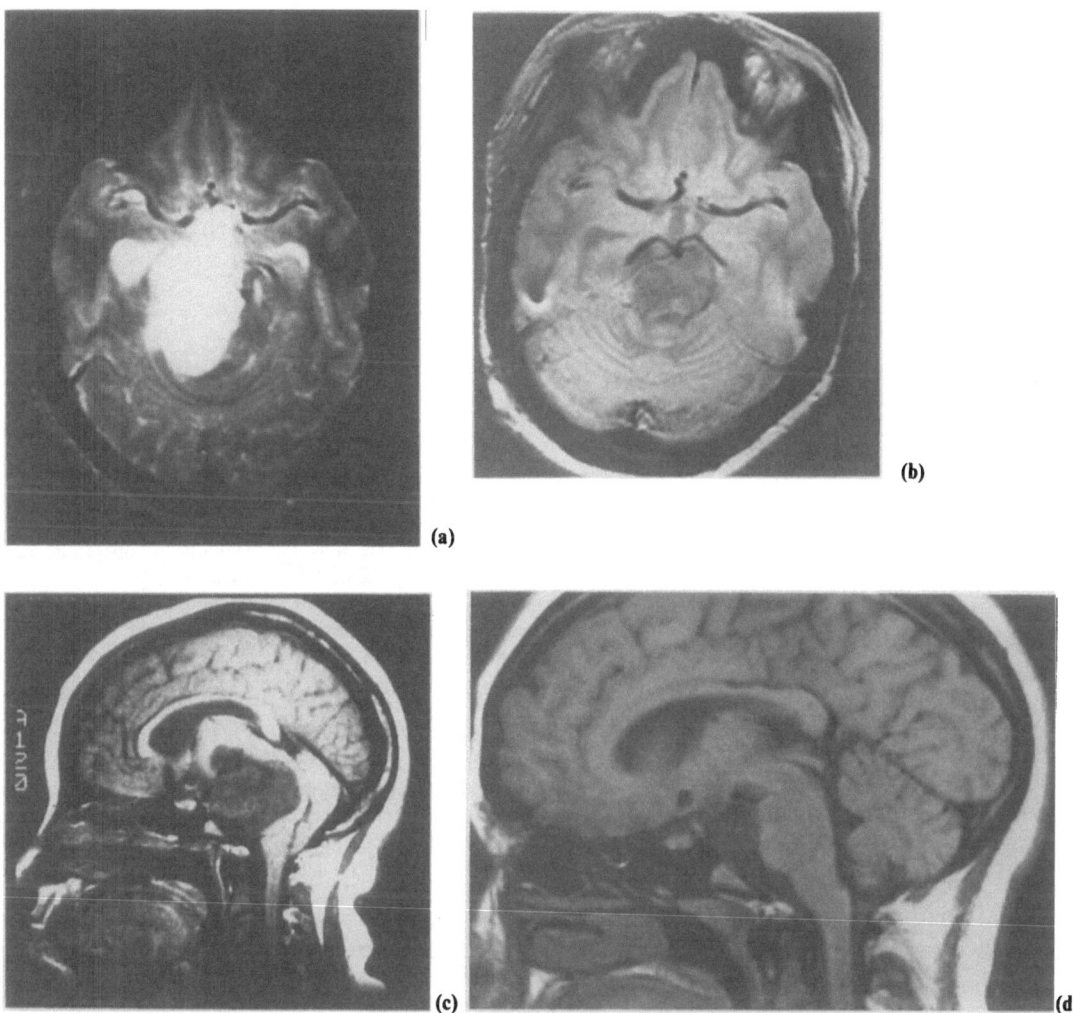

Fig. 4. MR images of a large epidermoid tumour with extensive supra- and infratentorial extensions, optimally managed through the petrosal approach. a) Preoperative axial view, b) postoperative axial view, c) preoperative sagittal view, d) postoperative sagittal view

Case Material

Our series consists of 33 patients: 21 with meningiomas, 7 with schwannomas, and 5 with epidermoid tumours. These were operated on during the years 1983 through 1989. There was no mortality. Total removal was achieved for all but 3 patients with meningiomas (Fig. 4). To date, there has been no recurrence in those having total removal. Because all the tumours in this series were slow-growing, the follow-up period is short. A longer follow-up is needed. Complications included hemiparesis and dysphasia from venous infarction of the temporal lobe in one patient, permanent facial nerve palsy in 2 patients, temporary facial nerve palsy in 3 patients, temporary lower cranial nerve palsy in 3 patients, loss of hearing in one patient, and decreased hearing in another. Hearing improved in one patient. Pulmonary embolism occurred in 5 patients, CSF leak in two, one of whom needed surgical repair, and a pseudo-meningocele, which subsided after spinal drainage, occurred in one.

Discussion

Approaches to the posterior cranial base fall into 3 main categories[1]. *Intradural* approaches include the suboccipital, subtemporal, frontotemporal, and combined suboccipital and temporal approaches. *Anterior extradural* approaches include the transoral, transcervical, transsphenoidal, transethmoidal, transmaxillotomy, and transbasal approaches. *Lateral approaches* include the infratemporal, transcochlear, petrosal, and transtemporal.

We found the petrosal approach as presented above to be superior for intradural tumours located in the clival and petroclival areas[3]. This approach has several advantages: the cerebellum and temporal lobes are minimally retracted, the operative distance to the clivus is shortened by 3 cm, the surgeon has a direct line of sight to the lesion and the anterior and lateral aspects of the brain stem, the neural and otological structures including the cochlea, the labyrinth and the facial nerves are preserved, the transverse and sigmoid sinuses as well as the vein of Labbé and the basal occipital veins are preserved, the tumour's blood supply is intercepted early in the procedure, multiple axes for dissection are provided, and dissection is performed along a longitudinal axis, alleviating the need for temporal lobe retraction.

Coagulation of the vein of Labbé or the basilar occipital vein leads to temporal lobe venous infarction with potentially devastating neurological deficits. Malis[8] has emphasized ligation of the sigmoid sinus lateral to the entrance of the vein of Labbé to preserve venous flow through the other side. Our technique, however, preserves the sinus and avoids injury to the vein. To date, we have not found it necessary to ligate and section the sinus. In fact, we believe sigmoid sinus ligation should be avoided. A fatal outcome has been reported subsequent to sigmoid sinus ligation.[7,10] Furthermore, not infrequently, the dominant draining vein of the temporal lobe enters the sinus further laterally than its usual anatomic location. If a tear occurs in the sinus wall, it is repaired with sutures or a patch graft. In our series, reconstruction of the sinus with venous graft was carried out in one case in which the sinus was injured beyond repair. Because of the potential risk to the sinus, the venous anatomy should be delineated preoperatively with digital angiography, confirming not only the patency of the opposite side, but the connection between the two sides at the torcula heropili.

Acknowledgement

The authors are grateful to Julie Hipp for her editorial assistance.

References

1. Al-Mefty O (1989) Surgery of the cranial base. Kluwer, Boston, pp 239–258
2. Al-Mefty O, Fox JL, Smith RR (1988) Petrosal approach for petroclival meningiomas. Neurosurgery 22: 510–517
3. Al-Mefty O, Schenk MP, Smith RR (1991) Petroclival meningiomas. In: Wilkins RH, Rengachary SS (eds) Neurosurgical operative atlas. Williams & Wilkins, Baltimore
4. Bailey P (1939) Concerning the technique of operation for acoustic neurinoma. Zentralbl Neurochir 4: 1–5
5. Fraenkel J, Hunt JR (1904) Contribution to the surgery of neurofibroma of the acoustic nerve. Ann Surg 40: 293–319
6. Hakuba A, Nishimura S, Tanaka K, Kishi H, Nakamura T (1977) Clivus meningioma: Six cases of total removal. Neurol Med Chir (Tokyo) 17: 63–77
7. Hitselberger WE, House WF (1966) A combined approach to the cerebellopontine angle. Arch Otolaryngol 84: 267–285
8. Malis LI (1985) Surgical resection of tumours of the skull base. In: Wilkins RH, Rengachary SS (eds) Neurosurgery, Vol 1. McGraw-Hill, New York, pp 1011–1021
9. Morrison AW, King TT (1973) Experiences with a translabyrinthine–transtentorial approach to the cerebellopontine angle: Technical note. J Neurosurg 38: 382–390
10. Symon L (1982) Surgical approaches to the tentorial hiatus. In: Krayenbühl H *et al* (eds) Advances and technical standards in neurosurgery, Vol 9. Springer, Wien New York, pp 69–112

Correspondence: Prof. O. Al-Mefty, M.D., Division of Neurological Surgery, Loyola University Medical Center, 2160 S. First avenue, Maywood, Illinois 60153, U.S.A.

Acta Neurochirurgica, Suppl. 53, 171–182 (1991)
© by Springer-Verlag 1991

Surgical Management of Clival Meningiomas

T. Javed and **L. N. Sekhar**

Department of Neurosurgery, Presbyterian-University Hospital, Pittsburgh, Pennsylvania, U.S.A.

Summary

The surgical management of intradural clival tumours is difficult due to the relative inaccessibility of the clivus through traditional neurosurgical approaches, and the intimate relationship of such tumours to critical neurovascular and brainstem structures. This report concentrates on the experience with clival menigiomas, which are the most common intradural clival tumours. Between July 1983 and July 1990, 52 patients with petroclival meningiomas underwent surgical excision of their tumours. A variety of skull base approaches were utilized to obtain wide tumour exposure with minimal brain retraction. Large or giant tumours required multiple approaches and staged removal of tumour. Tumour resection was evaluated by a standard protocol of postoperative MR or CT scans. Total tumour resection was achieved in 38 cases (73%), subtotal resection in 11 (21%) and partial resection in 3 (6%). Follow-up has ranged from 4 to 83 months. Two patients had recurrence of tumour requiring re-operation with one receiving additional external beam radiation. Two postoperative deaths occurred, one from pheumonia and another from infectious complications. The most common postoperative morbidity were lower cranial nerve palsy, aspiration peumonia and temporary hemiparesis.

Keywords: Clivus; meningioma; skull bases approaches; basilar artery.

Introduction

Surgery of clival tumours has traditionally been associated with a relatively high mortality and morbidity[2,39,18] due to the difficulty in obtaining adequate exposure, and due to the involvement of adjacent brainstem and neurovascular structures by tumour. Recent advances in imaging modalities have improved our anatomical understanding of tumour location and involvement of adjacent neurovascular structures. Modern skull base approaches are providing improved tumour exposure with minimal brain retraction. These factors, along with improvement in neuroanesthesia and critical care medicine, merit the re-evaluation of the surgical management

of these hitherto complicated lesions. The object of the present report is to describe the experience in the surgical management of 52 patients with clival meningiomas in order to evaluate the effect of recent advances in imaging technology, critical care medicine, and surgical techniques on outcome.

Materials and Methods

The hospital charts of 52 patients with meningiomas involving the clivus that were operated on at the University of Pittsburgh from July 1983 to July 1990, were reviewed. The majority of patients were operated by L.S. Three additional patients that were managed non-surgically were excluded from the present study. All patients underwent careful preoperative clinical examination and radiological evaluation with high resolution computerized tomography (CT) performed with a G.E. 9800 scanner using soft tissue and bone algorithms and 3 mm axial and coronal sections through the cranial base area preoperatively. After 1984, all patients underwent magnetic resonance imaging (MRI), using a T_1 and T_2 weighted images, and recently with intravenous enhancement. Cerebral angiography was performed preoperatively to evaluate tumour blood supply and to define vascular anatomy. Preoperative embolization was performed in cases where tumour blood supply was predominantly by the external carotid artery. Balloon test occlusion of the internal carotid artery (BTO-ICA) with clinical and qunatitative cerebral blood flow measurements was performed in cases where manipulation or sacrifice of the ICA was anticipated. Postoperative evaluation was performed by interview and neurological examination in a standardized format. CT or MRI scans according to a standard skull base protocol was performed postoperatively at 3–12 month intervals. Additional tests such as audiogram, brainstem, and somatosensory evoked potentials were performed as needed.

Operative Approaches

The safety of skull base surgery has been greatly enhanced by the introduction of intraoperative evoked potential and cranial nerve EMG monitoring (8). Muscle relaxants are avoided after induction of anesthesia if cranial nerve EMG monitoring is contemplated. Operative approaches can be divided into two major groups: *simple approaches*, which are adequate for small and

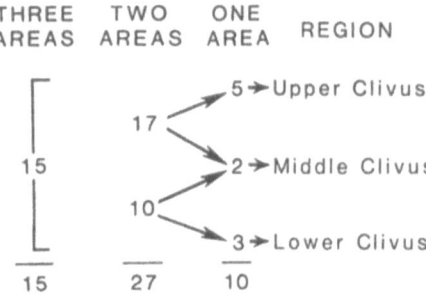

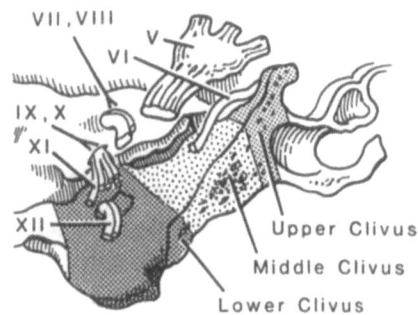

Fig. 1. Division of the clivus into upper, middle and lower clivus, and the areas of involvement by tumour

medium sized tumours, and *complex approaches*, which are more appropriate for large and giant tumours. In our experience, large or giant tumours, tumours encasing basilar artery and tumours that are technically more difficult to excise generally require complex approaches and staged tumour resection. The object of each approach is to obtain the widest tumour exposure with minimal amount of brain manipulation and retraction possible. The clivus can be divided into three segments: upper, middle and lower clivus. The *upper clivus* is defined as the area above the trigeminal root, the *midclivus* lies between the trigeminal and glossopharyngeal nerve roots, and the *lower clivus* is the area below CN IX (Fig. 1). *Centrolateral* tumours are defined as those whose epicenter is in the middle fossa or the petrous bone, where as *central tumours* have their epicenter in the clivus, with minimal extension laterally.

Simple Approaches

Frontotemporal/Anterior Subtemporal Approach with Zygomatic Osteotomy

This provides excellent exposure for tumours involving the tentorial notch and upper clival region. Tumour resection can be achieved by either a trans-Sylvian approach or utilizing an anterior subtemporal approach. In the latter approach, resection of the anterior 4 cm of the inferior temporal gyrus can be very helpful in obtaining adequate tumour exposure while at the same time minimizing temporal lobe

retraction. The removal of the petrous apex bone medial to the horizontal segment of the petrous ICA extends the lower reach of this approach. It is predominantly suited for tumours of the tentorial notch, with extension to the upper and mid-clivus, especially ipsilaterally.

Very Lateral Retrosigmoid Approach

This approach is one that most neurosurgeons are familiar with and provides excellent exposure for tumour removal from the petrous ridge region, the intradural jugular foramen area, foramen magnum region and centrolateral lesions involving the middle and lower clivus below the trigeminal root. It may be inadequate for the resection of tumour from the tentorial notch area. In addition, when the brainstem has been deeply indented by the tumour, particularly by the more centrally located tumours, dissection of tumour from midbrain and pons may be difficult through this approach. The anterior inferior cerebellar artery and CNs VIII, IX, and X are at greatest risk of injury during this operation. This approach is usually suitable for small and medium sized tumours of the mid or lower clival area.

Extreme Lateral Transcondylar Approach[17]

This approach is used for the management of lower clival/foramen magnum tumours with extension into the upper cervical spine and where the cerebral artery or cranial nerves 9–12 may be encased by the tumour. In this approach, a small retrosigmoid craniectomy is followed by a partial mastoidectomy up to the vertical segment of the facial canal, and the sigmoid sinus is unroofed to the point where it turns to join the jugular bulb. The posterior half of the occipital condyle is removed along with the lateral third of C_1 lamina. This exposes the extradural vertebral artery at the point of its entry through the dura. The dura is opened in a cruciate manner, and the vertebral artery is completely mobilized from C_1 to C_2 to the vertebro-basilar junction. This provides a very lateral exposure of the lower clivus, foramen magnum, and vertebral artery. The surgeon can look in front of the spino-medullary junction to see the opposite CNs XII, XI, X and IX bilaterally and the vertebro-basilar junction. This allows tumour removal without the need for brainstem or spinal cord retraction and reduces the risk of vertebral artery injury since it is completely exposed during the approach.

Frontotemporal Transcavernous Approach

This approach is used for tumours involving the cavernous sinus and the upper clival area, when removal of the intracavernous tumour is one of the goals of the operation. The use of this approach has been previously described[16]. Access to the upper clivus is obtained by working between the supraclinoid ICA and oculomotor nerve, between oculomotor nerve and trochlear nerve, or between trochlear nerve and VI. If intracavernous carotid is excised as a part of tumour resection (with or without ICA saphenous bypass grafting), access to the midclivus can be obtained by removal of the petrous apex, upper clivus, and sphenoid bone, and by working through the cavernous sinus. The major advantages of this approach are that the upper clivus and a portion of the mid-clivus can be approached through the middle cranial fossa without the need for posterior temporal lobe retraction, and that the tumour is devascularized very early in the operation.

Complex Approaches

Frontotemporal/Preauricular Infratemporal Approach (Fig. 2)

This provides both intra- and extradural exposure, the details of which have been previously described[15]. Briefly, following a preauricular incision and resection of the mandibular condyle, the petrous ICA is

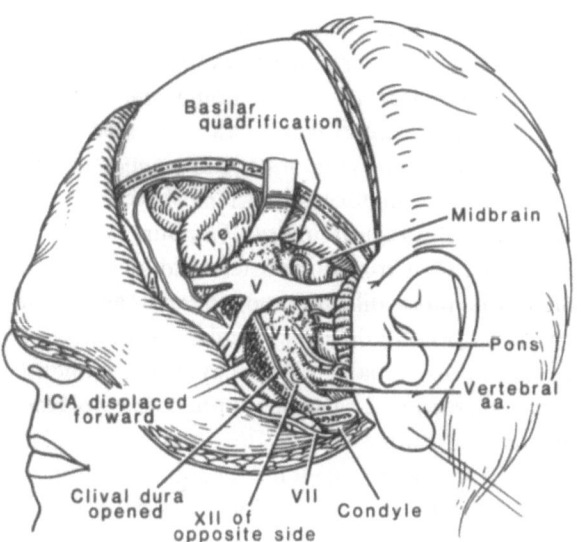

Fig. 2. The frontotemporal/preauricular infratemporal approach to clival meningiomas. The petrous ICA is unroofed and displaced anteriorly. Removal of petrous apex provides exposure from the tentorial notch down to CNs XII

unroofed in the carotid canal and is mobilized forward after displacing it out of the carotid canal or after dissecting it free of tumour. The region of the petrous apex and lateral clivus is then drilled away using a high-speed drill, being careful not to injure the cochlea and the facial nerve, which lie posterior, superior and slightly lateral to the genu of the petrous carotid artery. After opening the dura, tumour can be removed from the region of the tentorial notch and from the clivus below the trigeminal nerve. The sixth cranial nerve and the midbasilar artery, along with its branches and the pons, are readily exposed by this approach. This approach allows the downward extension of the subtemporal approach , inferiorly to CN XII. The ipsilateral cerebellopontine angle structures are not exposed.

Posterior Subtemporal/Presigmoid Approach (Fig. 3)

This approach has also been described by Al-Mefty, et al. and Samii[1,10], and is suitable for centrolateral, mid-clival and petrous apex lesions. Exposure of the upper clival region is possible, but may require considerable posterior temporal lobe retraction. Exposure of the lower clivus is limited by the sigmoid sinus and may only be obtained at the expense of division of the sinus or working posterior to it. We divide the sigmoid sinus only when there is cross circulation demonstrable angiographically, and the sinus is non-dominant. When the sigmoid sinus is divided, we reconstruct it at the end of the procedure.

Total Petrosectomy (Fig. 4)

The use of this approach for intradural neoplastic lesions has been previously described[6,11]. This approach is utilized for exposure of giant or very complex petroclival meningiomas and provides the best exposure possible by any single approach . After performing a temporal craniotomy, zygomatic osteotomy, and excision of the mandibular condyle, the entire petrous and upper cervical ICA is exposed and translocated anteriorly. The facial nerve is unroofed in its entire course through the petrous bone from the internal auditory canal to its exit through the stylomastoid foramen. By displacing the intrapetrous facial nerve posterio-inferiorly and petrous ICA forward, the entire petrous temporal bone is removed in a piecemeal fashion down to the jugular bulb inferiorly. In this manner, the widest possible exposure

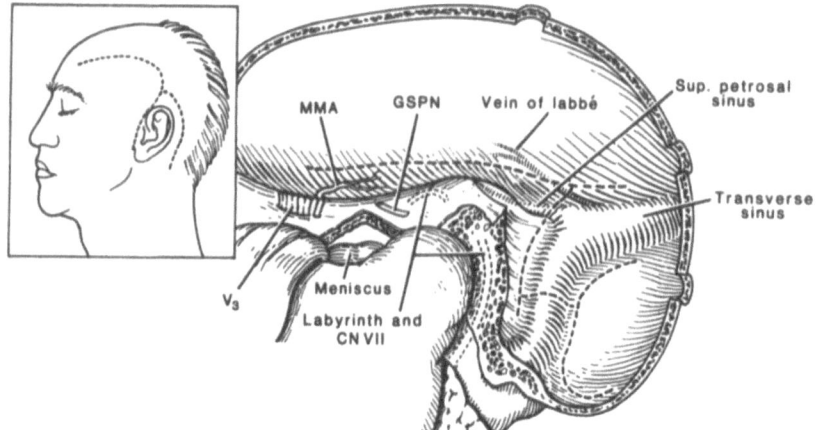

Fig. 3. The posterior subtemporal/pre-sigmoid approach exposes midclival and petrous apex lesions. Further working space can be obtained by division of the non-dominant sigmoid sinus

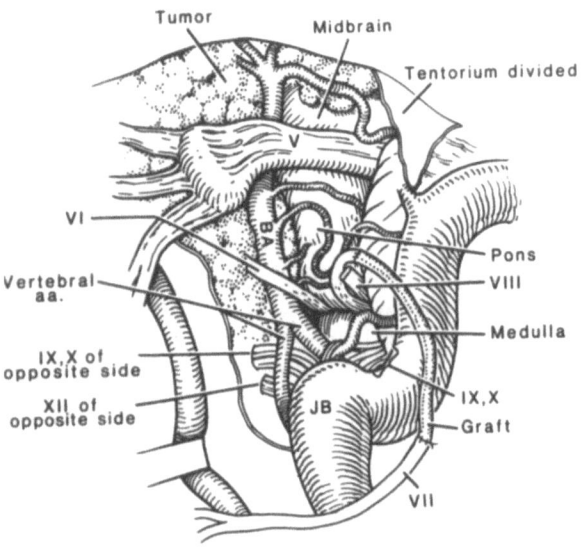

Fig. 4. Exposure of a large clival meningioma by a total petro-sectomy approach as utilized in patient E.M. The petrous ICA has been displaced forward and the facial nerve displaced postero-inferiorly, to improve exposure. The encased basilar artery is seen. Facial nerve graft was not necessary in this case

of the petroclival area is obtained with the exception of the ipsilateral lower clival area, which is limited by the jugular bulb and cranial nerves exiting through the jugular foramen. This approach can be combined with the extreme lateral approach to gain exposure of this blind area. The major disadvantage is the loss of hearing and prolonged facial paralysis from retraction which will recover to a House Grade 3 function, but never completely. This limits its use to patients who have severe hearing impairment ipsilaterally, have giant sized tumours, recurrent tumours, or tumours with considerable encasement of the basilar artery.

Technique of Tumour Resection

Even though excellent tumour exposure can be obtained by utilizing the skull base approaches described, it is important for the surgeon to use careful microsurgical techniques during tumour removal to reduce operative morbidity and to achieve good tumour resection. Some of the difficulties encountered during tumour resection include increased tumour vascularity, severe brainstem displacement, absence of an arachnoid plane between tumour and brainstem, scar from previous surgery, and neurovascular encasement. Tumour resection could be performed despite these problems.

The general principles of tumour resection include early tumour devascularization and debulking of tumour with the aid of bipolar cautery and suction. The Malis irrigation bipolar (Codman, Shurtley, etc) is very useful when dissecting tumour from encased vessels, cranial nerves and the brainstem. Tumour dissection from the brainstem is best performed in the arachnoid plane. When this arachnoid plane is absent, it is important to preserve brainstem pial membrane to prevent neurological injury. Tumour dissection from encased vertebro-basilar artery and its branches is often the most difficult and stressful aspect of tumour resection. In cases of vascular encasement, it is important to initially devascularize the tumour. Vascular dissection is best performed by working from areas of normal vessels to areas of vascular encasement. Encased cranial nerves are dissected in a plane parallel to the nerve with the aid of EMG monitoring.

Reconstruction of the skull base defect is performed in layers, initially closing dura primarily or with dural graft (fascia lata or pericranium). If the Eustachian tube is entered during the approach , this is packed with fat on both ends and sutured. Any exposed paranasal sinuses are exenterated and packed with fat and fascia. Larger defects are covered with a well vascularized muscle flap (usually a temporalis muscle flap).

Illustrative Cases

Patient #1 (O.C)

This 67-year-old woman presented with a ten year history of headaches and a recent onset of right hemiparesis, unsteady gait, slowness of speech and mentation. Axial and sagittal MRI showed

a giant left petroclival meningioma with left cavernous sinus involvement and cavernous ICA encasement (Fig. 5 a). Associated hydrocephalus was treated with a ventriculoperitoneal shunt, which resulted in some improvement of speech, gait and mentation, but the hemiparesis persisted.

She underwent resection of the upper half of the tumour initially, using a frontotemporal craniotomy, orbitozygomatic osteotomy, and trans-sylvian approach. At surgery, the upper basilar artery and its perforators, the posterior cerebral artery and posterior communicating artery were noted to be encased by tumour. The tumour was successfully dissected from these vessels. The remaining tumour was resected three weeks later using a presigmoid, infratemporal/subtemporal approach. Almost complete tumour resection except for a small fragment in the left cavernous sinus was achieved (Fig. 5).

Her postoperative course was complicated by ventricular arrhy-

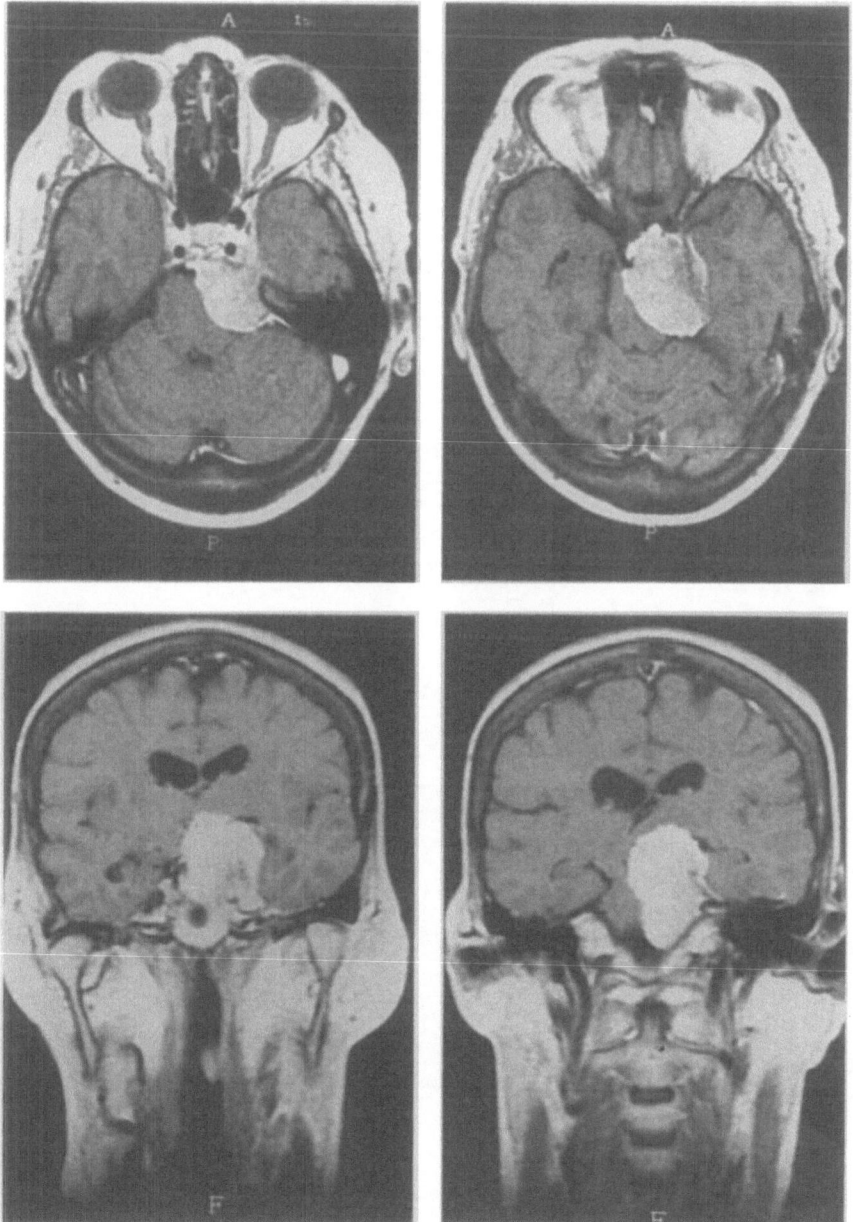

Fig. 5 a. Axial and coronal MRI with intravenous contrast of patient O.C. shows a giant petroclival meningioma with cavernous sinus involvement. There is encasement of the carotid and distal basilar artery. Marked brainstem displacement is apparent

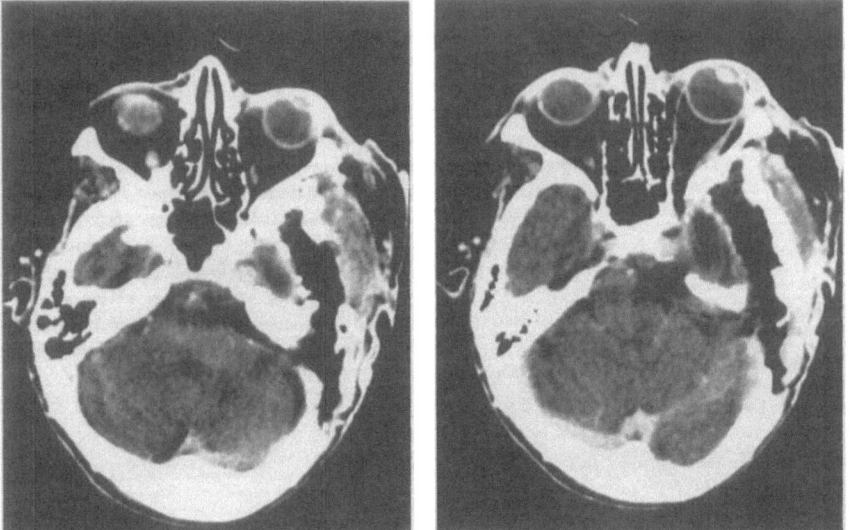

Fig. 5 b. Postoperative axial CT scan with contrast showing complete tumour resection except for a small remnant in left posterior cavernous sinus

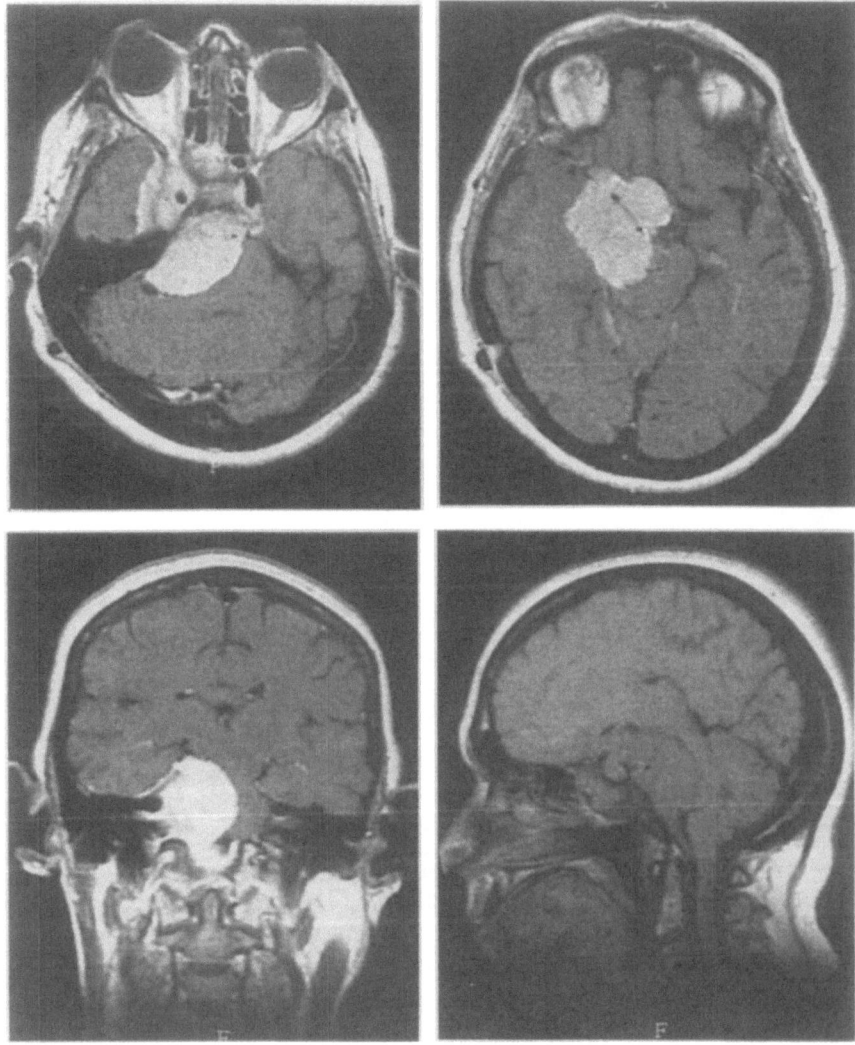

Fig. 6 a

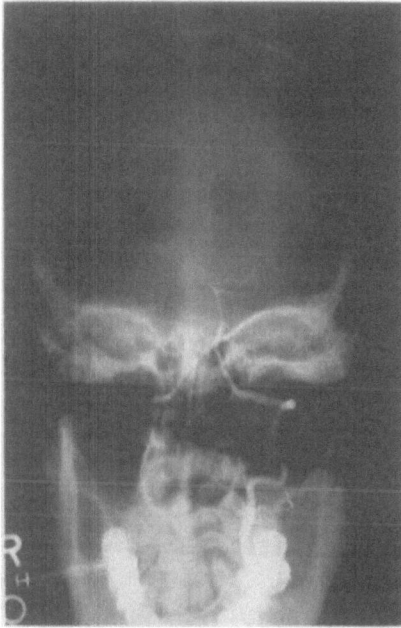

Fig. 6 b. AP view of vertebro-basilar circulation with left vertebral injection. The distal basilar artery is displaced to the left and is markedly narrowed by the encasing tumour. The posterior cerebral and superior cerebellar arteries are displaced superiorly

thmias requiring an extended stay in the intensive care unit. In follow-up six months later, she has a mild hemiparesis, but is ambulating independently.

Patient #2 (E.M.)

This 63-year-old women presented with gait ataxia and memory difficulty to her local neurosurgeon. CT scan showed a right petroclival meningioma and hydrocephalus. She underwent ventriculoperitoneal shunt with temporary symptomatic improvement. Three years later, she was referred to this institution with oculomotor paresis, gait ataxia and difficulty with mentation. MRI scans showed progression in tumour size with cavernous sinus involvement and encasement of ICA and upper basilar artery and its branches (Fig. 6 a). Cerebral angiography (Fig. 6 b) showed severe distal basilar artery stenosis from tumour encasement and displacement of basilar artery and its branches.

She underwent a frontotemporal craniotomy, orbitozygomatic osteotomy and trans-sylvian approach with resection of tumour from the supraclinoid ICA and its branches and the superior cavernous sinus. At the second stage of surgery, further attempts at tumour resection through a presigmoid subtemporal approach were unsuccessful due to limited tumour exposure obtained by this approach. Further exposure was obtained by performing a total petrosectomy. This provided excellent exposure for complete resection of tumour from the petroclival region, without incurring any injury to the encased basilar artery or its branches. postoperatively, she has anacusis on the right, facial paresis, and a resolving abulia.

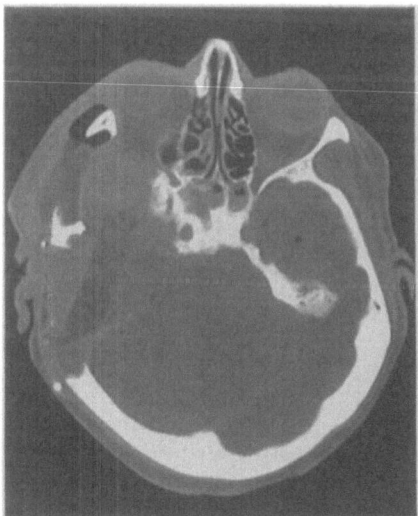 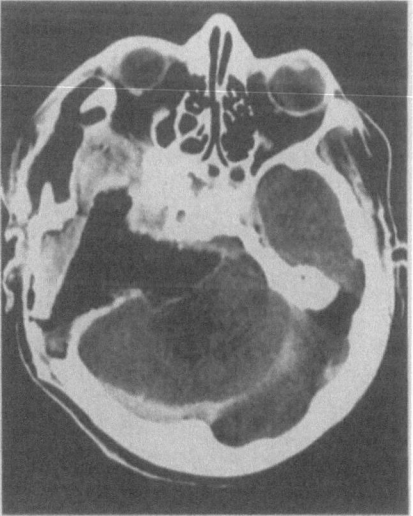

Fig. 6 c. Postoperative axial CT scans. The CT scan on the left shows the extent of bone removal performed and the exposure that can be achieved by the total petrosectomy approach. Encased CT scan on right shows complete tumour excision except small remnant in the right cavernous sinus

Fig. 6 a. Axial, coronal and sagittal MRI of patient E.M. shows a large right petroclival meningioma with tumour extension into the cavernous sinus, middle fossa, Meckel's cave internal auditory canal. This basilar artery is extremely narrowed by tumour encasement (*left upper*) and the encased P. Comm is apparent (*right upper*). The brainstem appears to be severely compressed by the tumour, but an arachnoid plane between tumour and brainstem is preserved

Postoperative CT scans with contrast (Fig. 6 c) shows complete tumour resection, except a small remnant in the right cavernous sinus. The remaining tumour will be treated with stereotactic radiosurgery if it shows evidence of growth in the future.

Patient #3 (M.B.)

This 61-year-old lady presented to her doctor with paresthesia of the left face and was found to have a small petroclival meningioma which was treated conservatively. Increasing headaches, neck pains, diplopia, gait ataxia and progression of trigeminal symptoms prompted repeat studies which showed marked increase in tumour size. The tumour was noted to be partially encasing the basilar artery and involving the cavernous sinus and sphenoid sinus (Fig. 7 a). The upper part of the tumour was initially resected through a frontotemporal and preauricular infratemporal approach, after saphenous vein graft replacement of the intracavernous ICA. Because of tumour involvement of the sphenoid sinus and a high risk of postoperative CSF leak from intracranial procedure to resect this portion of the tumour, we elected to resect tumour from the sphenoid sinus and pack this area with autologous fat through a transsphenoidal approach. Ten days later, the remaining tumour in the petroclival region was completely resected using a presigmoid infratemporal/subtemporal approach, and reconstruction of the abducens nerve was performed with a graft.

Postoperative CT scan with contrast shows complete tumour resection (Fig. 7 b). One month postoperatively, she is neurologically intact except for a left oculomotor paresis and abducens palsy.

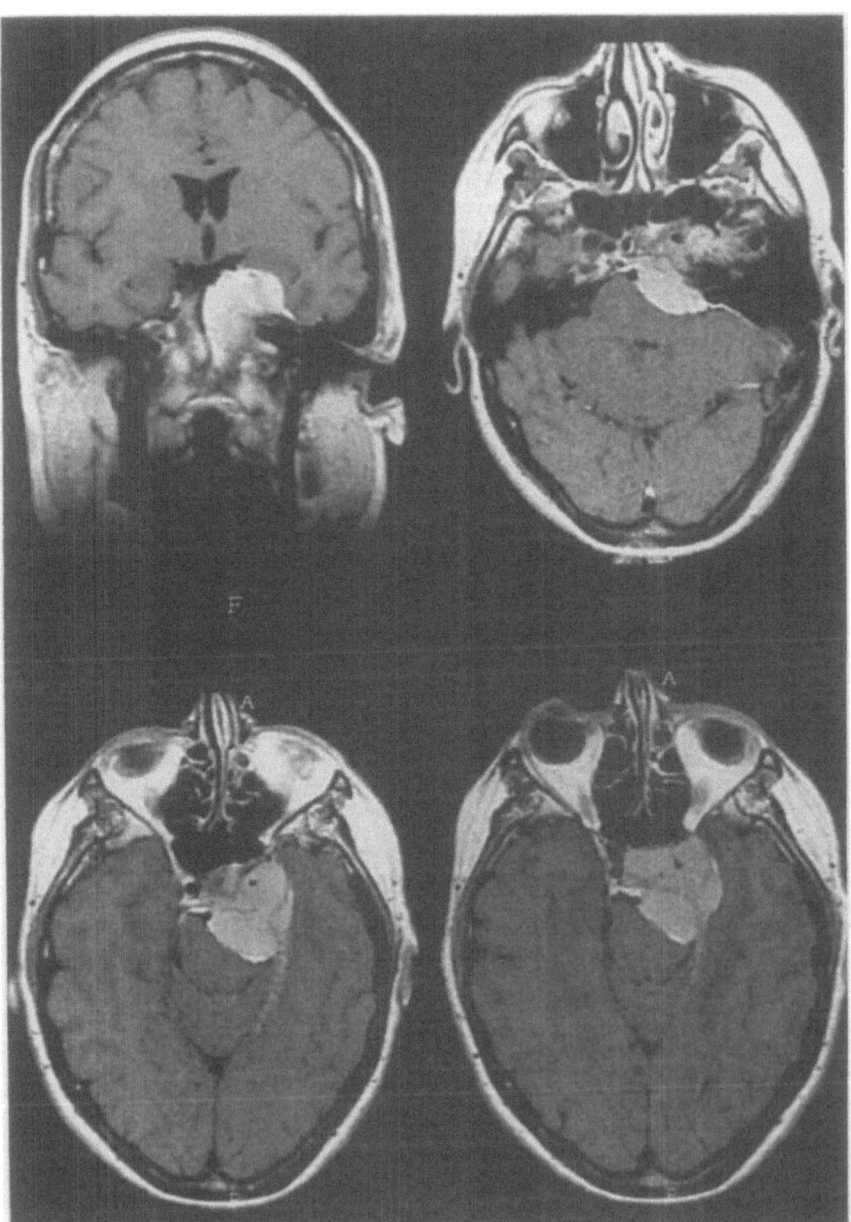

Fig. 7 a. MRI with enhancement in patient M.B. show large left petroclival meningiomas with tumour extension into the left cavernous sinus, Meckel's cave and internal auditory canal. The supraclinoid ICA is encased and narrowed by the tumour. The basilar artery is also encased, but not narrowed

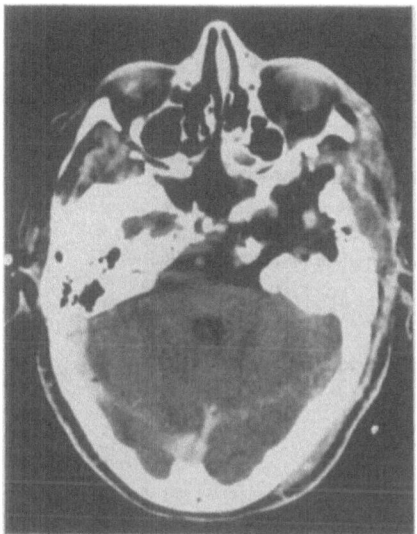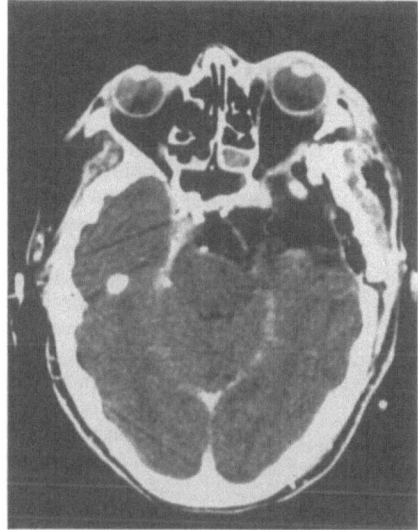

Fig. 7b. Postoperative axial CT scans with contrast showing complete tumour resection

Results

Of the total of 52 patients in this series, 44 were women and 8 men aged 24–73 years with an average of 51 (SD $+/-$ 12 years). Presenting symptoms in this group of patients (Table 1) were similar to those noted in previous reports[1,3,7,10,12,13,14]. Cranial nerves in close proximity to the tumour (V, VI, VII, VIII and IX, X complex) were most frequently involved with the trigeminal nerve being by far the most commonly involved cranial nerve. Other common neurological findings included dementia, gait ataxia and motor

deficits. Areas of clival involvement are summarized of Fig. 1.

The operative approaches utilized are listed on Table 2. A variety of different skull base approaches were utilized to obtain wide tumour exposure, with the retrosigmoid approach being the most frequently used (44%). 28 patients underwent a single operation with 24 requiring two or more staged opertions, usually by different approaches to effect tumour removal. Patients with large or more complex tumours (vascular encasement or scarring from previous surgery) generally required more than one operation. Extent

Table 1. *Clinical Presentation in 52 Patients with Petroclival Meningiomas*

	Cases No.	%
Headache	17	33
Seizures	3	6
Dementia	6	12
Motor weakness	7	13
Hemisensory loss	4	8
Gait ataxia	20	38
Limb ataxia	5	10
Cranial nerve problems:		
II Decreased vision	3	10
V Pain	12	23
Sensory loss	13	25
VII Weakness	5	10
VIII Tinnitus	5	10
IX, X Paresis	10	19
XII Dysarthria	2	4

Table 2. *Operative Approaches Used for Tumour Resection*

	Cases no.	%
Simple Approaches:		
Frontotemporal or subtemporal/transzygomatic	10	19
Frontotemporal/orbitozygomatic/transcavernous	19	36
Very lateral retrosigmoid approach (suboccipital)	23	44
Extreme lateral transcondylar-C_1 laminectomy	7	13
Complex Approaches:		
Frontotemporal/preauricular infratemporal approach	10	19
Posterior subtemporal/presigmoid transpetrous approach		
with sigmoid sinus division	3	6
without sigmoid sinus division	5	10
Total petrosectomy	6	12
Single operation	28	54
Two or more operations	24	46

Table 3. *Extent of Tumor Resection, Treatment of Residue and Recurrence*

	No.	%
Total excision	38	73
Subtotal excision (90% of tumour volume)	11	21
Partial excision (second planned operation refused)	3	6
Location of residual tumour (in more than one area in some patients)		
Clivus	10	19
Cavernous sinus	7	13
Treatment of residual tumour		
Observation (some awaiting second state surgery)	10	19
Gamma knife	4	8
Recurrence treatment		
Re-operation	2	4
+ External radiation	1	2

Table 4. *Complications of Surgery*

Complications	Cases no.	%
Death	2	4
Cerebral infarction (hemiparesis/worsening mental status)	3	6
Cerebral edema (hematoma)	4	8
Subdural hygroma/hematoma (operative drainage)	3	6
Temporary hemiparesis	7	13
Locked in syndrome	1	2
Cerebral abscess	1	2
Bulbar palsy (CNs IX, X) requiring tracheostomy	10	19
Aspiration pneumonia	7	13
CSF leaks	5	10
Meningitis	2	4
Wound infection	1	2
Diabetes insipidus	3	6
Hydrocephalus	3	6

* More than one complication occurred in each individual patient.

of tumour resection was based on operative findings and MRI/CT scans (with and without contrast) obtained 2–3 months postoperatively.

Total tumour excision was achieved in 38 cases (73%), subtotal excision in 11 (21%) and partial excision in 3 (6%) (Table 3). Small areas of residual tumour were usually found in the cavernous sinus (13%) and/or the clivus (17%). Residual tumour was treated by observation alone in 10 patients and gamma knife radiosurgery in 4. In many patients, residual tumour was left in areas because of the age of the patient or because of scar tissue from prior operation.

The follow-up period has ranged from 4 months to 83 months. Two recurrences occurred in patients who had an apparent total excision. One had a small recurrence at the margin of the previous resection and was successfully re-operated. The other had a sizable recurrence of a malignant meningioma which was treated by re-operation and external beam radiation.

Postoperative complications are summarized on Table 4. Operative deaths occurred in two patients. One patient with a large mid and lower clival tumour developed ipsilateral CNs IX, X and XII paralysis postoperatively, requiring tracheostomy for airway protection. She developed a massive pneumonia and died suddenly. The second patient with a giant petroclival meningioma with basilar artery encasement had a rather complicated postoperative course, including wound infection, sepsis and pulmonary aspiration requiring a tracheostomy. She was making good progress when she was found dead two months

postoperatively from pulmonary complications. Three patients sustained probable brainstem infarction. In one patient, occlusion of a tumour encased cerebellar artery during surgery resulted in a temporary hemiparesis and obtundation with eventual slight worsening of preoperative hemiparesis (Karnofsky preop 70; postop 60). In a second case of recurrent meningioma, single perforator occlusion led to dementia and hemiparesis (Karnofsky preop 70; postop 40). The third patient had five previous operations and radiation therapy and sustained superior cerebellar artery occlusion during our operation. This patient sustained a worsened hemiparesis (Karnofsky preop 50; postop 40). One patient sustained temporal lobe and cerebellar contusion after a posterior subtemporal and presigmoid transpetrous approach to the tumour. Re-operation to remove contused brain was followed by the development of a localized abscess. The patient had a prolonged convalescence after drainage of the abscess (Karnofsky preop 80; postop 70). Pulmonary complications were frequently related to cranial nerve IX, X dysfunction, and the incidence has been reduced by increasing use of tracheostomy.

Discussion

The natural history of most petroclival meningiomas is one of slow but relentless growth which, if left untreated, eventually leads to a fatal outcome[3,4]. Up until the 1970s, diagnosis of these tumours was difficult and surgical intervention carried an operative mortality of as high as 53%[18]. The introduction of the operating microscope to neurosurgery, advances in neuroanesthesia, and critical care medicine, paved the way towards aggressive surgical attack on these lesions. This has resulted in a more acceptable mortality of 0–17%[1,5,7,10,13,14,18].

Our results confirm previous reports[1,5,10,12,13], regarding the feasibility of total surgical excision (73%) with acceptable morbidity. It is important for the surgeon treating these difficult lesions to be familiar with all the different skull base approaches available to facilitate optimal tumour resection. Complete surgical excision of these benign tumours is best performed at first surgical attempt[1,10], due to absence of postsurgical scarring. We adhere to this basic surgical principle for the smaller tumours, but feel that the larger, more complex tumours are best resected by staging surgery. Frequently, a single approach does not provide adequate exposure of the whole tumour to facilitate safe tumour resection, and the time required for complete tumour resection may be beyond the endurance of both patient and the surgical team. We leave thin sheets of silastic between the tumor and brain interface to prevent adhesions and re-operate within two weeks.

Tumours encasing the vertebro-basilar artery and its branches were traditionally felt to be inoperable. We had 11 patients in this series with vertebro-basilar artery encasement, 6 of whom had gross total excision, 4 subtotal excision and 1 partial excision of their tumours. The successful resection of these tumours presents the greatest challenge to the neurosurgeon. The major difficulty lies in the preservation of every single perforator vessel coming off the basilar artery. Similarly, we do not feel that the absence of an arachnoidal plane precludes total tumour resection. The main cause of postoperative major morbidity is injury to the basilar artery branches. Injury to even a single perforator vessel can result in brainstem infarction. This occurred in 3 patients with single perforator injury (1 in a patient with basilar artery encasement). Development of techniques for reconstruction of these injured microvessels may reduce the incidence of this complication in the future. Dissection of tumour from encased vessels is facilitated by initial devascularization of the tumour and working from normal vessels to areas of encased vessels. Arterial injury to the major vessel can often be repaired by suture reanastomosis. Neurophysiological monitoring of cranial nerve III, VI, VII, VIII, IX or X, as well as brainstem evoked responses and somatosensory evoked responses, is critical in reducing mortality and morbidity.

The incidence of severe complications in this series has continued to decrease with increasing experience in surgical techniques. Our mortality of 4% compares favourably to other reported series[1,5,7,10,18]. However, it is difficult to compare results in different series because the operative difficulty of these tumours is variable and factors contributing to operative problems are not stated in most series. Complication rates are increased in patients with large or giant sized tumours, patients who have undergone multiple operations or received previous radiation therapy and the presence of vascular encasement.

The decision on the extent of surgical resection, and what to do with residual or recurrent tumour can be a difficult one, particularly in a patient with minimal symptoms. The patient's physiological age, general medical condition, and the surgeon's experience are factors that must be taken into consideration during decision making. Some of these tumours may remain dormant or grow very slowly over a long period of time before becoming severely symptomatic. In older patients, a subtotal tumour removal with observation or stereotactic radiosurgery of a small remnant is recommended. In Mayberg et al. series[7], only 4 (15%) of the 26 patients with subtotal removal had clinical progression and eventually died of their tumours. In Sekhar and Samii series[14], only 1 of the 5 patients known to have residual tumour clinically progressed to the point of requiring re-operation. In the present series, 2 patients with subtotally excised tumour experienced regrowth in the intradural or osseous areas. One underwent another operation with complete excision and the other underwent excision of the osseous areas and gamma knife radiosurgery for residual tumour in the cavernous sinus.

The slow growth pattern of these tumours also points out the importance of a lengthy follow-up for the evaluation of any form of treatment used. Even though major advances have taken place on the surgical front, further work needs to be done to develop adjuvant treatments for recurrent or residual tumour.

Conclusion

The surgical management of clival meningiomas continues to be a formidable technical challenge to the neurosurgeon. Present skull base approaches and application of microneurosurgical techniques have resulted in successful resection of tumours with an acceptable mortality and morbidity. Further work is needed to effectively treat residual tumour and recurrence. The follow-up has not been long enough to formulate any conclusions on the long-term results of radical surgical excision.

References

1. Al-Mefty O, Fox JL, Smith RR (1988) Petrosal approach for petroclival meningiomas. Neurosurgery 22: 510–517
2. Campbell E, Whitfield RD (1948) Posterior fossa meningiomas. J Neurosurg 5: 131–153
3. Cherrington M, Schneck SA (1966) Clivus meningiomas. Neurology 16: 86–92
4. Cushing HW, Eisenhardt L (1938) Meningiomas: their classification, regional behaviour, life history and surgical end results. Ch C Thomas, Springfield, Ill., pp 3–387
5. Hakuba A, Nishimura S, Taneka K, Kish H, Nakamura T (1977) Clivus meningioma. Six cases of total removal. Neurol Med Chir 17: 63–77
6. House W, Hitselberger W (1976) The transcochlear approach to the skull base. Arch Otolaryngol 102: 334–342
7. Mayberg MR, Symon L (1986) Meningiomas of the clivus and apical petrous bone. Report of 35 cases. J Neurosurg 65: 160–167
8. Moller RA (1987) Electrophysiological monitoring of cranial nerves in operations in the skull base. In: Sekhar LN, Schramm VL (eds) Tumors of the cranial base, diagnosis and treatment. Futura Publishing Co., Mount Kisco, NY, pp 123–132
9. Russell JR, Bucy PC (1953) Meningiomas of the posterior fossa. Surg Gynecol Obstet 96: 183–1953
10. Samii M, Ammirati M, Mahran A, Bini W, Sepehrnia A (1989) Surgery of petroclival meningiomas: report of 24 cases. Neurosurgery 24: 12–17
11. Sekhar LN, Estonillo R (1986) Transtemporal approach to the skull base: An anatomical study. Neurosurgery 19: 799–808
12. Sekhar LN, Jannetta PJ (1987) Petroclival and medial tentorial meningiomas. In: Sekhar LN, Schramm VL (eds) Tumors of the cranial base, diagnosis and treatment. Futura Publishing Co., Mount Kisco, NY, pp 623–640
13. Sekhar LN, Jannetta PJ, Burkhart L et al (1990) Meningiomas involving the clivus: a 6-year experience with 41 patients. Neurosurgery 27: 764–781
14. Sekhar LN, Samii M (1986) Petroclival and medial tentorial meningiomas. In: Scheuremann H, Schurmann K, Helms J (eds) Tumors of the skull base, extra and intracranial surgery of skull base tumours. Walter de Gruyter, Berlin, pp 141–158
15. Sekhar LN, Schramm VL, Jones NF (1987) Subtemporal-preauricular infratemporal foassa approach to large lateral and posterior cranial base neoplasms. J Neurosurg 66: 488–499
16. Sekhar LN, Sen CN, Jho HD, Janecka IP (1989) Surgical treatment of intracavernous neoplasms: a four year experience. Neurosurgery 24: 18–30
17. Sen, Sekhar LN (1990) An extreme lateral approach to intradural lesions of the cervical spine and foramen magnum. Neurosurgery 27: 197–202
18. Yaşargil MG, Martara RW, Curcic M (1980) Meninginomas of basal posterior cranial fossa. In: Krayenbühl H et al (eds) Advances and technical standards in neurosurgery, Vol 7. Springer, Wien New York, pp 3–115

Correspondence: Prof. L. N. Sekhar, M.D., Department of Neurosurgery, Presbyterian University Hospital, DeSoto at O'Hara Streets, Pittsburgh, PA 15213, U.S.A.

Acta Neurochirurgica, Suppl. 53, 183–192 (1991)

Extradural Petrous Bone and Petroclival Neoplasms

L. N. Sekhar, Sh. Pomeranz, and **Ch. N. Sen**

Department of Neurosurgery, University of Pittsburgh School of Medicine, Presbyterian-University Hospital, Pittsburgh, Pennsylvania, U.S.A.

Summary

Extradural petroclival tumours are composed of a spectrum of histological and anatomical configurations dictating a variety of surgical approaches. The experience with 68 such tumours operated at the University of Pittsburgh is presented, emphasizing the basal subfrontal and lateral approches. 85% of these tumours are benign or low-grade malignaneies, with 62% of these totally resected, resulting in a 5.4% recurrence rate. The operative mortality was 1.5% and major morbidity 3%. Well-planed surgery based on precise anatomical knowledge and imaging is the basis of treatment for petroclival tumours.

Keywords: Cranial base surgery; petroclival tumours.

Introduction

The petroclival region is surgically challenging due to its depth in the cranial base and its proximity to the brain stem, cranial nerves (CN) V–XI, and the vertebro-basilar and carotid arteries. Many operative approaches have been developed with the aim of combining relative ease, maximal exposure and minimal risk to the surrounding structures. Different approaches are often required for lesions in close proximity in the petroclival region. This necessitates knowledge of petroclival anatomy, imaging modalities, and each of the surgical approaches. We define petroclival lesions as those infiltrating solely the clivus or the clivus and the petrous bone. In this paper, the experience with 68 extradural petroclival neoplasms operated upon between 1983 and 1990 in the Department of Neurological Surgery, University of Pittsburgh is presented. All the operations were performed under the direction of neurosurgeons LNS or CNS.

Surgical Anatomy of the Petroclival Region

The clivus, composed of parts of the sphenoid and occipitial bones and extending from the dorsum sella to the foramen magnum (Fig. 1), is the midline anterior aspect of the posterior cranial fossa. The petrous temporal bone is pyramid-shaped, with the apex pointing anteromedially and abutting the clivus at the petro-occipital synchondrosis. The base of the petrous pyramid is on the lateral surface of the skull, underlying the external ear. Posteriorly and inferiorly, the petrous temporal bone is connected to the squamous occipital bone[14]. The petrous bone separates the middle and posterior cranial fossas laterally[15].

The internal cartoid artery (ICA) enters the petrous bone via the carotid canal and exits into the cavernous sinus. The Eustachian tube passes from the middle ear to the nasopharynx, anterio-inferio-medially, just

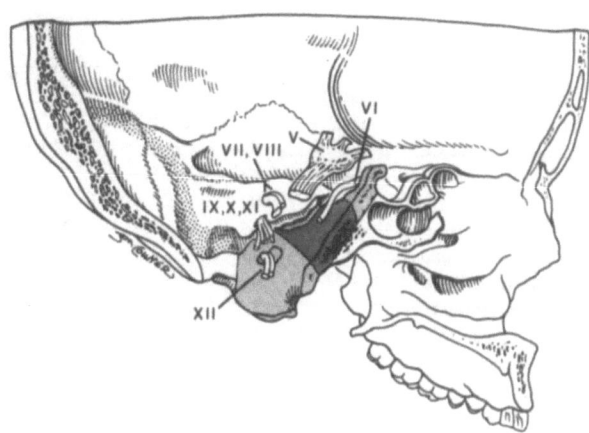

Fig. 1. Lateral scheme of the clivus divided into superior, medial and inferior thirds with the relationships of CN V–XII

lateral to the bend of the ICA from its petrous vertical to horizontal segment.

The intracranial clivus and petrous bone are lined with bilayered dura. Within the dural layers are the superior and inferior petrosal and sigmoid sinuses, located respectively along the petrous ridge, at the inferior-posterior petrosal base and along the posterior-lateral base of the petrous bone. The clival dura contains a rich plexus of veins.

CN XII exits the cranium via the hypoglossal canal at the inferio-lateral aspect of the clivus, the occipital condyle being inferio-medial to the canal. The jugular foramen is at the posterior aspect of the petroclival junction, containing the proximal internal jugular vein, and CNs IX-XI. The cavernous sinus lies anterior to the petroclival junction and communicates posteriorly with the clival venous plexus and petrosal sinuses.

The vertebrobasilar arterial complex lies on the clival dura, anterior to the brain stem. The lateral aspect of the brain stem and the anterior aspect of the cerebellar hemispheres abut the posterior petrous region.

Anterior to the clivus are the oro and nasopharynx inferiorly and superiorly the sphenoid sinus and pituitary gland.

The clivus may be divided into an upper region which lies above the petrous apex and CNs V and VI, a middle region below the petrous apex and above the jugular foramen pars nervosa, (between CNs VII and XI) and a lower region, which lies below the pars nervosa of the jugular foramen[24] (Fig. 1).

Neoplasms of the Petroclival Region

One classification of petroclival lesions is based on their intra or extradural location, some tumours being both intra and extradural. The histology of the 68 extradural petroclival tumours operated at our institution between 1983-90 is listed in Table 1. 59% of these tumours were low-grade malignancies, primarily chordomas and chondrosarcomas. Menin-

Table 1. *Extradural Petroclival Neoplasms Operated 1983–1990 Histology and Disease Status*

	Total	NED	AWD	DOD	DOC
Benign Lesions					
Cholesterol granuloma	3	3	–	–	–
Epidermoid cyst	1	1	–	–	–
Chondroblastoma	1	1	–	–	–
Neurilemmoma IX, X	4	4	–	–	–
Meningioma	4	2	–	1	1
Glomus jugulare	4	4	–	–	–
Teratoma, benign	1	1	–	–	–
Craniopharyngioma	2	1	–	1	–
	20	17	–	2	1
Low Grade Malignancies					
Chordoma	18	9	8	1	–
Chondrosarcoma	11	5	6	–	–
Cardiac myxoma (metastatic)	1	1	–	–	–
Pituitary adenoma (invasive)	5	4	1	–	–
Adenoid cystic Ca	5	2	2	1	–
	40	21	17	2	–
High Grade Malignancies					
Squamous cell Ca	4	–	–	4	–
Adenocarcinoma	1	–	–	1	–
Basal cell carcinoma	1	1	–	–	–
Osteogenic sarcoma	2	1	1	–	–
	8	2	1	5	1

NED = No evidence of disease; AWD = Alive with disease; DOD = Dead of disease; DOC = Dead, other cause.

giomas, which comprise 61% of the intradural petroclival tumours[20] were only 6% of the extradural lesions in this region.

Operative Approaches to the Petroclival Region

The plethora of useful operative approaches to the extradural petroclival region is listed in Table 2[24]. This multitude of approaches attests to the adage that difficult problems breed multiple solutions.

Approaches through the pharynx and/or facial sinuses[1,2,4,5,11,16,17,18] traverse potentially contaminated fields. Planned or inadvertent opening of the dura with these approaches can have a significant potential for CSF infection, especially in consideration of the frequent difficulties in closing the wounds. Blood vessels that are exposed may rupture catastrophically due to the infectious process.

Though giving a relatively direct view of the clivus, the anterior approaches are limited laterally by the optic nerves and internal carotid arteries. In case of injury to the ICA, control and repair are difficult via an anterior approach. Obviously, the anterior approaches cannot address lesions that are predominantly petrosal. In the Derome transbasal[7] and the basal subfrontal[19,24] approaches, an adequate cranial

base reconstruction can be attained by rotating down a galeal-pericranial flap[27]. The advantage of the basal subfrontal approach, in which a biorbital osteomy is performed, over the Derome approach, is that less frontal lobe retraction is required to attain the same cranial base exposure.

The lateral and anterolateral approaches to the petroclival region in general provide a wider exposure in more shallow operative field of the petroclival region than the anterior approaches[6,19,21,22,29]. The ipsilateral internal carotid artery can usually be controlled proximal and distal to the tumour, and, if necessary, repaired or graft-replaced[23].

Petroclival neoplasms crossing the midline will often require a combination of approaches that may be performed in one or more steps to completely resect the lesion. Combining the basal frontal with a lateral approach, either the transylvian transcavernous or the preauricular subtemporal-infratemporal, will provide the needed exposure to resect large anterolateral tumours. The operative field will include the sphenoethmoid sinuses, all of the midline clivus with the middle and lower clivus across midline to the opposite petrous apex, the ipsilateral petrous apex, the ipsilateral petrous ICA, the ipsilateral cavernous sinus, and the medial contralateral cavernous sinus.

In addition to combining a basal frontal and a lateral approach, a combination of two ipsilateral approaches can be useful. The subtemporal preauricular infratemporal approach combined with the frontotemporal transcavernous approach gives access to virtually all of unilateral petroclival lesions without destroying the vestibulocochlear mechanism and good immediate facial nerve function. The extreme lateral transcervical approach[25,28] is often combined with the subtemporal-infratemporal approach for lesions which involve the lower clivus, foramen magnum, occipital condyle, the jugular foramen and the C_1 area. The occasional bilateral resection about the occipital condyles, for a tumour such as a foramen magnum chordoma, will require fusion of the occiput to the upper cervical vertebra[25]. Approaches through the petrous bone (transcochlear[10] translabryinthine[13], total petrosectomy[24]) are destructive to the inherent structures. The exposure of the intrapetrous course of the facial nerve, and its mobilization or reconstruction is an integral part of the transpetrosal approach[9]. The presigmoid and posterior subtemporal petrosal approach (Al-Mefty, Samii) provides a narrow entry between the sigmoid sinus and petrous bone, and is more useful for intradural neoplasms.

Table 2. *Extradural approaches to the petroclival region*

Anterior
Transbasal (derome)
Basal subfrontal (modified transbasal)
Transethmoidal
Transsphenoidal
Transoral
Bilateral maxillotomy (Le Fort I osteotomy)
Unilateral maxillotomy approach (Cocke–Robertson) (Janecka)

Lateral
Subtemporal-preauricular infratemporal (Sekhar)
Postauricular transtemporal (infratemporal/Fisch)
Transcochlear (House)
Total petrosectomy
Extended middle fossa (House)
Transcervical (Stevenson)
Extreme lateral (Sen–Sekhar)

Combined Anterior and Lateral
Basal subfrontal
or
Transethmoidal   + subtemporal-infratemporal

or
Transsphenoidal

Combined Lateral
Frontotemporal-infratemporal   +   subtemporal-transcavernous
  subtemporal-infratemporal   +   extreme lateral

Preoperative Evaluation and Treatment

After a medical history, otological, neurological, and general physical examination, all patients undergo thin cut axial and coronal computerized tomography (CT) with soft tissue and bone algorithms and magnetic resonance imaging (MRI) in the T_1 and T_2 sequences and with intravenous gadolinium. Cervical and four-vessel cerebral angiograms are performed. If the ICA is encased by tumour or may be significantly manipulated during the operation, a balloon test occlusion (BTO) of the ICA is performed with a follow-up stable xenon CT cerebral blood flow evalution[8]. Any hearing deficits are further tested as well as preoperative somatosensory evoked potentials (SSEP) and contralateral brain stem evoked responses (BSER).

Anesthesia, Monitoring and Positioning

General endotracheal anesthesia is performed with an inhalation agent to allow intraoperative neurophysiological monitoring. SSEPs and BSERs are routinely monitored. The contralateral BSER is a sensitive indicator of excessive ipsilateral temporal lobe retraction, presumably due to brain stem compression. If an attempt is made to dissect the facial nerve from tumour or within the petrous bone, intraoperative facial monitoring is utilized. CN III, VI, X, XI, and XII may also be monitored if necessary with percutaneous electrodes in the respective muscles. An intraoperative electroencephalogram is monitored to follow burst suppression if barbiturate of etomidate coma is include to protect the brain. A constant intravenous infusion of thiopental at 2mg/kg/hour appears to relax the brain and minimizes the need for inhalation anesthetic agents, which may cause brain swelling in excessive doses.

A lumbar subarachnoid drain is usually inserted if CSF drainage will be required for brain relaxation.

Operative Approaches

Frontotemporal Transcavernous Approach

When the cavernous sinus is involved extensively by the tumour, the opening of the cavernous sinus and tumour removal allows the complete resection of the tumour when combined with other extradural approaches described here. In addition, the surgeon can also work through the cavernous sinus to remove tumours of the petrous apex-clivus junction.

Subtemporal, Transzygomatic, Transpetrous Apex Approach

For tumours of the upper and midclivus bulging posteriorly and compressing the brainstem and basilar artery, this intradural approach is used. A temporal craniotomy is combined with a zygomatic osteotomy including the condylar fossa. The tumour is approached subtemporally and removed after opening the clival dura. The exposure can be extended lower down the clivus by removing the petrous apex, medial to the horizontal segment of the petrous ICA. This approach does not allow radical removal of the tumour in the

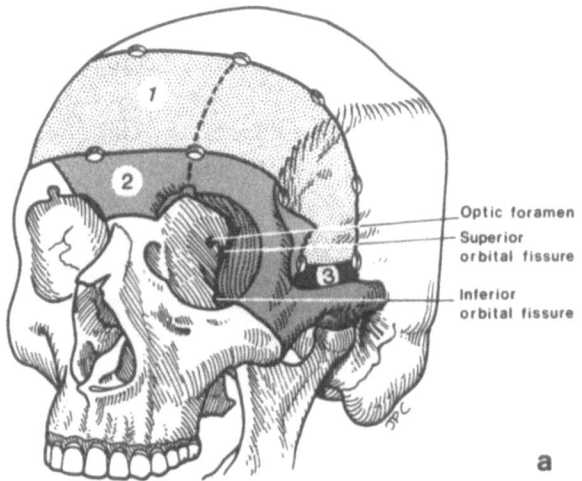

Fig. 2a. Extent of craniotomy, orbitozygomatic osteotomy and temporal craniotomy. Dotted lines indicate where the craniotomy can be stopped if only a unilateral subfrontal approach is chosen. (With permission, Ref. 24)

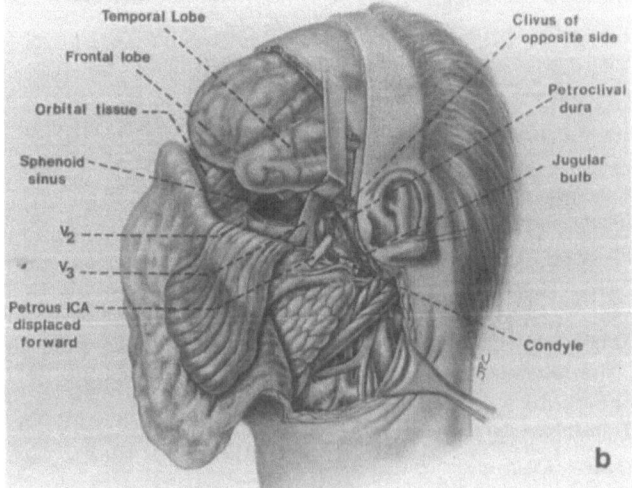

Fig. 2b. Exposure achieved from a subtemporal-infratemporal approach. (With permission, Ref. 24)

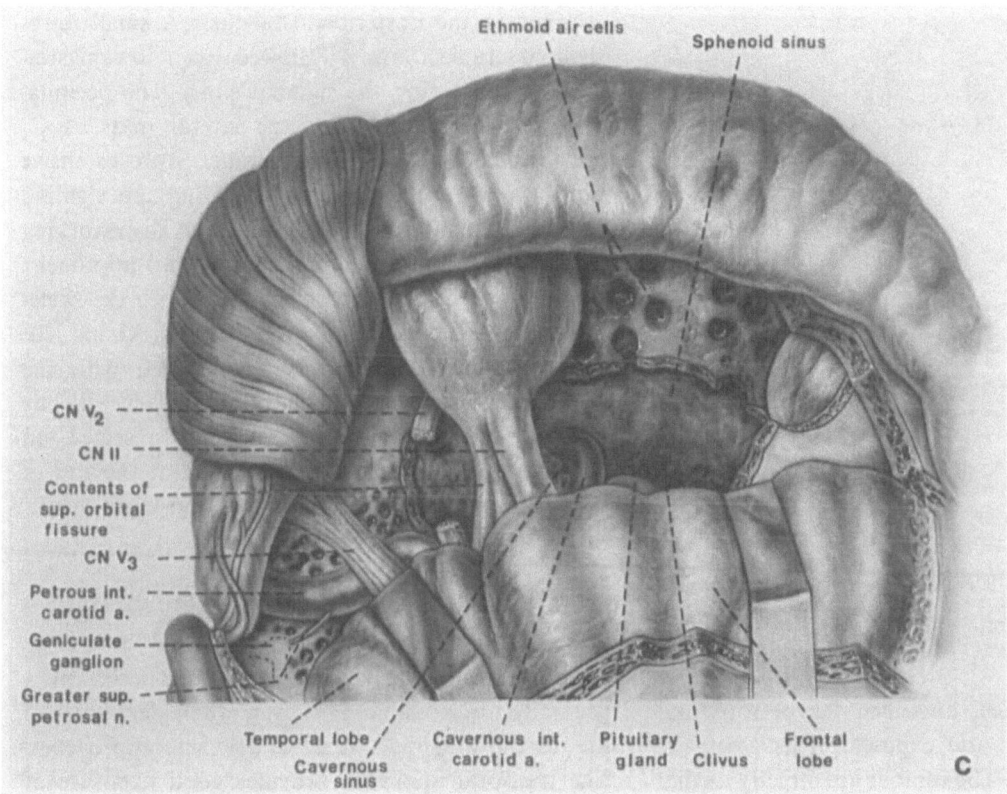

Ethmoid air cells Sphenoid sinus

CN V₂

CN II

Contents of sup. orbital fissure

CN V₃

Petrous int. carotid a.

Geniculate ganglion

Greater sup. petrosal n.

Temporal lobe / Cavernous int. Pituitary Frontal
Cavernous carotid a. gland Clivus lobe
sinus

c

Fig. 2 c. Exposure achieved from a subfrontal approach. (With permission, Ref. 24)

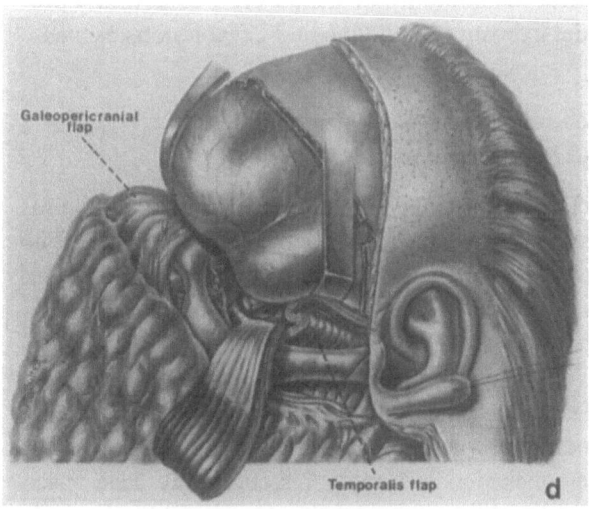

Galeopericranial flap

Temporalis flap d

Fig. 2 d. The galeofrontalis flap. A portion of the temporalis muscle is also being used to cover the petrous internal carotid artery. (With permission, Ref. 24)

clivus, but allows the careful dissection of tumour from the critical structures from a lateral perspective.

Basal (Extended) Frontal Approach

This is a modification of Derome's transbasal approach. A bifrontal craniotomy is combined with a bilateral orbito-fronto-ethmoidal osteotomy. The optic nerves are bilaterally unroofed and the sphenoid sinus is opened widely. Tumour removal is performed from the clivus from the base of the dorsum sellae down to the foramen magnum. Both cavernous sinuses are decompressed medially by removal of the body of the sphenoid bone. Some of the petrous apices can be also removed, but lateral exposure is limited by the optic nerves, cavernous sinuses, petrous internal carotid arteries, and the hypoglossal nerves. If the tumour involves the dura, it can be resected with it, and a small patch graft applied. Further reconstruction of the tumour cavity is performed with an anteriorly based pericranial or galeofrontalis flap, with autologous fat tucked inside the flap to fill the dead space.

Subtemporal-Infratemporal Approach

In this approach, a bicoronal incision is extended inferiorly in front of the pinna of the ear. The upper branches of the facial nerves are lifted up in the flap along with the parotid tissues and the deep fascia. A temporal craniotomy is combined with a zygomatic osteotomy, including the condylar fossa. The mandibular condyle is resected. An extradural middle fossa

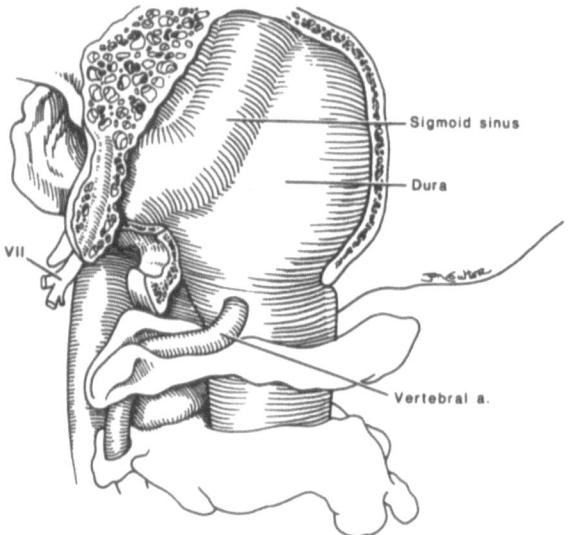

Fig. 3. Scheme of extreme lateral approach at the craniocervical junction

dissection is performed, and then the petrous and upper cervical ICA are exposed. The artery is completely mobilized. The tumour lies directly medial to the ICA and V_3 and is removed. Occasionally, V_3 is divided to further extend the exposure across the midline. V_3 is reattached with epineural sutures at the conclusion of tumour resection. The cartilaginous Eustachian tube is closed with sutures and autologous fat, and the posterior end of the Eustachian tube is closed with autologous fat. After tumour resection, a portion of the temporalis muscle or the entire muscle may be used as a flap to close the dead space created by tumour removal. This approach allows the removal of tumours occupying the petrous apex and the lateral aspect of the clivus. The division of V_3 or the combination with basal frontal approach allows the removal of tumour from almost the entire extradural clival area except the occipital condyle and the jugular foramen area.

Extreme Lateral, Transcondylar Approach

This approach is well suited for lower clival foramen magnum and C_1 lesions which involve the occipital condyles. With the patient in the lateral position, an L-shaped incision is made in the retroauricular area and the semispinalis, splenius capitis, sternomastoid, and oblique muscles are reflected down from the occipital and mastoid bones, and the C_1 transverse process. The vertebral artery is freed up extradurally in the C_1 area, and if necessary from C_2 transverse

foramen to the posterior fossa dura. A small retrosigmoid craniectomy is followed by a low mastoidectomy unroofing the sigmoid sinus. The occipital condyle and, if necessary, the lateral mass of C_1 are resected to expose the tumour. More extensive exposure can be obtained by ligating the sigmoid sinus and the internal jugular vein, and then working through the jugular bulb (transjugular approach). Tumour can be resected extradurally with the skeletonization and preservation of CNs IX, X, XI and XII. This approach can be nicely combined with the subtemporal and infratemporal approach. If one occipital condyle has been completely resected, an occiput to C_1–C_2 fusion is performed at the end of the operation using titanium plates and bone chips.

Transmaxillary and Trans-Oral Approaches

These approaches are sparingly used by us for tumour resections since radical tumour resection is generally not possible. However, when debulking of the tumour alone is a goal, we use these approaches. The transoral approach provides good exposure of midline lesions in the lower clival and C_1–C_3 area, whereas the transmaxillary approach (using a unilateral maxillotomy or a Le-Fort I osteotomy) provides exposure of midline mid-clival lesions as well.

General Principles of Tumour Resection and Reconstruction

The majority of extradural clival and petroclival tumours are removed in a piecemeal fashion. The ease of removal depends upon tumour consistency and vascularity. Any involved arteries must be dissected from a normal to an abnormal area. If the dura is involved by tumour, it is resected and repaired with a fascia lata patch. The bone around the tumour must be drilled away circumferentially for at least 1 cm. At the conclusion of tumour resection, any dead space must be obliterated, and the dura and blood vessels protected, preferably by using tissues with vascularity. If any cranial nerves or arteries are injured, immediate reconstruction is performed by resuture or with interposition graft.

Postoperative Management

A subcutaneous closed drainage system is maintained to gravity for the two days. Wide spectrum antibiotics, which are started at the initiation of surgery, are continued for two days postoperatively. Elastic stockings, sequential compression stockings, and low-dose subcutaneous heparin are utilized post-operatively as prophylaxis against deep vein thrombophlebitis until the patient is ambulating. A CT scan is performed on the day following surgery and periodically thereafter. If the ICA was dissected during surgery a postoperative angiogram of that vessel is performed to visualize any vessel damage. The mainstay of long-term postoperative imaging is the comparison of serial nonenhanced and enhanced MRIs since the wide resections, flaps, fat, and postoperative changes often make single readings difficult to interpret

Adjuvant Therapy

Radiation therapy has been utilized for cranial base chordomas and chondrosarcomas[3,26]. The definitive role of this therapy is yet to be defined[3,26]. Obviously for high-grade malignancies adjuvant therapy is an important part of their multi-modality treatment.

Complications

The complications incurred with the 68 patients operated for extradural petroclival tumours are listed in Table 3. One patient died of wound infection causing bilateral ICA rupture. This patient had an

Table 3. *Extradural Petroclival Neoplasms, 1983–1990 Operative Complications*

Death (infection, bilateral ICA rupture)	1
Cerebral infarct	
Delayed ICA occlusion, moderate recovery	1
Basilar perforator occlusion, no recovery	1
Basilar perforator injury, thalamic hemorrhage, recovering	1
Temporal hemiparesis, internuclear ophthalmoplegia (recovered)	1
Pneumocephalus 2° to postoperative spinal fluid drainage	2
Subdural hematoma, chronic (related to above)	2
Cerebrospinal fluid leakage (all reoperated)	
Eustachian tube	2
wound	2
Ethmoid sinus	1
Sphenoid sinus	5
Hydrocephalus, needing shunt	3
Infection	
Wound (excluding above case)	1
Meningitis (CSF leak associated)	2
Pharyngo-tympanic fistula (reoperation)	1

Cranial nerve palsies	Temporary	Permanent
CN III	5	–
CN IV	5	–
CN V	2	–
CN VI	10	–
CN VII	12	–
CN IX, X	6	4
CN XII	3	1

Outcome of operative complications	
Died	1
Mild disability, died of disease	1
Severe disability, living	2

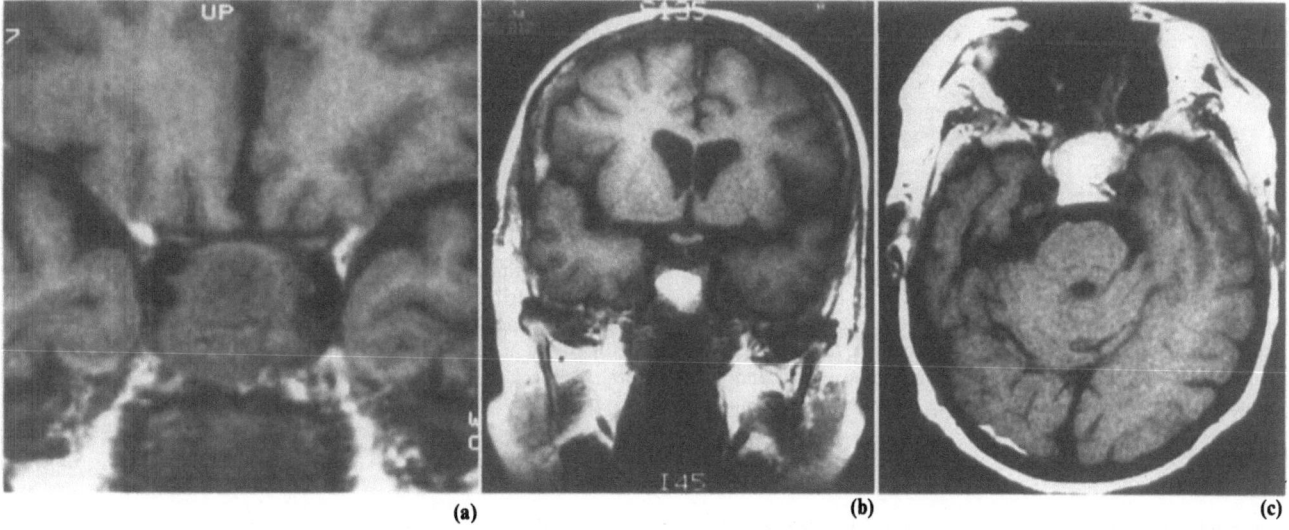

(a)   (b)   (c)

Fig. 4. H. P. 72-year-old woman with a sellar turcica and sphenoclival chordoma. She underwent tumour resection via a subfrontal transbasal approach. a) Preoperative coronal T_1 weighted nonenhanced MRI demonstrating the tumour in the upper clivus-sphenoid sinus region, extradural up to the cisterns of the optic nerves. The optic nerves themselves can be seen superolateral to the tumour. b) Postoperative coronal T_1 weighted nonenhanced MRI demonstrating fat that was placed following complete tumour resection. c) Postoperative axial T_1 weighted nonenhanced MRI

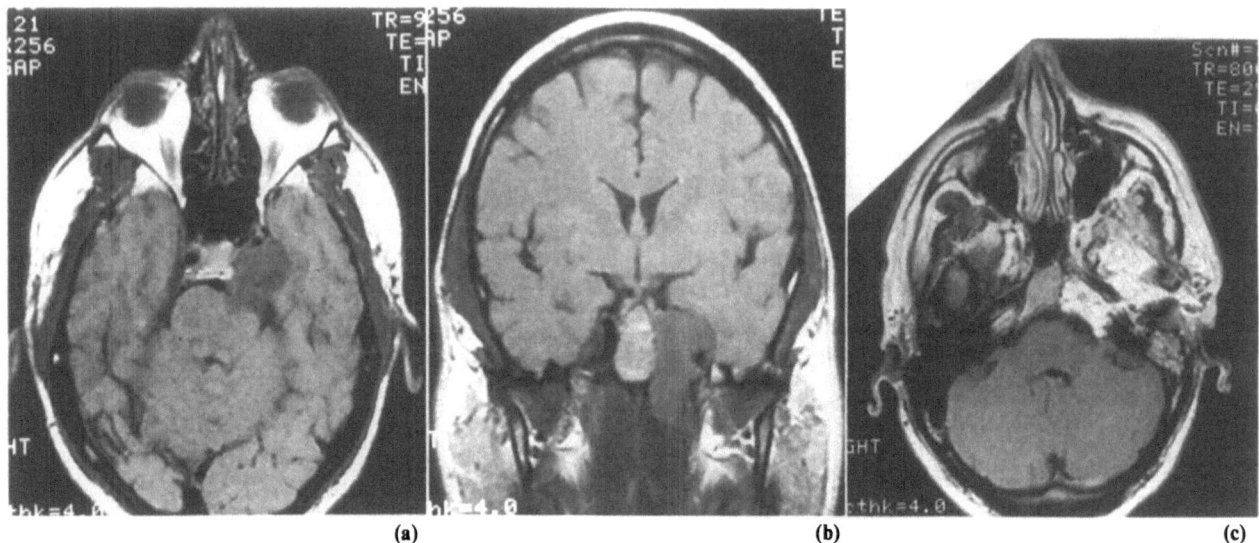

(a)   (b)   (c)

Fig 5. D. Z., 35 year-old man with diplopia, secondary to left abducens paresis. a) Preoperative axial nonenhanced T_1 weighted MRIs demonstrating the left petroclival chordoma extending into the cavernous sinus. b) Preoperative coronal MRI demonstrating tumour extent. The tumour was resected via a left frontotemporal craniotomy; subtemporal, preauricular-infratemporal approach. c) Postoperative nonenhanced T_1 weighted MRI demonstrating no residual tumour with fat in the tumour bed and subtemporal

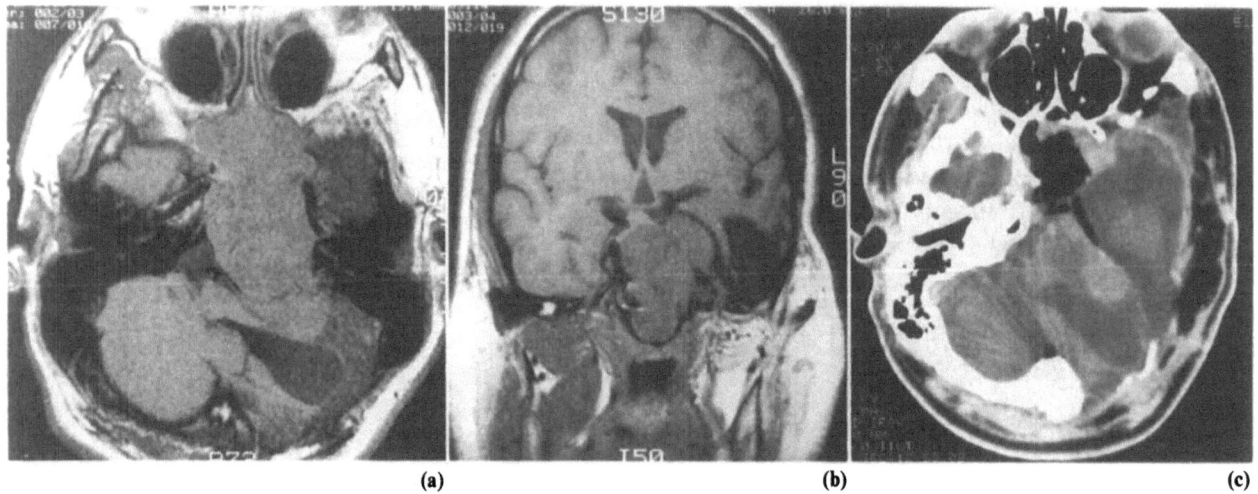

(a)   (b)   (c)

Fig. 6. K. P., 32-year-old man who 14 and 8 years previously underwent a left suboccipital craniectomy and left temporal craniotomy for a subtotal neurilemmoma resection. a), b) Axial and coronal nonenhanced T_1 weighted MRI demonstrating a large recurrent petroclival tumour with brainstem compression and displacement. Through a bifrontal craniotomy with subfrontal approach, left infra-temporal and subtemporal approach, and left neck exploration, the tumour was excised with a dural pericranial graft. Tumour resection was completed by a follow-up left retromastoid craniectomy, subtemporal and transtemporal approach with subtotal petrous bone resection. c) Contrast enhanced axial CT scan demonstrating the degree of bone and tumour resection

extensive squamous cell carcinoma with bilateral ICA encasement. In retrospect, this patient was not suitable for operation. Three patients had cerebral infarcts with substantial resultant neurosurgical deficits. Six patients had CSF leaks, 1 through the wound, 2 through the Eustachian tube, and three via the facial air sinuses. one patient had a pneumocephalus and one had a subdural hematoma that was evacuated. Four patients had wound infections. A total of twenty-eight cranial nerves were temporarily paretic

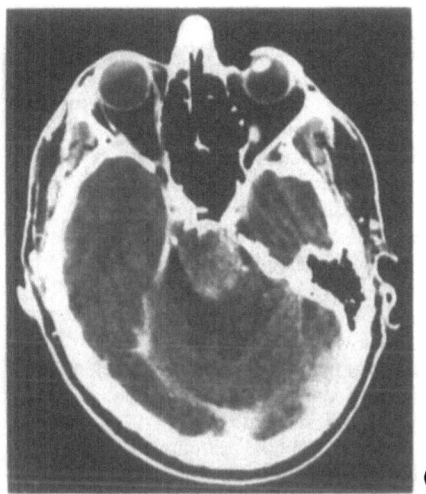

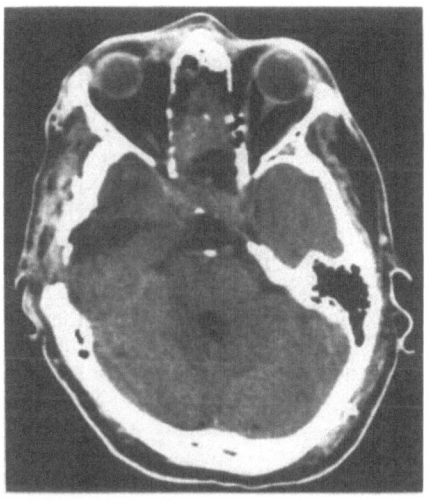

Fig. 7. R.V., 41-year-old with right abducens paresis. a) Axial contrast enhanced T_1 weighted MRI demonstrating a midline clivus chordoma compressing the brainstem and involving the posterior cavernous sinus bilaterally. b) Nonenhanced sagittal MRI demonstrating the tumour. Through a one-stage subfrontal transbasal and preauricular subtemporal–infratemporal approach complete tumour resection was attained. c) Postoperative nonenhanced axial CT demonstrating tumour resection and pericranial flap

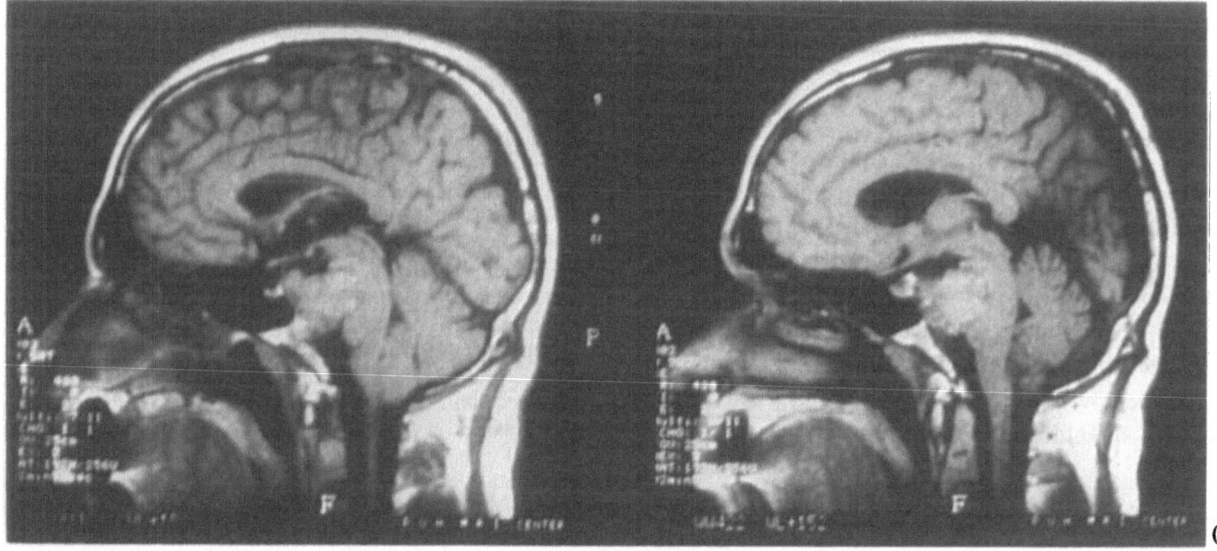

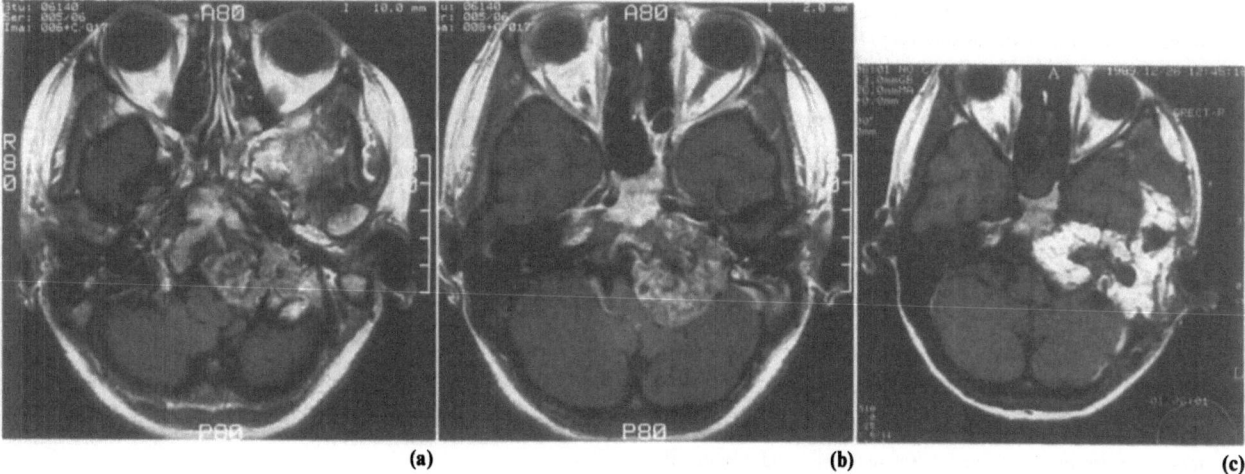

Fig. 8. A. G., 17-year-old woman who two years previously underwent a transoral partial chordoma resection due to left abducens paresis, dysphagia and swallowing difficulties. a), b) Contrast enhanced T_1 weighted MRI demonstrating middle and posterior fossa tumour extent. The patient underwent a three stage tumour resection via a temporal craniotomy, mastoidectomy, and retromastoid craniectomy, with a subtemporal infratemporal, presigmoid trans-temporal, and extreme lateral-transcondylar approaches. c) Postoperative axial nonenhanced T_1 weighted MRI demonstrating fat implanted following tumour resection

(several patients having multiple cranial nerves involved). Four patients had permanent cranial nerve deficits, three being CN IX and/or X.

Outcome

Table 1 lists the number of recurrences in accordance with histological groupings. Of the 37 benign and low-grade malignancy patients with total resection there were two recurrences in our follow-up of 6 months to 7 years; whereas, of the 23 with partial resection there were 10 recurrences. Of the eight malignant tumours six recurred.

Figures 4–8 demonstrate the pre- and postoperative imaging of four representing patients with extradural petroclival tumours that underwent surgery at the University of Pittsburgh between 1983–1990.

Conclusion

Extradural petroclival tumours include a spectrum of histological types and anatomical configurations with multiple surgical approaches available. Experience and knowledge of the surgical anatomy of this region is essential to attain optimal surgical results. The selection of the appropriate approach(es) can yield complete resections in a high percentage of these cases with an acceptably low morbidity rate.

References

1. Al-Mefty O, Fox JL, Smith RR (1988) Petrosal approach for petroclival meningiomas. Neurosurgery 22: 27
2. Archer DJ, Young S, Uttley D (1987) Basilar aneurysms: a new transclival approach via maxillotomy. J Neurosurg 67: 54
3. Austin-Seymour M, Munzenrider J, Goiten M, et al (1989) Fractionated proton radiation therapy or chordoma and low-grade chondrosarcoma of the base of the skull. J Neurosurg 70: 13–17
4. Cocke EW, Robertson JH, Robertson JT, et al (1990) The extended maxillotomy and subtotal maxillectomy for excision of skull base tumors. Arch Otolaryngol Head Neck Surg 116: 92–104
5. Crockard HA, Bradford R (1985) Transoral transclival removal of a schwannoma anterior to the craniocervical junction. J Neurosurg 62: 293
6. Goldenberg RA (1984) Surgeon's view of the skull base from the lateral approach. Laryngoscope 94: 1–21
7. Derome PJ, Visot A, Monteil JP, Maestro JL (1987) Management of cranial chordomas. In: Sekhar LN, Schramm VL Jr (eds) Tumors of the cranial base: diagnosis and treatment. Futura, New York, pp 607–622
8. Erba SM, Horton JA, Latchaw RE, et al (1988) Balloon test occlusion of the internal carotid artery with xenon CT cerebral blood flow imaging. AJNR 9: 533
9. Fisch U, Kumar A (1985) Infratemporal surgery of the skull base. In: Rand RW (ed) Microsurgery, 3rd ed. CV Mosby, St. Louis
10. House WF, Hitselberger WE (1976) The trans-cochlear approach to the skull base. Arch Otolaryngol 102: 334
11. Janecka IP, Sen CN, Sekhar LN, Arriaga (in press) Facial translocation. A new approach to the cranial base. Otolaryngol Head Neck Surg
12. Jones NF, Schramm VL, Sekhar LN (1987) Reconstruction of the cranial base following tumour resection. Br J Plast Surg 40: 155
13. King TT, Morrison AW (1990) Primary facial nerve tumors within the skull. J Neurosurg 72: 1–8
14. Lang J (1987) Middle cranial base anatomy. In: Sekhar LN, Schramm VL, Jr (eds) Tumors of the cranial base: diagnosis and treatment. Futura, New York, p 313
15. Lang J (1987) Posterior cranial base anatomy. In: Sekhar LN, Schramm VJ, Jr (eds) Tumors of the cranial base: diagnosis and treatment. Futura, New York, pp 441–460
16. Miller E, Crockard HA (1987) Transoral transclival removal of anteriorly placed meningiomas at the foramen magnum. Neurosurgery 20: 966
17. Mullan S, Naunton R, Hekmat-panah J, Vailati G (1966) The use of an anterior approach to ventrally placed tumors in the foramen magnum and vertebral column. J Neurosurg 24: 536
18. Sano K, Kinko M, Saito I (1966) Vertebro-basilar aneurysms, with special reference to the transpharyngeal approach to the basilar artery aneurysm. Brain Nerve (Tokyo) 18: 1197
19. Sekhar LN, Janecka IP, Jones NF (1988) Subtemporal-infratemporal and basal subfrontal approach to extensive cranial base tumors. Acta Neurochir (Wien) 92: 83
20. Sekhar LN, Jannetta PJ, Burkhart LE, et al (in press) Meningiomas involving the clivus: a 6-year experience with 38 patients. J Neurosurg
21. Sekhar LN, Schramm VL Jr, Jones NF (1987) Operative management of large neoplasms of the lateral and posterior cranial base. In: Sekhar LN, Schramm VL Jr (eds) Tumors of the cranial base: diagnosis and treatment. Futura, New York, pp 655–682
22. Sekhar LN, Schramm VL Jr, Jones NF (1987) Subtemporal-preauricular infratemporal fossa approach to large lateral and posterior cranial base neoplasms. J Neurosurg 67: 488
23. Sekhar LN, Schramm VL Jr, Jones NF, et al (1986): Operative exposure and management of the petrous and upper cervical internal carotid artery. Neurosurgery 19: 967
24. Sekhar LN, Sen CN (1989) Anterior and lateral basal approaches to the clivus. Contem Neurosurg 11: 1–8
25. Sen CN, Sekhar LN (in press) An extreme lateral approach to intradural lesions of the cervical spine and foramen magnum. Neurosurgery
26. Sen CN, Sekhar LN, Schramm VL Jr, et al (1989) Chordoma and chondrosarcoma of the cranial base: an 8-years experience. Neurosurgery 25: 931–941
27. Snyderman CH, Janecka IP, Sekhar LN, et al (1990) Anterior cranial base reconstruction: role of galeal and pericranial flaps. Laryngoscope 100: 49
28. Yasui T, Hakuba A, Kim SH, et al (1989) Trigeminal neurinomas: operative approach in eight cases. J Neurosurg 71: 506–511

Correspondence: Prof. L. N. Sekhar, M. D., F.A.C.S., Department of Neurosurgery, Presbyterian-University Hospital, DeSoto at O'Hara Streets, Pittsburgh, PA 15213, U.S.A.

Acta Neurochirurgica, Suppl. 53, 193–198 (1991)
© by Springer-Verlag 1991

Facial Translocation Approach to the Cranial Base

I. P. Janecka[1], D. W. Nuss[1], and Ch. N. Sen[2]

[1]Center for Cranial Base Surgery, Department of Otolaryngology, University of Pittsburgh, and [2]Department of Neurosurgery, Presbyterian University Hospital, Pittsburg, PA 15213, U.S.A.

Summary

Facial translocation is a new approach which has been developed for surgical management of extensive lesions of the anterolateral cranial base, including the nasopharynx, sphenoid sinus, clivus, infratemporal fossa, superior orbital fissure, and cavernous sinus. Temporary displacement of the craniofacial skeleton allows direct, wide access to this complex anatomic area, while giving the surgeon a high degree of control over critical neural and vascular structures.

Keywords: Facial translocation; anterolateral cranial base; nasopharynx; sphenoid sinus; clivus; infratemporal fossa; superior orbital fissure; cavernous sinus.

Introduction

Surgery of the cranial base is technically difficult because of the complex relationships of intracranial and extracranial anatomy. In the surgical treatment of cranial base lesions, successful outcome depends upon the adequacy of operative exposure and upon the surgeon's ability to protect critical neural and vascular structures.

Facial translocation is a new approach to the cranial base which provides wide surgical access and enhanced safety in the operative management of skull base disorders. Through systematic disassembly of facial soft tissues and the craniofacial skeleton, a broad surgical field can be achieved with unhindered access extending from the ipsilateral geniculate ganglion to the contralateral eustachian tube, and from the superior orbital fissure to the level of the hard palate. With this exposure, the surgeon has greater access to the basicranium and improved control of vital neurovascular structures.

This versatile method has been used in the management of benign and malignant tumours as well as complex cerebrospinal fluid fistulae. It has been particularly useful for approaching lesions in the difficult regions of the nasopharynx, clivus, sphenoid sinus, infratemporal fossa, and cavernous sinus.

Method

Facial incisions (Fig. 1 a and b) are designed to provide an "open book" exposure of the underlying skeletal framework. A modified Weber-Ferguson incision (lateral rhinotomy with optional lip-split) is made, and then extended horizontally across the medial canthus and into the inferior fornix of the conjunctiva. It then continues through the lateral canthus and horizontally across the temporal region at the level of the zygomatic arch. These incisions are carried down to the maxilla, inferior orbital rim, and zygomatic arch, respectively, so that the entire cheek including skin, subcutaneous tissue, and muscle are elevated from the bone in the subperiosteal plane. The resulting cheek flap is based on the facial and inferior labial vessels, and is, therefore, well-vascularized.

The horizontal incision then joins a hemicoronal incision, which is carried down to the level of the deep temporal fascia, exposing the temporalis muscle. The resulting superior skin flap is then elevated forward to reveal the frontotemporal skull and the superior and lateral orbital rims, again in the subperiosteal plane. This flap is vascularized by the supraorbital vessels, which remain intact. The orbito-zygomatico-maxillary skeleton is now completely accessible for craniofacial osteotomies, which will allow temporary translocation of the anterior face of the maxilla, malar eminence, zygomatic arch, orbital floor and lateral wall, and superior and lateral orbital rims, all in one segment (Fig. 2).

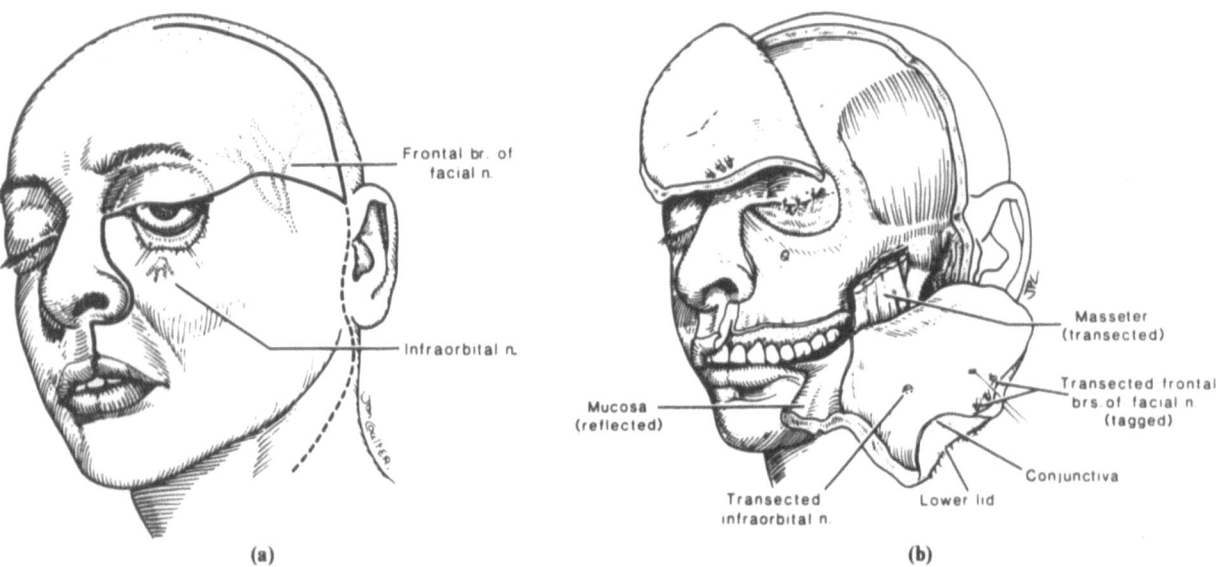

Fig. 1. Facial translocation: initial exposure. a) Incisions. The lip-splitting portion of the incision is optional. b) Soft tissue flaps developed, craniofacial skeleton exposed

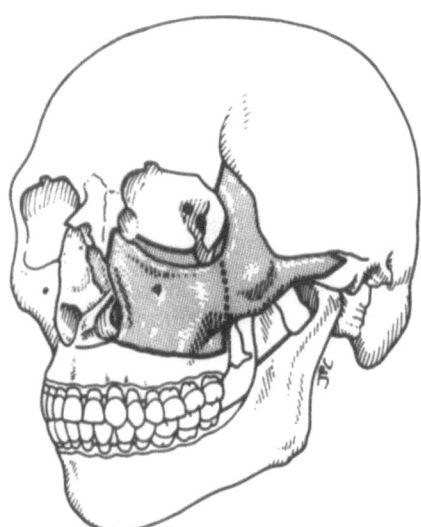

Fig. 2. Osteotomies for translocation of orbitozygomaticomaxillary skeleton

Next, the temporalis muscle is detached from its origin along the temporal fossa and reflected inferiorly, based on its primary vascular supply, the deep temporal vessels from the infratemporal fossa. The coronoid process of the mandible may be outfractured to enhance this rotation. At this point, the surgical field of view includes the nasopharynx, posterior wall of the maxilla, pterygoid plates and muscles, infratemporal fossa, and the subtemporal surface of the greater sphenoid wing (Fig. 3).

A frontotemporal craniotomy is now performed,

and the foramina ovale, spinosum, and rotundum are identified, as well as the superior orbital fissure. By dissecting medially between the maxillary (V2) and mandibular (V3) branches of the trigeminal nerve, the sphenoid sinus can be entered; the clivus and nasopharynx can be exposed just inferior to the sinus (Fig. 4). If necessary, the internal carotid artery (ICA) may now be identified at its entrance to the carotid canal and decompressed throughout its petrous course, up to the cavernous sinus. Along the floor of the middle fossa, the greater superficial petrosal nerve can be traced posterolaterally to locate the geniculate ganglion, a useful guide to the position of the intratemporal facial nerve.

Because of the depth and breadth of this exposure, the surgeon has three-dimensional visualization of the anterolateral skull base from intracranial and extracranial perspectives. Thus, the surgical objective – resection of tumour or repair of CSF fistula – can be accomplished more readily and more safely.

Once that objective has been accomplished, the reconstructive phase of the operation is begun. Re-establishment of the critical barriers separating the brain and the carotid artery from the oro-nasopharynx is most important. If dura has been violated then it must be repaired, either primarily or using grafts of pericranium or fascia. If possible, the dural repair should be insulated from oro-nasal contamination by interposing vascularized tissue such as a galeopericranial flap or the temporalis muscle.

The temporalis muscle, which has an excellent arc

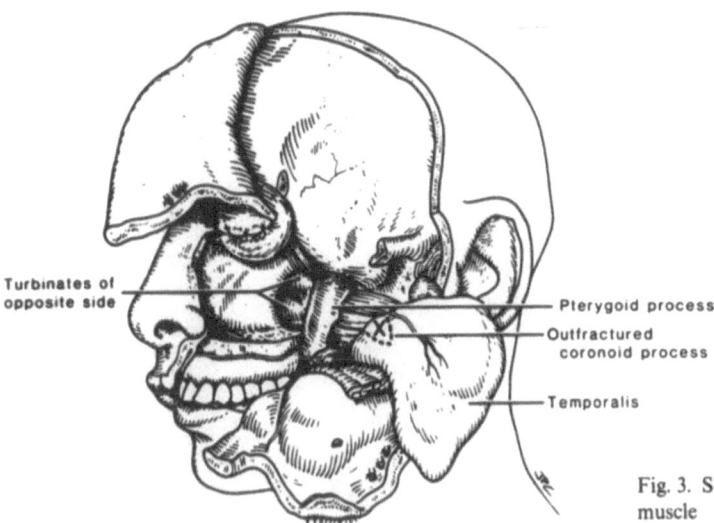

Fig. 3. Surgical field after osteotomies and reflection of temporalis muscle

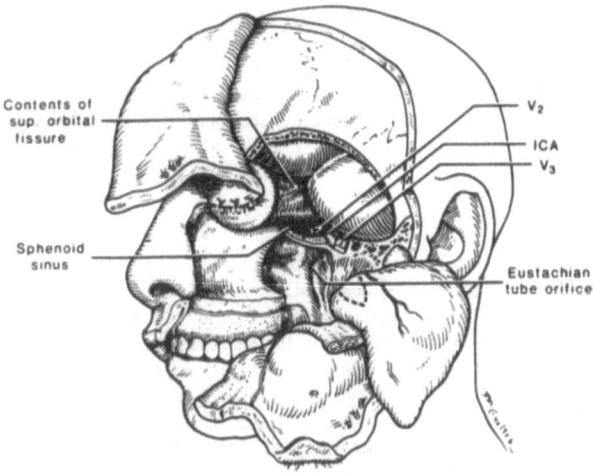

Fig. 4. Final operative exposure after frontotemporal craniotomy and skull base dissection

of rotation about its vascular pedicle, is also used to obliterate any openings into the sphenoid sinus or nasopharynx, and to fill in the space of the previous maxillary sinus.

The orbito-zygomatico-maxillary skeleton which was previously translocated is now replaced in its anatomic position, and secured using either 2–0 braided nylon sutures (placed through multiple drill-holes) or titanium miniplates.

The facial soft tissues are reapproximated beginning with the medial canthal tendon, which is secured to the lacrimal bone for stability. The upper and lower lacrimal canaliculi are stented with silicone tubings which are passed into the nasal cavity and left in place for approximately four weeks postoperatively. The

lateral canthal tendon is likewise attached to the lateral orbital rim.

The orbicularis oculi muscle and inferior fornix conjunctiva are repaired, and a temporary suture tarsorrhaphy (two horizontal mattress sutures over 5 mm lengths of silicone band) is placed to align and support the eyelids for approximately 7 to 10 days. If the infraorbital nerve has not been resected for oncologic or other reasons, it may be repaired either primarily or with a nerve graft.

The frontal branches of the facial nerve, which are always multiple at the level of the zygoma, are primarily repaired. This repair is greatly facilitated if, at the beginning of the approach phase, they are located using electromyography and tagged so they can be easily located during the reconstructive phase.

The facial skin and subcutaneous tissues are then carefully reapproximated. A stent is placed in the ipsilateral nasal cavity, where it remains for 7 to 10 days.

Clinical Cases

Patient 1: Spontaneous CSF Fistula

A 65-year-old male presented with a complaint of copious clear nasal discharge. He had previously been in good health and denied any history of trauma or prior surgery. On physical examination, the rhinorrhea was reproducible whenever the patient leaned forward. There were no other abnormalities evident.

A computed tomographic (CT) scan revealed an air-fluid level in the sphenoid sinus, and a focal defect in the lateral wall of the sinus in continuity with the middle cranial fossa (Fig. 5). A metrizamide CT-cisternogram confirmed this defect as the site of the CSF fistula.

The facial translocation approach was used to expose the anterolateral skull base, where a 1 cm defect was observed along the greater sphenoid wing (Fig. 6). This defect communicated with

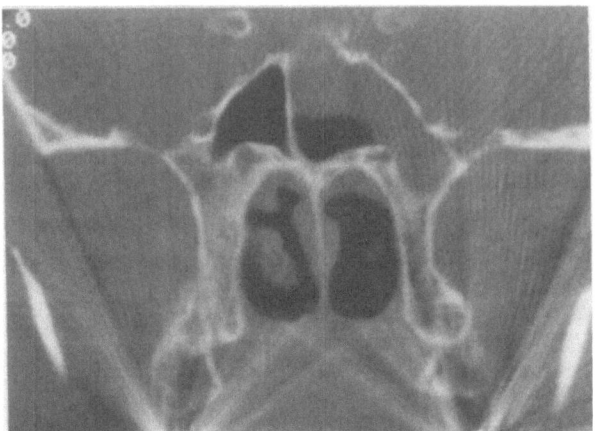

Fig. 5. Coronal CT scan of patient 1 showing fluid in left sphenoid sinus. Note focal defect in lateral wall of sinus in contact with middle cranial fossa

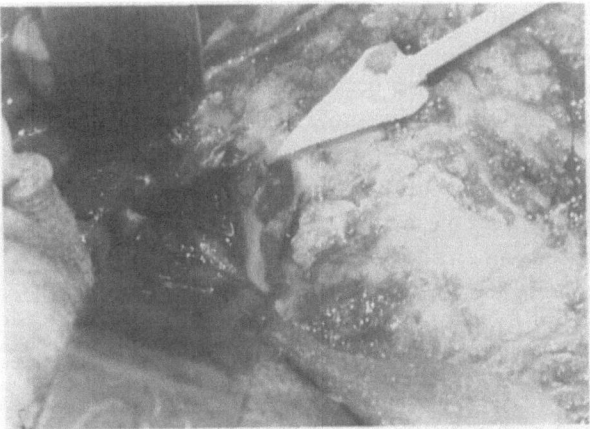

Fig. 6. Operative photograph of patient 1 showing focal defect in greater wing of sphenoid. This defect was contiguous with the middle cranial fossa and the sphenoid sinus as shown by CT. (Upper retractor displaces orbital contents anteriorly; lower retractor displaces pterygoid muscles posteriorly. Orientation similar to that in Fig. 3)

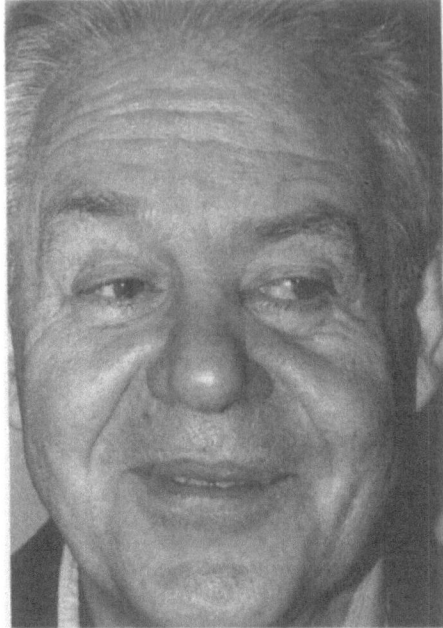

Fig. 7. Patient 1, nine months after left facial translocation operation. Note acceptable aesthetic result and return of frontalis function. (The lip-splitting portion of the incision was not used in this patient)

the middle cranial fossa as well as the sphenoid sinus. Biopsies of the area were unremarkable and failed to demonstrate neoplastic or inflammatory changes. The sinus was opened and stripped of its mucosa, and the dural defect was closed. The temporalis muscle was used to obliterate the sphenoid sinus and also to cover the exposed subtemporal dura.

The patient made an uneventful recovery and has been followed for 15 months without evidence of further CSF leakage. He has returned to his previous occupation. The frontal branches of the facial nerve have recovered, and his esthetic appearance is good (Fig. 7).

Patient 2: Juvenile Angiofibroma

A 17-year-old boy presented with progressive swelling of the cheek. Magnetic resonance (MR) scan (Fig. 8) showed extensive tumour in the nasopharynx, sphenoid sinus, infratemporal fossa, pterygopalatine fossa, superior orbital fissure, and cavernous sinus. Transnasal biopsy confirmed the diagnosis of angiofibroma.

Using the facial translocation approach, the orbito-zygomatico-maxillary skeleton was displaced, giving access to the lateral infratemporal fossa, where the internal maxillary artery was identified and ligated, decreasing the vascularity of the tumour. Working from above and below the skull base, the tumour was delivered from the cavernous sinus, and was then dissected free from its remaining attachments extracranially. The resection included the entire tumour, the face of the sphenoid sinus, the pterygoid plates, the nasopharyngeal wall, and the posterior maxilla. The temporalis muscle was used to reconstruct the nasopharyngeal wall and to obliterate the sphenoid and maxillary sinuses and the operative defect.

The postoperative recovery was uncomplicated and the patient was discharged from the hospital within one week. He was able to return to school and to resume his usual activities within one month. Sixteen months later, he remains asymptomatic and is free of recurrence both clinically and radiographically (Fig. 9).

Discussion

The anterolateral cranial base is an anatomically complex region. It may be difficult to approach surgically because of vital neural and vascular structures (e.g. carotid artery, optic nerve, facial nerve) encased within the craniofacial skeleton.

A number of operative approaches to portions of the anterolateral cranial base have been described[1-11], all of which have certain advantages but also disadvantages. One significant disadvantage common to many of these approaches is that of limited surgical exposure,

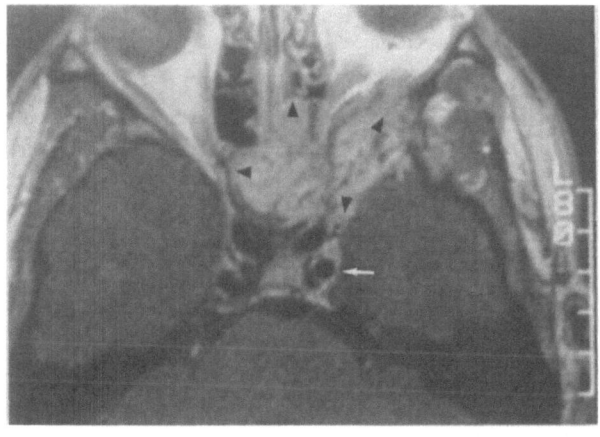

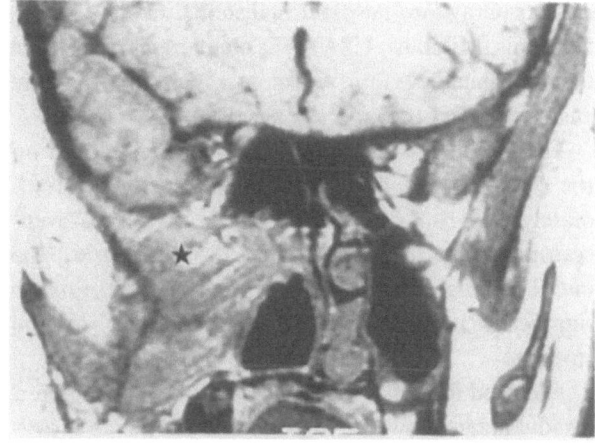

(a)

(a)

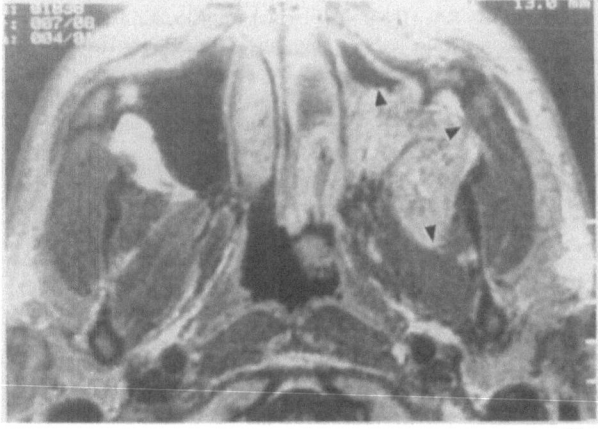

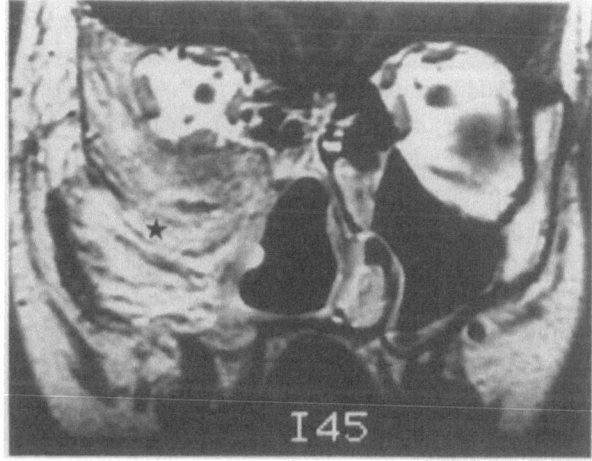

(b)

(b)

Fig. 8. Preoperative T1-weighted axial MR scan, patient 2.
a) Extensive angiofibroma (*arrowheads*) in sphenoid sinus, superior orbital fissure, and cavernous sinus, anterior to internal carotid artery (*arrow*). b) Tumour in infratemporal fossa

Fig. 9. Postoperative T1-weighted coronal MR scan of patient 2. a) At level of sphenoid sinus, showing no evidence of tumour and reconstruction of middle fossa floor with temporalis muscle flap (*). b) More anterior section demonstrating no evidence of tumour. Temporalis flap (*) fills previous maxillary sinus

which restricts the surgeon's visualization as well as his control over important structures.

Because it displaces the craniofacial skeleton, the facial translocation approach overcomes these disadvantages. It provides a direct approach to the skull base and results in a unified surgical field that is multidimensional and broadly accessible, with the benefits of intra- and extracranial exposures combined. Thus, lesions involving the sphenoid sinus, clivus, superior orbital fissure, cavernous sinus, infratemporal fossa, and nasopharynx may be dealt with directly and with maximal control over important neurovascular structures.

The facial translocation has now been used in over 25 patients[12] for management of cranial base lesions. It represents a safe alternative to other approaches and has been especially useful for dealing with

transcranial tumours in which there is significant extracranial extension. It has also been invaluable in the repair of complex CSF fistulae which failed other methods of repair.

Of course there are some disadvantages as well. The transection of the frontal branches of the facial nerve results in a temporary paralysis of the ipsilateral forehead. These nerves must be identified and repaired if function is to be restored. Return of function may then be expected within 6 to 9 months[13].

The nasolacrimal system must be stented as part of the reconstructive phase of the operation to prevent dacryostenosis and epiphora. This, however, is greatly simplified by the use of commercially available nasolacrimal stents with pre-attached wire passers (Crawford nasolacrimal stents, Jedmed Corp., St. Louis, Missouri, USA). The stents remain in place for approximately four weeks, at which time they are easily removed through the nasal cavity.

The eyelids must be temporarily sutured closed on the operated side and must remain so for approximately 7 to 10 days postoperatively, to help prevent ectropion and to support the lower lid during the initial healing. This is well tolerated and presents no significant problem for either the patient or the surgeon.

The need for facial incisions might be considered a disadvantage. However, cosmesis has not been a problem except in children in whom the incisions may remain red or hyperpigmented for several months. In adult patients, all of the incisions fall into esthetic skin tension lines, and are difficult to detect once they are healed. Additionally, the use of the inferior fornix incision rather than a subciliary skin incision has the effect of breaking the continuity of visible incisions, improving the esthetic result.

When considering these relatively minor disadvantages, it is helpful to do so with the perspective of the surgeon faced with a patient who has an extensive tumour or other lesion of the cranial base. Within this context, the great advantages of the facial translocation approach – wide exposure, improved visualization, and enhanced safety – are clearly more important.

References

1. Krespi YP, Sisson GA (1984) Transmandibular exposure of the skull base. Am J Surg 148: 534–8
2. Obwegeser HL (1985) Temporal approach to the TMJ, the orbit, and the retromaxillary-infracranial region. Head Neck Surgery 7: 185–99
3. Kennedy DW, Papel ID, Holliday M (1986) Transpalatal approach to the skull base. ENT J 65: 125–33
4. Holliday MJ, Nachalas N, Kennedy DW (1986) Uses and modifications of the infratemporal fossa approach to skull-base tumors. ENT J 65: 101–6
5. Holliday MJ (1986) Lateral transtemporal-sphenoid approach to the skull base. ENT J 65: 153–62
6. Biller HF, Lawson W (1986) Anterior mandibular-splitting approach to the skull base. ENT J 65: 134–41
7. McGuirt WF, Browne JD (1986) An anterolateral approach to the anterior skull base: case report of a malignant schwannoma of the pterygomaxillary space. Otolaryngol Head Neck Surg 95: 873
8. Sekhar LN, Schramm VL, Jones NF (1987) Subtemporal-preauricular infratemporal fossa approach to large lateral and posterior cranial base neoplasms. J Neurosurg 67: 488–99
9. Sofferman RA (1988) The septal translocation procedure: an alternative to lateral rhinotomy. Otolaryngol Head Neck Surg 98: 18–250
10. Gates GA (1988) The lateral facial approach to the nasopharynx and infratemporal fossa. Otolaryngol Head Neck Surg 99: 321–5
11. Fisch U, Mattox D (1988) Microsurgery of the skull base G Thieme, New York, Thieme Medical Publishers Inc., Stuttgart, pp 382–386
12. Janecka IP (in press) Facial translocation approach to cranial base: Clinical experience. Presented before American Academy of Otolaryngology – Head and Neck Surgery annual meeting, San Diego, CA, 1990
13. Nuss DW, Janecka IP (in press) Frontal branch of facial nerve in cranial base surgery. Presented before the North American Skull Base Society annual meeting, Los Angeles, CA, 1990

Correspondence: Prof. I. P. Janecka, M.D., F.A.C.S., Department of Otolaryngology, University of Pittsburgh, Eye & Ear Institute, 203 Lothrop Street, Suite 500, Pittsburgh, PA 15213, U.S.A.

Acta Neurochirurgica, Suppl. 53, 199–203 (1991)
© by Springer-Verlag 1991

Midfacial Split for Access to the Central Base

I. P. Janecka[1], **D. W. Nuss**[1], and **Ch. N. Sen**[2]

[1]Center for Cranial Base Surgery, Eye and Ear Institute, Department of Otolaryngology, University of Pittsburgh, and [2]Department of Neurosurgery, Presbyterian-University Hospital, Pittsburgh, Pennsylvania, U.S.A.

Summary

The technique of the madfacial split for access to the central cranial base is described. It provides – using bilateral facial osteotomies and soft tissue mobilization – a unified surgical field extending in the sagittal plane from the anterior cranial fossa floor and sphenoid sinus to the level of the fourth cervical vertebral body. In the axial plane, the periphery of the surgical access may extend to the jugular fossae and the hypoglossal canals. Experiences and results in eight patients are presented.

Keyword: Midfacial split; central craninal base; tumour; technique; results.

Introduction

The central compartment of the cranial base – the clivus, sphenoid sinus, nasopharynx, craniovertebral junction, and deep infratemporal fossa – has been difficult to reach with a single surgical approach. A number of techniques have been described for the purpose of exposure of the central skull base, including transsphenoidal[1,2], transmaxillary[3,4], transoral[5], transpalatal[6], transmandibular[7,8], and infratemporal[9,10] approaches. Although each of these has advantages, and can provide exposure of some portions of the central cranial base, it occasionally becomes necessary to have broader exposure encompassing the entire central compartment.

The midfacial split, utilizing bilateral facial osteotomies and soft tissue mobilization, provides a unified surgical field extending in the sagittal plane from the anterior cranial fossa floor and sphenoid sinus to the level of the fourth cervical vertebral body. In the axial plane, the periphery of the surgical access may extend to the jugular fossae and the hypoglossal canals.

Method

Aftrer the induction of gereral anesthesia via an oral endotracheal tube, the entire face is prepared and draped in sterile manner. Alternatively, a trancheotomy may be done first, especially when lower cranial nerve dysfunction is present or anticipated. The nasal cavities are packed with strip gauze impregnated with vasoconstrictor (such as epinephrine or oxymetazoline). The incision is marked and infiltrated with xylocaine 1/2% containing epinephrine 1:200,000. This incision consists of a median rhinotomy with supraobital extensions and continues inferiorly as a paramedian lip split with extension into the superior gingivolabial sulcus (Fig. 1).

The nasal portion of the incision bivalves the nose, allowing displacement of the external cartilages laterally, and exposing the cartilaginous septum (Fig. 2). The muco-perichondrium of one side of the septum is elevated from the cartilage for a distance of approximately two centimeters, and a vertical incision through the entire septum at this level releases the anterior cartilaginous septum from its attachment to the posterior septum. The septum is similarly detached from the floor of the nose and from the undersurface of the nasal bones, and the septal flaps (with the anterior septal cartilage still attached on one side) are then reflected laterally. The mucosa of the lateral pyriform apertures is then incised to expose the bony margins of the nasal fossa.

At the lower end of the columella, the incision is brought inside the sill of the nostril, and continues downward along the philtrum of the lip. At the vermilion, a horizontal notch is made for improved

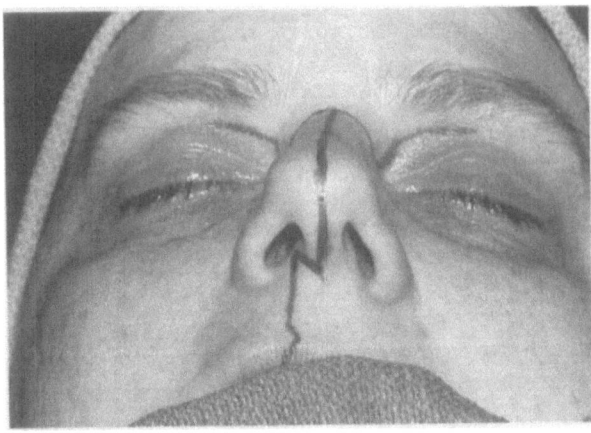

Fig. 1. Incisions for midfacial split approach to central cranial base

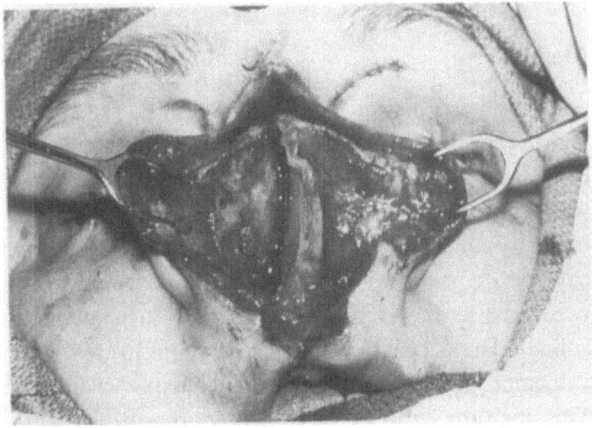

Fig. 2. External nose bivalved, showing lateral displacement of tip cartilages, and exposing the nasal septum

cosmesis, and the lip is then divided vertically. The gingivolabial sulcus is incised bilaterally to expose the lower maxillae. Next, the facial soft tissues are elevated from the nasomaxillary bones until the infraorbital nerves are seen.

The upper end of the nasal incision is extended horizontally below the eyebrows, exposing the superior and medial orbital rims. Elevation of the periorbita reveals the anterior ethmoid foramen, which serves as a guide to the position of the frontoethmoid suture line; the anterior ethmoid artery is then coagulated with bipolar current and divided. Inferiorly, the nasolacrimal duct is identified, retracted upward, and transected as distally as possible in an oblique manner to discourage late stenosis. This orbital dissection gives access to the superior, medial, and inferior walls and facilitates subsequent osteotomies.

At this point, the facial skeleton is exposed from the superior orbit to the inferior maxilla, and from one infraorbital foramen to the other (Fig. 3), and osteotomies are now begun (Fig. 4). Axial bone cuts are made from the medial orbit on one side to the other, through the nasion, taking care to stay below the frontoethmoid suture so as to avoid injury to the cribriform plate and forntal lobes. A second cut is made across the lower maxilla as in Lefort I osteotomy. Vertical cuts are then made just medial to the infraorbital nerves bilaterally, including the medial orbital floor, and extending down to the Lefort I cut. The osteomies in the medial and inferior orbit are then connected using either an angled reciprocating saw blade or a fine curved osteotome. Next, a midline nasal osteotomy is made, and the two bony segments – each consisting of the anterior maxilla, inferomedial orbital rim and floor, and nasal bone – are mobilized from the underlying medial maxillary walls using stout scissors. These segments are now removed and

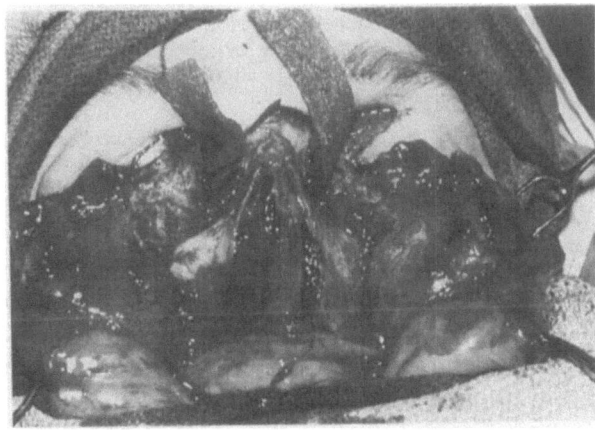

Fig. 3. Exposure of nasomaxillary skeleton after mobilization of soft tissues. Cotton pledgets are placed in each orbit after indentification, coagulation, and division of anterior ethmoid arteries. Alveolar ridge and tongue is seen inferiorly (patient is edentulous)

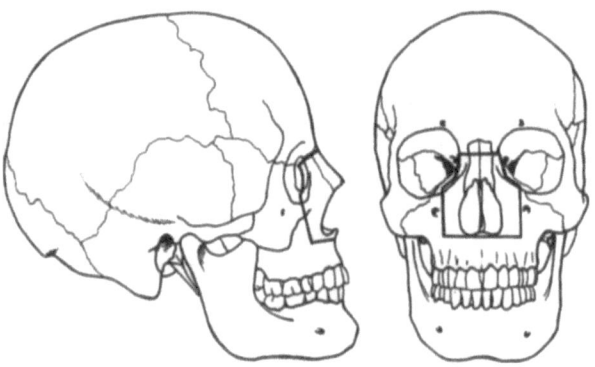

Fig. 4. Nasomaxillary osteotomies

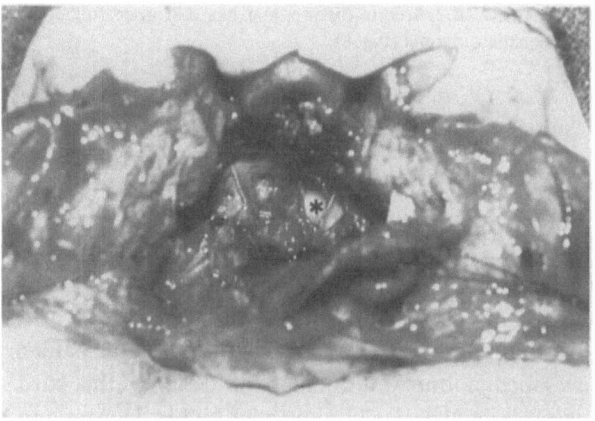

Fig. 5. Surgeon's view after osteotomies and displacement of nasal septum. In this case, the sphenoid sinus has been opened, revealing the mucosa of its posterior wall (*). Direct access to adjacent clivus and entire nasopharynx is also achieved

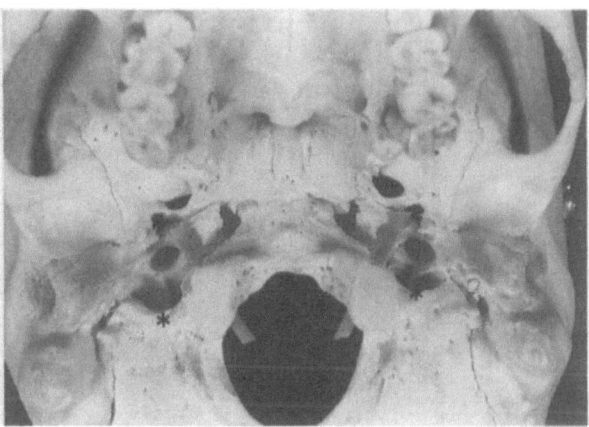

Fig. 6. Dry skull showing relationship of clivus to jugular foramen (*) and hypoglossal canal (probe)

preserved in moist gauze for reconstruction later in the procedure.

With the nasal cavities and maxillary sinuses now widely exposed, the madial maxillary walls are resected, and the remaining nasal septum is either resected or dislocated to one side, providing direct access to the nasopharynx, sphenoid sinus, and clivus (Fig. 5).

For more inferior exposure, the hard palate is split in the midline as well, and each half is separated from the pterygnoid plates using as osteotome. Each hemipalate (still attached to its vascular pedicle) is then rotated laterally and retracted. The soft palate is also divided in the midline, giving access to the entire oronasopharynx and C1-C2 area.

If futher inferior and/or lateral exposure is needed, a parasymphyseal mandibular split is added. Perilingual dissection (preserving the lingual and hypoglossal nerves) opens the parapharyngeal space, and the retropharyngeal space is then entered by elevation of mucosa with pharyngeal muscles to expose the prevertebral fascia. This layer may be split in an "L" shape (in the midline with a horizontal cut at the level of the mesopharynx). Wide exposure of the craniovertebral junction and upper cervical vertebrae is thus achieved.

Following indentification of the atlanto-occipital and the petro-occipital junctions in relation to the clivus, further lateral dissection may be carried out by elevation of the prevertebral muscles and eustachian tube along the inferior aspect of the petrous bone. Dissecting in this plane, the jugular fossa and the hypoglossal canal may be exposed (Fig. 6).

After the oncological or reparative work at the central cranial base has been completed, the reconstruction is begun by replacing the anterior nasomaxillary bony segshments. Fixation may be accomplished using sutures, wire, or miniplates. (We prefer to avoid using ferrous metals because of imaging scatter on postoperative CT and MRI studies, and because of potential problems with altered dosimetry is patients receiving radiation therapy. However, plates made of titanium or Vitallium are acceptable.)

Soft tissues are reappoximated. The nasolacrimal ducts are replaced into their anatomic positions and need not be stented as long as they have been transected distally. The anterior nasal septum, still attached to the muco-perichondrium on one side, is replaced in the midline and is secured by mattress sutures to the muco-perichondrim of the opposite side. Silicone-tube nasal stents are placed to support the septum and to help maintain a patent nasal airway during the first postoperative week.

The medial canthal tendons are fixed with sutures to the nasal bones to prevent telecanthus. Subcutaneous tissues and skin are meticulously reapproximated and an adhesive nasal dressing is placed.

If the palate has been divided, it is replaced and secured using minifixation plates along the Lefort osteotomy line. Similarly, if mandibulotomy has been performed, reconstruction using plates is preferred.

Illustrative Case

A 56 year old female with a two year history headaches was found to have a mass originating from the posterior nasal septum and vomer. Biopsy relvealed a chondroid neoplasm, and diagnostic imaging (Fig. 7) confirmed involvement of the sphenoid rostrum, posterior nasal septum, vomer, and both medial maxillary walls.

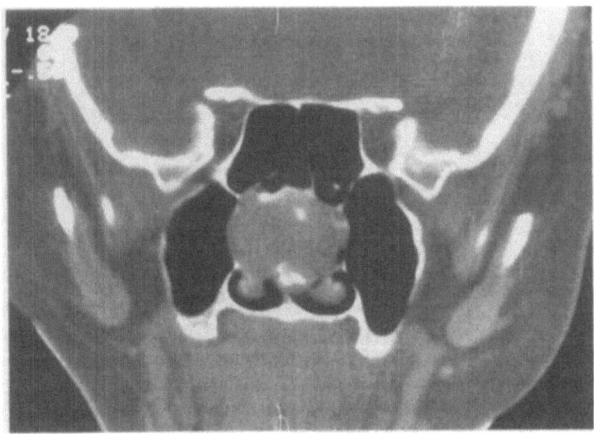

Fig. 7. Coronal CT scan showing 3x3 cm chondrosarcoma of vomer and sphenoid rostrum. Note extension to both medial maxillary walls

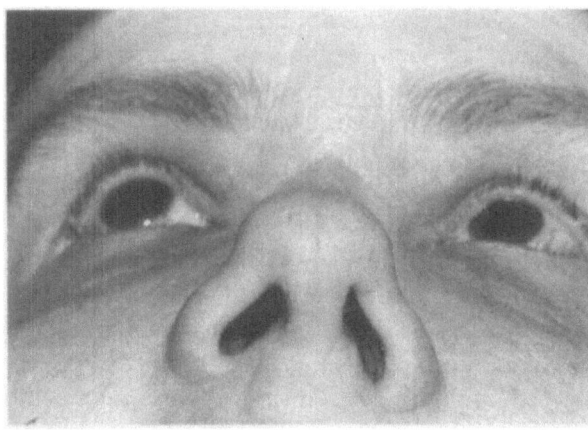

Fig. 8. Patient one year following midfacial split for resection of chondrosarcoma

Using the midfacial split approach, the septum, medial maxillary walls, and sphenoid rostrum and floor were resected. The anterior nasomaxillary complex was replaced and the patient healed primarily and without complication. On pathologic examination of the specimen, the diagnosis of low-grade chondrosarcoma was made. Margins of resection were clear. One year following surgery,

she remains well, is free of disease, and has had good functional and cosmetic outcome (Fig. 8).

Results

The midfacial split approach has been used, to variable extent, in eight patients to date. Indications for surgery are listed in Table 1. Primary healing of the facial bones and soft tissues was observed in all patients with two exceptions. One patient, who was edentulous and underwent a median split of the palate, developed a one centimeter fenestrum of the hard palate which was easily obturated by his denture and required no treatmet. The second patient developed CSF leak which required re-exploration. Subsequent healing was uneventful. Soft palate function was preserved in all patients in whom there was no preoperative dysfunction. Mild to moderate nasal crusting was observed in all patients for several weeks following surgery, but resolved with saline nasal irrigation, and no patient required further intervention. All facial incisions have healed with asethetically satisfactory results.

Discussion

Lesions that affect the midline of the cranial base have been difficult to approach surgically because of their deep location and relationship to the facial skeleton and soft tissues which restrict access. Transsphenoidal, transmaxillary, transoral, trans-palatal, and transmandibular approaches all provide access to the central cranial base, but each has anatomic limitations which compromise the ultimate exposure. The infratemporal approach gives good unilateral exposure of the lateral and paracentral skull base, with the added benefit of direct control of the carotid artery, but at the midline the visualization is often inadequate.

Table 1. *Midfacial Split for Access to Central Cranial Base*

Patients	Diagnosis	Site	Healing
J. A.	Adenocarcinoma	Midface	Primary
R. C.	Neuroblastoma	Midface	Primary
B. F.	Melanoma	Nasopharynx	Primary
D. H.	Chondrosarcoma	Nasopharynx	Primary
C. M.	Mucoepidermoida Ca	Infratemporal fossa	Secondary (CSF leak)
V. McP.	Carcinoma (Ca)	Nasopharynx	Primary
M. B.	Carcinoma	Nasopharynx	Primary
D. M.	Arteriovenous Malformation	Spinal cord	Secondary (1 cm Palatal opening)

The midfacial split, by disassembling the anterior facial skeleton, essentially combines the benefits of the transsphenoidal, transmaxillary, transoral, and trans-mandibular approaches, thereby providing a unified surgical field with improved access to the entire midline of the cranial base as well as the craniocervical junction. This technique has been used clinically with good functional and aesthetic results and few complications.

References

1. Hardy (1969) Transsphenoidal microsurgery of the normal and pathological pituitary. Clin Neurosurg 16: 185–216
2. Hardy J (1976) Transsphenoidal neurosurgery of intracranial neoplasm. In: Thompson RA, Green JR (eds) Advances in Neurology Series, Vol 15. Raven Press, New York, pp 261–274
3. Hamberger CA, Hammer G, Norlen G, Sjogren B (1961) Transantrosphenoidal hypophysectomy. Arch Otolaryngol 74: 2–8
4. Brown DH (1989) The Lefort I maxillary osteotomy approach of surgery of the skull base. J Otolaryngol 18 (6): 289–92
5. Crockard HA (1985) The transoral approach to the base of the brain and upper cervical cord. Ann Royal Coll Surg Eng 67: 321–325
6. Kennedy DW, Papel ID, Holliday M (1986) Transpalatal approach to the skull base. ENT Journal 65: 125–133
7. Biller HF, Lawson W (1986) Anterior mandibular-splitting approach to the skull base. ENT Journal 65: 134–141
8. Krespi YP, Sisson GA (1984) Transmandibular exposure of the skull base. Am J Surg 148: 534–538
9. Fisch U, Pilsbury HC (1979) Infratemporal fossa approach to lesions in the temporal bone and base of skull. Arch Otolaryngol 105: 99–107
10. Holliday MJ (1980) Lateral transtemporal-sphenoid approach to the skull base. ENT Journal 65: 153–162

Correspondence: Prof. I. P. Janecka, M. D., F.A.C.S., Department of Otolaryngology, University of Pittsburgh, Eye and Ear Institute, 203 Lothrop Street, Suite 500, Pittsburgh, PA 15213, U.S.A.

Subject Index

Georg Emil Cold

Cerebral Blood Flow in Acute Head Injury

The Regulation of Cerebral Blood Flow and Metabolism During the Acute Phase of Head Injury, and Its Significance for Therapy

(Acta Neurochirurgica / Supplementum 49)

1990. 16 figures. VIII, 64 pages.
Cloth DM 98,-, öS 686,-
Reduced price for subscribers
to "Acta Neurochirurgica":
Cloth DM 88,20, öS 617,40
ISBN 3-211-82224-0

Prices are subject to change without notice

During the last decade a multitude of studies concerning the dynamic changes in cerebral blood flow (CBF), cerebral metabolic rate of oxygen ($CMRO_2$), and intracranial pressure (ICP) in the acute phase after head injury have been published. These studies have been supplemented with studies of cerebral autoregulation, CO_2 reactivity and barbiturate reactivity. Other investigations include studies of cerebrospinal fluid pH, bicarbonate, lactate and pyruvate.

In this book experimental and clinical studies of the dynamic changes in CBF, $CMRO_2$, CO_2 reactivity and barbiturate reactivity are reviewed. The author's own clinical studies of the dynamic changes in CBF and cerebral metabolism are summarized and discussed, and the therapeutical implication as regards the use of artificial hyperventilation, sedation with barbiturate and mannitol treatment are discussed.

J. D. Pickard, G. Maira, Ch. E. Polkey, T. Trojanowski (eds.)

Neurosurgical Aspects of Epilepsy

Proceedings of the Fourth Advanced Seminar in Neurosurgical Research of the European Association of Neurosurgical Societies, May 17–18, 1989, Bresseo di Teolo, Padova, Italy

(Acta Neurochirurgica / Supplementum 50)

1990. 19 figures. VIII, 144 pages.
Cloth DM 160,-, öS 1120,-
Reduced price for subscribers
to "Acta Neurochirurgica":
Cloth DM 144,-, öS 1008,-
ISBN 3-211-82227-5

Prices are subject to change without notice

The surgical treatment of epilepsy in an expanding area of endeavour and an expertise that remains underutilised in many countries. This book includes the contributions that were discussed and modified accordingly at the Fourth Advanced Seminar in Neurosurgical Research held on May 17th–18th, 1989, in Padua, Italy. It presents current reviews of the epileptic focus, the pathological focus, membrane electrophysiology of epileptiform activity, pathophysiology of acute brain damage, neuropathology, epidemiology of drug resistant epilepsy, adverse effects of antiepileptic drugs and postmarketing surveillance, controversies in post-traumatic epilepsy and epilepsy following neurosurgical intervention, role of prophylactic therapy, principles of surgery of epilepsy and selection criteria including electrophysiology, psychometry, neuroradiology, nuclear medicine, the long term results of the various surgical techniques and discussion of why so few patients are operated on for epilepsy despite cogent arguments in its favour, particularly when considered in the context of cost benefit analysis and rehabilitation. The book provides ready access to a wide range of literature not readily available elsewhere and the editors' wish is that further research into intractable epilepsy be facilitated.

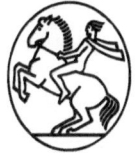

Springer-Verlag Wien New York

Sachsenplatz 4–6, P.O. Box 89, A-1201 Wien · Heidelberger Platz 3, D-1000 Berlin 33
175 Fifth Avenue, New York, NY 10010, USA · 37-3, Hongo 3-chome, Bunkyo-ku, Tokyo 113, Japan